INTRODUCTION TO
Physical Therapy
Second Edition

Michael A. Pagliarulo, PT, EdD

Associate Professor
Department of Physical Therapy
Ithaca College
Ithaca, New York

With 104 illustrations

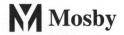 Mosby

An Affiliate of Elsevier Science

St. Louis   London   Philadelphia   Sydney   Toronto

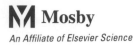

An Affiliate of Elsevier Science

Acquisitions Editor: Andrew Allen
Manuscript Editor: Amy Norwitz
Production Manager: Mary Stermel
Illustration Specialist: Lisa Lambert
Book Designer: Marie Gardocky Clifton

INTRODUCTION TO PHYSICAL THERAPY, SECOND EDITION

NOTICE

Physical Therapy is an ever-changing field. Standard safety precautions must be followed, but as new research and clinical experience broaden our knowledge, changes in treatment and drug therapy may become necessary or appropriate. Readers are advised to check the most current product information provided by the manufacturer of each drug to be administered to verify the recommended dose, the method and duration of administration, and contraindications. It is the responsibility of the treating physician, relying on experience and knowledge of the patient, to determine dosages and the best treatment for each individual patient. Neither the Publisher nor the editor assumes any liability for any injury and/or damage to persons or property arising from this publication.

Permissions may be sought directly from Elsevier's Health Sciences Rights Department in Philadelphia, USA: phone: (+1)215-238-7869, fax: (+1)215-238-2239, email: healthpermissions@elsevier.com. You may also complete your request on-line via the Elsevier Science homepage (http://www.elsevier.com), by selecting 'Customer Support' and then 'Obtaining Permissions'.

Mosby, Inc.
An Affiliate of Elsevier Science
11830 Westline Industrial Drive
St. Louis, Missouri 63146

Printed in the United States of America.

Library of Congress Cataloging-in-Publication Data

Introduction to physical therapy/[edited by] Michael A. Pagliarulo.—2nd ed.
p.   cm.
Rev. ed. of: Introduction to physical therapy/Michael A. Pagliarulo. 1996. Includes
bibliographical references and index.
ISBN 0–323–01057–1
1. Physical therapy. I. Pagliarulo, Michael A. II. Pagliarulo, Michael A. Introduction to
   physical therapy.
[DNLM: 1. Physical Therapy. WB 460 I616 2001]
RM700.P34 2001
615.8′2—dc21   00–068119

International Standard Book Number 0–323–01057–1

03 04 05 9 8 7 6 5 4 3

This book is dedicated to my father, Anthony, for his sense of responsibility and work ethic and my mother, Louise, for her complete unselfishness and commitment to our family.

As Italian immigrants to the United States with limited educational backgrounds, they survived the hard times of the Depression and World War II through perseverance and fortitude. I am grateful to their values, sense of pride in achievement, and insistence on advanced education.

MICHAEL A. PAGLIARULO

Contributors

Barbara C. Belyea, PT, MS

Clinical Assistant Professor/Director, Department of Physical Therapy, Ithaca College, Ithaca, New York

Physical Therapy for Musculoskeletal Conditions

Susan E. Bennett, PT, EdD, NCS

Clinical Associate Professor and Director, Physical Therapy; Clinical Assistant Professor of Neurology, State University of New York at Buffalo; Clinical Research Associate, Rehabilitation Medicine, Kaleida Health, Buffalo General Hospital, Buffalo, New York

Current Issues

Ray A. Boone, PT, MEd

Adjunct Associate Professor, Department of Physical Therapy, Ithaca College—Rochester Campus, Rochester, New York

Physical Therapy in Cardiopulmonary Conditions

Cheryl A. Carpenter, PTA, MEd

Instructor and Academic Coordinator of Clinical Education, The Metropolitan Community Colleges—Penn Valley Campus, Kansas City, Missouri

The Physical Therapist Assistant

Jennifer E. Collins, PT, BS, MPA

Assistant Director and Assistant Professor, Department of Physical Therapy, University of Findlay, Findlay, Ohio

Physical Therapy for the Older Adult

Hilary B. Greenberger, PT, MS, OCS

Associate Professor, Department of Physical Therapy, Ithaca College; Staff Physical Therapist, Cornell University, Ithaca, New York

Physical Therapy for Musculoskeletal Conditions

Michael A. Pagliarulo, PT, EdD

Associate Professor, Department of Physical Therapy, Ithaca College, Ithaca, New York

Physical Therapy: Definition and Profession; Roles and Employment Settings; American Physical Therapy Association

Shree Pandya, PT, MS

Assistant Professor, Department of Neurology and Department of Physical Medicine and Rehabilitation, University of Rochester Medical School, Rochester, New York
Physical Therapy for Neuromuscular Conditions

Angela Easley Rosenberg, PT, DrPH

Instructor, Division of Physical Therapy; Training Director, Center for Development and Learning, University of North Carolina, Chapel Hill, North Carolina
Physical Therapy for Pediatric Conditions

Laurie A. Walsh, PT, BS, JD

Associate Professor, Department of Physical Therapy, Daemen College, Amherst, New York
Laws, Regulations, and Policies

R. Scott Ward, PT, PhD

Associate Professor, Division of Physical Therapy, University of Utah; Staff, Intermountain Burn Center, University of Utah Health Sciences Center, Salt Lake City, Utah
Physical Therapy for Integumentary Conditions

Preface

It is amazing how much this profession has changed in the short period since the first edition of this text was published in 1996. External forces, such as managed care, and internal forces, such as the move toward the clinical doctorate, have had extensive impact on practice and education. I am eager to see this second edition become available to continue to provide accurate and current descriptions of the profession and practice of physical therapy.

In view of the success of the first edition, the purpose and fundamental content of this text remain unchanged. Like the first edition, this text was designed to present an introduction and broad background on the profession (Part I) and practice (Part II) of physical therapy. The introductory nature of the content continues to focus on the student beginning a PT, PTA, or health-related educational program. Nevertheless, major updates and revisions were made to describe the current conditions within our profession. All chapters were revised to reflect the concepts and terminology of the *Guide to Physical Therapist Practice*, particularly the elements of the Patient/Client Management Model. For example, all chapters in Part II continue to open with a general description and presentation of common conditions in the practice area; however, subsequent revised topic headings are principles of examination; principles of evaluation, diagnosis, and prognosis; and principles of direct intervention. These chapters close with case studies and summaries. A chapter on integumentary conditions was added, and the sequence of the chapters in Part II was changed to follow the *Guide*. The chapter on current issues was extensively updated to describe the impact of managed care and movement toward the clinical doctorate. Demographic information and policy documents were updated to incorporate data and revisions current as of summer 2000. The chapter on Laws, Regulations, and Policies was rewritten by a physical therapist with a JD credential to ensure accurate information as it affects our profession. The Special Topics chapter from the first edition was omitted and essential portions were incorporated into existing chapters. Finally, learning objectives were added to each chapter to provide a set of expectations for the reader.

As an instructor, I expect and welcome feedback. Comments from those who have used the first edition were very helpful to guide this revision. I believe this edition will continue to provide the reader with a comprehensive description of our exciting profession. I look forward to comments for future enhancements.

MICHAEL A. PAGLIARULO

Acknowledgments

Perhaps nontraditionally, I will begin my thanks by expressing my gratitude, admiration, and love for my family. Tricia, my wife, and Michael, David, and Elisa, our children, were always supportive of this work. Their questions demonstrated a genuine interest in this project, and their endorsement was an inspiration.

In addition to my family, the success of this text is in large measure due to the contributors. Experts in their respective areas, they have been responsive to my requests and have ensured that their chapters contain current and accurate information. I welcome to this edition Laurie A. Walsh and R. Scott Ward, who have written chapters on legal issues and integument, respectively. It has been a rewarding experience to work with all the contributors. Personnel within the Harcourt Health Sciences umbrella have continued to provide support and guidance, particularly Mary Tatum in her thorough review of the manuscript and helpful comments. I also offer special thanks to Gina White for her perseverance and success with computer graphics. (Thank goodness she still speaks to me.)

MICHAEL A. PAGLIARULO

Contents

Part I

Profession

Physical therapy is knowledge. Physical therapy is clinical science. Physical therapy is the reasoned application of science to warm and needing human beings. Or it is nothing.[7]
Helen J. Hislop, PT, FAPTA

Physical Therapy: Definition and Profession

Michael A. Pagliarulo

KEY TERMS

OBJECTIVES   After reading this chapter, the reader will be able to

- Define physical therapy
- Describe the components of the model of disablement
- Describe the characteristics of a profession
- Describe a brief history of the profession of physical therapy in the United States and the major factors that influenced its growth and development

The profession of **physical therapy** has evolved in two decades of rapid growth. Although it has received substantial publicity, confusion remains regarding its unique characteristics. For example, how does physical therapy differ from occupational or chiropractic therapy? This chapter's first purpose, then, must be to present and define this profession.

To define physical therapy thoroughly, it is essential to also present a brief history of its development. A review of the past will demonstrate how the profession has responded to societal needs and gained respect as an essential component of the rehabilitation team. It will also link some current trends and practices with past events.

DEFINITION   Part of the confusion regarding the definition of physical therapy results from the variety of legal definitions seen from state to state. Each state has the right to define this field and regulate the practice of physical therapy in its jurisdiction. These definitions are commonly included in legislation known as a "practice act," which pertains to a specific profession. (Practice acts in physical therapy are further described in Chapter 5.)

To limit this variety, the Model Definition of Physical Therapy for State Practice Acts was created by the Board of Directors of the American Physical Therapy Association (APTA) and was recently amended to more accurately reflect the scope of practice (Box 1–1).[9]

This definition identifies several activities inherent to the practice of physical therapy. First and foremost, physical therapy begins with an examination to determine the nature and status of the condition. Findings from the examination are interpreted to establish a diagnosis, prognosis, and plan of care. Interventions are then administered and modified in accordance with the patient's responses. The interventions used focus on musculoskeletal, neuromuscular, cardiopulmonary, and integumentary disorders. Other activities also important for effective practice include consultation, education, and research. Finally, it should be noted that physical therapists also provide preventive services to maintain health and wellness (see Chapter 2 for a more detailed description of the activities of a physical therapist).

A fundamental aspect of the definition is that physical therapy is "provided by or under the direction and supervision of a physical therapist." This qualification is further stipulated in a section of another policy (adopted by the House of Delegates of the APTA) specifying that physical therapists and physical therapist assistants working under the direction of a physical therapist are the *only* individuals who provide physical therapy (Box 1–2).[14]

Another basic feature of the definition is that it anchors examination and intervention to the concept of disablement. In the **disablement model**, the

Box 1–1

Model Definition of Physical Therapy for State Practice Acts

Physical therapy, which is the care and services provided by or under the direction and supervision of a physical therapist, includes:

1. examining (history, systems review, test and measures) individuals with impairments, functional limitations, and disability or other health-related conditions in order to determine a diagnosis, prognosis, and intervention; tests and measures may include the following:
   - aerobic capacity and endurance
   - anthropometric characteristics
   - arousal, attention, and cognition
   - assistive and adaptive devices
   - community and work (job/school/play) integration or reintegration
   - cranial nerve integrity
   - environmental, home, and work (job/school/play) barriers
   - ergonomics and body mechanics
   - gait, locomotion, and balance
   - integumentary integrity
   - joint integrity and mobility
   - motor function
   - muscle performance
   - neuromotor development and sensory integration
   - orthotic, protective, and supportive devices
   - pain
   - posture
   - prosthetic requirements
   - range of motion
   - reflex integrity
   - self care and home management
   - sensory integrity
   - ventilation, respiration, and circulation
2. alleviating impairment and functional limitation by designing, implementing, and modifying therapeutic interventions that include, but are not limited to:
   - coordination, communication and documentation
   - patient/client-related instruction
   - therapeutic exercise (including aerobic conditioning)
   - functional training in self care and home management (including activities of daily living and instrumental activities of daily living)
   - functional training in community and work (job/school/play) integration or reintegration (including instrumental activities of daily living, work hardening, and work conditioning)

Box continued on following page

- manual therapy techniques (including mobilization and manipulation)
- prescription, application, and, as appropriate, fabrication of assistive, adaptive, orthotic, protective, supportive, and prosthetic devices and equipment
- airway clearance techniques
- wound management
- electrotherapeutic modalities
- physical agents and mechanical modalities
3. preventing injury, impairment, functional limitation, and disability, including the promotion and maintenance of fitness, health, and quality of life in all age populations.
4. engaging in consultation, education, and research.

From Model Definition of Physical Therapy for State Practice Acts, BOD 03-00-17-39. Alexandria, VA, American Physical Therapy Association, 2000.

focus is on functional abilities that result from a medical condition, unlike in the medical model, which focuses on treating the ailment. Several versions of this model exist and were well described by Jette.[8] This concept is fundamental in the *Guide to Physical Therapist Practice*, a pivotal document describing a new approach to patient care, and is based on the scheme presented by Nagi.[5, 11, 12] As described in the *Guide*, the process of disablement includes impairment, functional limitations, and disability. **Impairment** is loss or abnormality of a body function or structure at the cellular, tissue, organ, or system level. Impairment causes **functional limitation,** which is a decreased ability of a *person* to perform a task without regard to the context or environment. A **disability** occurs if the functional limitation restricts activity in a particular context or environment. Through the examination, the physical therapist determines the presence and extent of impairment, functional limitation, and disability before establishing a plan of care. (A similar model of disablement developed by the World Health Organization is described in Chapter 11.)

Box 1–2

Position on Provision of Physical Therapy Interventions and Related Tasks

It is the position of the American Physical Therapy Association that physical therapists are the only professionals who provide physical therapy interventions. Physical therapist assistants are the only paraprofessionals who provide selected physical therapy interventions under the direction and at least general supervision of the physical therapist.

From Position on Physical Therapy Intervention, HOD 06-00-17-28. Alexandria, VA, American Physical Therapy Association, 2000.

Newer terminology in this definition also reflects the health promotion and consultative areas of service. Traditionally, physical therapists have provided care to **patients**—individuals who have disorders that require interventions to improve their function.[5] **Client** is the term used to refer to an individual who seeks the services of a physical therapist to maintain health or a business that hires a physical therapist for consultation. These areas of involvement have become more significant in the recent evolution of the profession.

PHYSICAL THERAPY AS A PROFESSION

The model definition provides a comprehensive description of the *practice* of physical therapy. A companion document addresses the *profession* of physical therapy, which was adopted by the House of Delegates (policymaking body) of the APTA in 1983 and recently revised (Box 1–3).[15]

Two significant features of this position statement that embellish the model definition are that physical therapy is a profession and that it promotes optimal health and function. The latter feature—promotion of optimal health and function—is a goal established with patient/client/family input. Optimal function may meet or exceed the level before injury or disease or may be severely diminished as a result of impairment. The former feature of this position statement—that physical therapy is a profession—warrants further discussion.

Figure 1–1 lists the characteristics of a **profession** as a hierarchy.[10] The first characteristic, a lifetime commitment requiring an individual's dedication to the profession, may seem formidable. The second characteristic, a representative organization, provides standards, regulations, structure, and a vehicle for communication. In physical therapy, this characteristic is fulfilled by the APTA. The third characteristic, specialized education, ensures competency to practice. For example, all licensed physical therapists must have a minimum of a 4-year baccalaureate degree, and all physical therapist assistants must have an associate degree. The fourth characteristic, service to clients, is obvious in physical

Box 1–3

Position on Physical Therapy as a Health Profession

Physical therapy is a health profession whose primary purpose is the promotion of optimal health and function. This purpose is accomplished through the application of scientific principles to the processes of examination, evaluation, diagnosis, prognosis, and intervention to prevent or remediate impairments, functional limitations and disabilities as related to movement and health.

Physical therapy encompasses areas of specialized competence and includes the development of new principles and applications to meet existing and emerging health needs. Other professional activities that serve the purpose of physical therapy are research, education, consultation and administration.

From Position on Physical Therapy as a Health Profession, HOD 06-99-19-23. Alexandria, VA, American Physical Therapy Association, 1999.

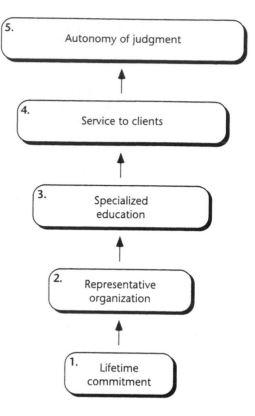

Figure 1–1. Hierarchy of the criteria to define a profession.

therapy and provides a direct benefit to society. Finally, the last feature, autonomy of judgment, applies regardless of whether the therapist practices in a jurisdiction where a physician's referral is required by law. Independent and accurate judgment is inherent in every evaluation, plan of care, and discharge plan conducted by the physical therapist. This last criterion is frequently used to distinguish a professional from a technician (an individual who requires supervision).

As a profession, physical therapy emulates the criteria listed in Figure 1–1. Such was not always the case, and evolution of the profession has entailed significant change and varying degrees of recognition from other professions. The next section provides a brief overview of the history of physical therapy.

HISTORICAL DEVELOPMENT

Examining the origin and development of the profession and practice of physical therapy in the United States will serve to explain some of the current characteristics and conditions. It will also demonstrate how certain positions have changed over time. The reader is referred to resources at the end of this chapter for more detailed historical accounts.

Origins of Physical Therapy

Granger described how physical measures were used in ancient civilizations to relieve pain and improve function.[4] Massage was used by the Chinese in 3000

BC, described by Hippocrates in 460 BC, modified by the Romans, and accepted as a scientific procedure in the early 1800s. Techniques of muscle re-education developed from this evolution. Hydrotherapy was practiced by the Greeks and Romans through the use of baths and river worship. Finally, electrotherapy developed with the introduction of electricity and electrical appliances beginning in the 1600s.

More modern techniques of physical therapy were practiced extensively in Europe before being used in the United States, particularly in England and France. It took the outbreak of polio epidemics and World War I to bring these techniques to the United States.

Impact of World War I and Polio

It is unfortunate that the impetus to develop physical therapy in this country was the response to widespread suffering; at the same time, such an origin demonstrates the direct humanitarian motivation that serves as its foundation. First came the epidemics of polio (poliomyelitis or infantile paralysis) in 1894, 1914, and 1916, which left tens of thousands of children paralyzed and in need of "physical therapy." Subsequently, at the outbreak of World War I, the Surgeon General of the United States sent a group of physicians to England and France to learn about physical therapy techniques so that those wounded in war could be better managed. As a result, the Division of Special Hospitals and Physical Reconstruction was created in 1917.[2] This Division was responsible for training and managing **reconstruction aides** (exclusively women) who would provide physical reconstruction to those injured in war. These women were the forerunners of the profession and practice of physical therapy in the United States (Fig. 1–2).

During this period, polio epidemics were occurring in Vermont. A statewide program known as the "Vermont Plan" was developed to study the cause and

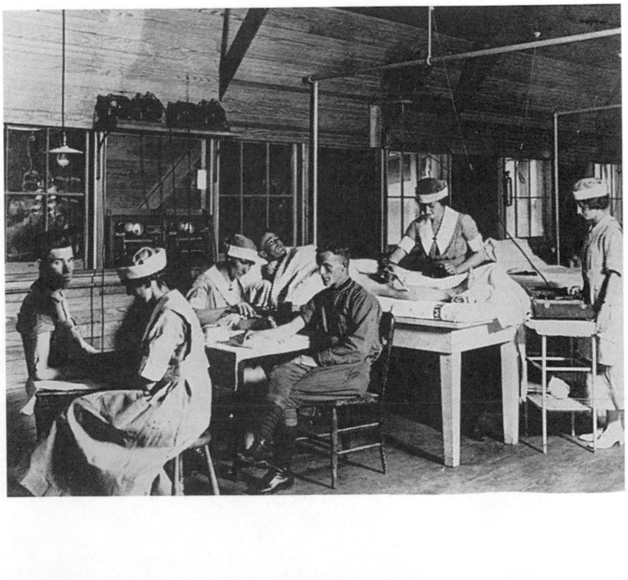

Figure 1–2. Reconstruction aides treating soldiers wounded in World War I at Fort Sam Houston, Texas, in 1919. (Reprinted from Historical Photograph Packet with permission from the American Physical Therapy Association.)

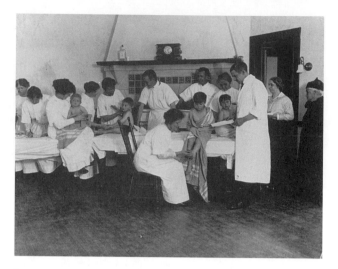

Figure 1–3. Physical therapists and physicians working together to evaluate and treat children at a poliomyelitis clinic in New England in 1916. (Reprinted from Historical Photograph Packet with permission from the American Physical Therapy Association.)

effects of the disease. This plan included health care teams that conducted field visits to provide care for children with polio.[3] These teams consisted of orthopaedic surgeons, public health nurses, **physiotherapists** (commonly known as "physicians' assistants"), brace makers, and stenographers. Physiotherapists became involved in making accurate measurements to determine muscle strength and providing therapy through exercise and massage (Figs. 1–3 and 1–4).

Post–World War I Period

Even when the war ended, the need for physical therapy continued. Attention shifted from preserving a fighting force to maintaining a working force. Hu-

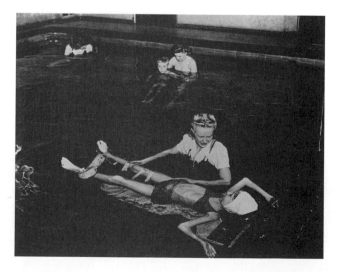

Figure 1–4. Aquatic therapy was very effective for individuals who had polio. (Reprinted from Historical Photograph Packet with permission from the American Physical Therapy Association.)

manitarian interests and the labor requirements of an industrial society resulted in a focus on "crippled children."[13] As the reconstruction aides moved into civilian facilities to address these needs, their titles and practices were plagued by confusion and ambiguity. The time had come to establish a clear identity through a national organization.

The origin of the first national organization representing "physical therapeutics" is traced to a meeting suggested by a military physician. This meeting materialized on January 15, 1921, at Keen's Chop House in New York City and was attended by 30 reconstruction aides and 5 physicians. Accomplishments of the first meeting included creation of a national organization, the **American Women's Physical Therapeutic Association,** and election of the first president, Mary McMillan.[1] The organization's first constitution indicated that it was established to maintain high standards and provide a mechanism to share information (Box 1–4).

Mary McMillan was the overwhelming choice for president (Fig. 1–5). Trained in England, she is credited with becoming the first "physical therapist" in the United States.[3] As a reconstruction aide, she was stationed at Walter Reed General Hospital in Washington, DC, and was appointed head reconstruction aide in 1918. Later, while at Reed College in Portland, Oregon, she also participated in the largest of seven emergency training programs for reconstruction aides (over 200 students).

Under the leadership of Miss McMillan, the new organization took immediate action. Two membership categories were established: charter members (reconstruction aides) and active members who "shall be graduates of recognized schools of **physiotherapy** or physical education, who have had training and experience in massage and therapeutic exercise, with some knowledge of either electrotherapy or hydrotherapy."[6] An official journal, *P.T. Review,* was established and first published in 1921. Annual meetings were initiated in

---

BOX 1–4

Founding Objectives of the American Women's Physical Therapeutic Association

1. To establish and maintain a professional and scientific standard for those engaged in the profession of physical therapeutics.
2. To increase efficiency among its members by encouraging them in advanced study.
3. To disseminate information by the distribution of medical literature and articles of professional interest.
4. To make available efficiently trained women to the medical profession.
5. To sustain social fellowship and intercourse upon grounds of mutual interest.

From Beard G: Foundations for growth: A review of the first forty years in terms of education, practice, and research. Phys Ther Rev 1961;41:843–861.

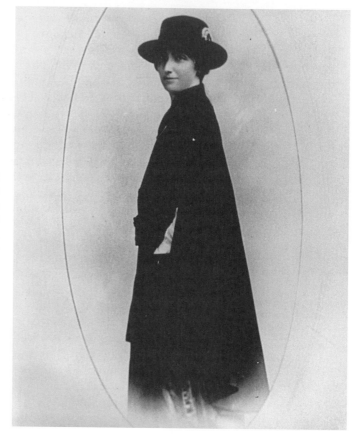

Figure 1–5. Mary McMillan, the founding president of the American Women's Physical Therapeutic Association (precursor to the American Physical Therapy Association), was elected in 1921. (Reprinted from Historical Photograph Packet with permission from the American Physical Therapy Association.)

conjunction with annual meetings of the American Medical Association (AMA) to capitalize on their programs and gain recognition. The name of the organization was changed in 1922 to the **American Physiotherapy Association (APA).** Two males were admitted in 1923. In 1926, the journal was retitled *Physiotherapy Review.*

Two issues developed that involved physicians and took decades to resolve. The first pertained to identity. Physicians perceived these practitioners to be technicians or aides and suggested that this distinction be reflected in their title. Members of the APA believed that they had a more professional status and objected to that reference. This issue was not resolved until the 1940s, when physicians established physical medicine as a medical specialty. These physicians were known as **physiatrists,** and the term "physical therapist" (without adding "technician" or "aide") became acceptable thereafter.[13]

The second issue was more substantive and involved education requirements. No standard educational program existed for a physiotherapist; therefore, the APA developed a suggested curriculum and published it in 1928. It was a 9-month program (1200 total clock hours). Entrance requirements included graduation from a school of physical education or nursing.[1] In contrast, most of the students in the 14 training programs for reconstruction aides were physical education teachers or graduates of physical education schools. A committee of the APA visited all institutions offering educational programs for physiotherapists and published a list of 11 approved programs in 1930.

The action by the APA did not fully resolve this issue. Greater recognition of education programs and standards was required, so the APA sought assistance from the AMA in 1933. Consequently, the Council on Medical Education and Hospitals of the AMA inspected 35 schools of physiotherapy. Based on this inspection, as well as input from the APA and other related organizations, the AMA adopted the *Essentials of an Acceptable School for Physical Therapy Technicians* in 1936. Entrance requirements and length of program remained essentially unchanged; however, the curriculum was stated in detail, and other characteristics were stipulated (institutional affiliation, faculty, resources, clinical facilities). Thirteen schools were approved by the AMA in 1936.[1]

Impact of World War II and Polio

Once again, national and global tragedies combined to expand the need for physical therapy, and as before, the profession responded. To meet the demands of the war, eight emergency courses (6 months in length) were authorized to be offered among the 15 approved full-length programs in physical therapy. These shortened courses were discontinued in 1946 when war-related demands for services dropped.

Unfortunately, the need to address individuals with polio continued. In response to repeated epidemics, the **National Foundation for Infantile Paralysis** (often referred to as the **Foundation**) was established in 1938 for research, education, and patient services.[2] Physical therapists continued to provide vital services for children who were affected by the disease.

The Foundation was a source of substantial support for the profession and practice of physical therapy. Catherine Worthingham, a past president of the APA, accepted the position of Director of Professional Education on the staff of the Foundation in 1944. In the same year, the first national office of the APA was established in New York City, and the first executive director was hired. Both these actions were made possible by a grant from the Foundation. In that same year, a permanent headquarters and staff for the APA made it possible to create the House of Delegates to serve as the policymaking body of the organization. Other grants from the Foundation provided (1) scholarships to recruit and retain physical therapy students and faculty, (2) funds to create a consultant to recruit and assign physical therapists for emergency work relating to polio, and (3) financial support for training in techniques fostered by Sister Kenny for individuals with polio (early application of moist heat to permit mobilization and prevent contractures).

Post–World War II Period

The U.S. Army recognized the need to retain physical therapists in an organized unit to provide service to military personnel. As a result, the Women's Medical

Specialist Corps was established in 1947. It consisted of physical therapists, occupational therapists, and dietitians. A physical therapist, Emma Vogel, became the first chief of the Corps and was accorded the rank of colonel.[2] Later, in 1955, the Corps became the Army Medical Specialist Corps to allow men and women to serve with commissions in the military.[1]

A major breakthrough in the treatment of polio occurred during this period with the introduction of gamma globulin and the Salk vaccine. Finally, this disease could be controlled. Physical therapists then played prominent roles during field trials of these medications, which began in 1951.

Name clarification continued as the term "physiatrist" became recognized as the title given to physicians who practiced physical medicine. **Physical therapists** could now practice "physical therapy." This role clarification was reflected in the new name for the national organization, the American Physical Therapy Association, in 1947 and a new title for the journal, *Physical Therapy,* in 1962. It was also demonstrated in the title of the new *Essentials,* which extensively revised the original document of 1936. The new title, *Essentials of an Acceptable School of Physical Therapy,* no longer referred to technicians. It was adopted by the AMA in 1955 and used to approve new and existing educational programs for over 20 years. The new *Essentials* established minimum curricular standards, including a program length of 12 months.

1960s Through 1980s

This three-decade period was characterized by growth and recognition in education, practice, and research. Societal issues of this period included an aging population, health promotion, and disease prevention. Federal legislation funded health care for a variety of populations, which increased the demand for physical therapy. The profession responded with several actions.

First, policy statements were adopted by the APTA in the 1960s to clarify the preparation and use of physical therapist assistants and aides (see Chapter 3). These positions were necessary to meet the growing demands for services.

The headquarters of the APTA was relocated to Washington, DC, in 1971 to establish stronger political involvement. Executive operations were further strengthened when the office building was purchased in Alexandria, Virginia, in 1983.

New education programs were developed in an attempt to keep pace with the demand; curricular evolution was inherent as health care in general expanded. This period opened with an APTA policy declaring the baccalaureate degree as the minimum educational requirement for a physical therapist (1960). By the late 1970s, it became clear that a postbaccalaureate degree would be necessary to master the knowledge and skills required for competent practice. Consequently, a critical policy adopted by the APTA in 1979 (amended in 1980) stated that new and existing programs in physical therapy must award a postbaccalaureate degree by December 31, 1990 (see Chapter 6). This requirement had a major impact on curricular development.

This period also involved evolution of the historical link between the AMA and the APTA (formerly APA) regarding approval (accreditation) of educational programs. The APTA became more actively involved in the accreditation process. In 1974, it adopted the *Essentials of an Accredited Educational Program for the Physical Therapist,* which represented a dramatic departure from the prescriptions in the 1955 *Essentials.*[13] In 1977, the APTA became recognized by the U.S. Office of Education and Council on Postsecondary Education as an accrediting agency. Standards for Accreditation of Physical Therapy Educational Programs was adopted by the APTA in 1979. In 1983, after contesting the value of the AMA in the accreditation process, the APTA became the sole agency for accrediting physical therapist and physical therapist assistant education programs. This recognition marked the maturity of the profession.

Growth and development in the areas of practice and research resulted in new organizational units and opportunities. The American Board of Physical Therapy Specialties was created by the APTA in 1978 to provide a mechanism to receive certification and recognition as a clinical specialist in a certain area. Direct access became legal in 20 states by 1988.[13] A policy was adopted by the APTA in 1984 to recognize diagnosis in physical therapy. Regarding research, the Foundation for Physical Therapy was initiated in 1979 to promote and support research in the profession.

1990s

This decade opened with continual changes in practice, education, and research, but a sense that external forces not favorable to the profession were developing. New reimbursement patterns began to cause serious limitations in the practice environment. Through managed care, insurance companies restricted the number of covered physical therapy visits and funding levels for each service. The limited clinical research available was inadequate to convince third-party payers to reverse the trend. Job availability and salaries plateaued and then declined in some facilities. This unfavorable situation was compounded by the continued proliferation of education programs. One study predicted a surplus of physical therapists by the end of the decade.[16]

Through the course of this period, the APTA took a strong leadership role in addressing the issues. Extensive legislative lobbying and rallying public sentiment resulted in governmental intervention that protected patients' rights and lifted some of the funding caps. Clinical research to support evidence-based practice was given priority on the research agenda. The *Guide to Physical Therapist Practice* was developed to clearly define the roles and services of a physical therapist based on a disablement model.[5] The dramatic shift to postbaccalaureate education gave rise to several national conferences that resulted in *A Normative Model of Physical Therapist Professional Level Education* to provide guidance to these programs. Subsequently, a new document entitled *Evaluative Criteria for the Accreditation of Physical Therapist Education Programs* was adopted. Similar activities were conducted to refine the role and education of the physical therapist assistant. A separate deliberative body was created for the physical therapist assistant, the Representative Body of the National Assembly. The period ended with consideration of a vision document that described new directions to the year 2020, including the provision of services by doctors of physical therapy.

Several of the issues identified in this final period continue to evolve. The profession and practice of physical therapy remain responsive to societal needs. Subsequent chapters in Part I and, in particular, Chapter 6 provide further description.

Summary _____

Physical therapy is a profession that enjoys a proud heritage. From the reconstruction aides of World War I to the independent practitioner of today, physical therapists continue to provide services to reduce pain, improve function, and maintain health. This chapter provided a definition of physical therapy as a preamble to the remainder of the text. The history of the profession was traced from its origins in World War I. The influence of poliomyelitis and world wars, relationships with the AMA, development of the APTA, and recognition as a profession were described. In the decades following World War II, growth and development were paramount features of the profession until managed care and other health care cost control forces took hold in the 1990s. The millennium ended with positive changes in reimbursement patterns for physical therapy and a vision for practice in the year 2020.

References

1. Beard G: Foundations for growth: A review of the first forty years in terms of education, practice, and research. Phys Ther Rev 1961;41:843–861.
2. Davies EJ: The beginning of "modern physiotherapy." Phys Ther 1976;56:15–21.
3. Davies EJ: Infantile paralysis. Phys Ther 1976;56:42–49.
4. Granger FB: The development of physiotherapy. Phys Ther 1976;56:13–14.
5. Guide to Physical Therapist Practice. 2nd ed. Phys Ther 2001;81:9–744.
6. Hazenhyer IM: A history of the American Physiotherapy Association. Physiother Rev 1946;26(1):3–14.
7. Hislop HJ: The not-so-impossible dream. Phys Ther 1975;55:1069–1080.
8. Jette A: Physical disablement concepts for physical therapy research and practice. Phys Ther 1994;74:380–386.
9. Model Definition of Physical Therapy for State Practice Acts, BOD 03-00-17-39. Alexandria, VA, American Physical Therapy Association, 2000.
10. Moore WE: The Professions: Roles and Rules. New York, Russell Sage Foundation, 1970.
11. Nagi S: Some conceptual issues in disability and rehabilitation. *In* Sussman M (ed): Sociology and Rehabilitation. Washington, DC, American Sociological Association, 1965.
12. Nagi S: Disability concepts revisited: Implications for prevention. *In* Pope A, Tarlov A (eds): Disability in America: Towards a National Agenda for Prevention. Washington, DC, National Academy Press, 1991.
13. Pinkston D: Evolution of the practice of physical therapy in the United States. *In* Scully RM, Barnes ML (eds): Physical Therapy. Philadelphia, JB Lippincott, 1989.
14. Position on Provision of Physical Therapy Interventions and Related Tasks, HOD 06-00-17-28. Alexandria, VA, American Physical Therapy Association, 2000.
15. Position on Physical Therapy as a Health Profession, HOD 06-99-19-23. Alexandria, VA, American Physical Therapy Association, 1999.
16. Vector Research Inc: Executive Summary, Workforce Study. Alexandria, VA, American Physical Therapy Association, 1997.

Suggested Readings _____

American Physical Therapy Association: Healing the Generations: A History of Physical Therapy and the American Physical Therapy Association. Lyme, CT, Greenwich Publishing Group, 1995.
Comprehensive and detailed description of the history and evolution of the profession and practice of physical therapy in the United States.

The beginning: Physical therapy and the APTA. Alexandria, VA, American Physical Therapy Association, 1979.
Excellent anthology of selected articles that describe the history of physical therapy and the APTA.

Hazenhyer IM: A history of the American Physical Therapy Association: 2. Formative years, 1926–1930. Physiother Rev 1946;26(2):66–74.
Describes the pertinent issues confronting the profession during this period, including the first published curriculum and a review of educational programs, controversy over technicians versus professionals, legislation to regulate practice, and growth of the journal.

Hazenhyer IM: A history of the American Physical Therapy Association: 3. Coming of age, 1931–1938. Physiother Rev 1946;26(3):122–129.
Continues description of issues in previous article as they evolved during this prewar period.

Hazenhyer IM: A history of the American Physical Therapy Association: 4. Maturity, 1939–1946. Physiother Rev 1946;26(4):174–184.
In this final article in the series, the author describes issues involving membership rights, chapter organizations, further curricular changes, impact of the National Foundation for Infantile Paralysis, activities in military service, and the journal.

Mathews JS: Professionalism in physical therapy: Current Patterns and Future Directions. *In* Mathews JS (ed): Practice Issues in Physical Therapy. Thorofare, NJ, Slack, 1989.
Comprehensive review of aspects that contribute to physical therapy as a profession and to physical therapists as professionals.

REVIEW QUESTIONS _____

1. How does the APTA's "definition" of physical therapy differ from its "philosophical statement"?

2. Describe the practice versus profession of physical therapy, and identify the documents that describe each.

3. Define "profession" and apply its five characteristics to physical therapy. Is it a profession?

4. How did polio and World Wars I and II affect the origin and evolution of physical therapy in the United States?

All *physical therapists, regardless of title or position, function in multiple capacities, shifting from one to another as the situation demands. For example, the clinician serves as a teacher, a supervisor, a negotiator, a clinician researcher, an advocate, and a business administrator. Physical therapists in other positions not only share those functions but may assume additional ones as well.*
Geneva R. Johnson, PT, FAPTA

Roles and Employment Settings

Michael A. Pagliarulo

ROLES IN THE PROVISION OF PHYSICAL THERAPY
    Primary, Secondary, and Tertiary Care
    Team Approach
    Prevention and Wellness
    Patient/Client Management Model
OTHER PROFESSIONAL ROLES
    Consultation
    Education
    Critical Inquiry
    Administration
EMPLOYMENT CHARACTERISTICS
    Demographics
    Employment Facility
SUMMARY

KEY TERMS

assessment

diagnosis

direct access

ergonomics

evaluation

examination

functional capacity evaluation

goals

history

informed consent

intervention

plan of care

prevention	Standards of Practice for Physical Therapy
primary care	systems review
prognosis	tertiary care
screening	tests and measures
secondary care	work-conditioning program
SOAP note	work-hardening program

OBJECTIVES   After reading this chapter, the reader will be able to

- Describe the roles of the physical therapist in primary, secondary, and tertiary care
- Describe the roles of the physical therapist in prevention and wellness
- Describe the components of the patient/client management model
- Describe general features of tests and measures and direct interventions used in physical therapy
- Describe other professional roles of the physical therapist in the areas of consultation, education, critical inquiry, and administration
- List and describe the demographic characteristics of physical therapists

In the past two decades, the demand for and recognition and reimbursement of services provided by physical therapists and physical therapist assistants have evolved dramatically. This transformation has resulted from several trends and outside influences, including the aging population, federal legislation entitling children in public schools to health care, a burgeoning public interest in personal fitness, and actions taken by insurance companies and the government to contain the rising cost of health care. Physical therapists and physical therapist assistants have had to adapt to these rapid and extensive changes. At times, these paradigm shifts have been frustrating to comprehend and accommodate. A quote from a Putnam Investments advertisement aptly summarizes these sentiments: "You think you understand the situation, but what you don't understand is that the situation just changed."[12]

Our profession has succeeded and will continue to succeed. We have followed several of the "ground rules" proposed by Price Pritchett, including becoming a quick-change artist, accepting ambiguity, and holding ourselves accountable for our individual actions.[12] To provide a framework to understand the profession of physical therapy in this context of change, this chapter will examine the varied and shifting roles of the physical therapist, the breadth of services provided, and the variety of employment settings where these services exist. Recent data will be presented to describe current demographic information and employment activities and conditions.

2

ROLES IN THE PROVISION OF PHYSICAL THERAPY

The primary role of a physical therapist involves direct patient care. While physical therapists engage in many other activities and in some cases no longer participate in clinical practice, patient care remains the foremost employment activity. For this reason, the **Standards of Practice for Physical Therapy** is perhaps the foremost core document approved by the House of Delegates of the American Physical Therapy Association (APTA). The Standards and their accompanying criteria, approved by the Board of Directors of the APTA, identify "conditions and performances that are essential for provision of high-quality physical therapy" (Fig. 2–1).[14] They address not only the provision of services but also other professional roles, including administration, education, and research. A description of these roles is presented later and in the following section.

Primary, Secondary, and Tertiary Care

Individuals who seek health care may move through multiple levels of specialization. The first level of care is called **primary care** and is defined as that level of health care delivered by a member of the health care system who is responsible for the majority of the health needs of the individual.[6] This level of care is generally provided by the first person in contact with the recipient, but not necessarily so. Family and community members may provide care at this level. **Secondary care** is provided by clinicians on a referral basis, that is, after the individual has received care at the primary level. In **tertiary care**, the service is provided by specialists who are frequently employed in facilities that focus on particular health conditions. These services may also be provided on a referral basis.

Physical therapists are engaged in practice at all three of these levels. Commonly, physical therapy is delivered by referral as secondary or tertiary care. In the latter case, the service may be provided in a highly specialized unit, such as a burn care center. However, the entry point for an individual seeking physical therapy services is shifting to primary care and is described as **direct access** (sometimes also known as "autonomous practice" or "patient's choice"). Burch described the preferred use of the phrase "direct access" in contrast to "practice without referral," which implies no regard or interest in the critical services provided by practitioners in other disciplines.[3] Direct access, currently legal in 33 states, refers to the direct accessibility of physical therapists to anyone seeking those services without the stipulation of referral from another health care provider. In this role, the physical therapist serves as a "gatekeeper" for further health care services. (For more information on direct access and the role of gatekeeper, see Chapter 6.)

Team Approach

Regardless of the level of care provided, the physical therapist works in collaboration with other health care professionals, including physicians, nurses, occupational therapists, dentists, social workers, speech-language pathologists, and orthotists/prosthetists. As the public seeks the services of other health care

Standards of Practice for Physical Therapy

The physical therapy profession is committed to providing an optimum level of service delivery and to striving for excellence in practice. The House of Delegates of the American Physical Therapy Association, as the formal body that represents the profession, attests to this commitment by adopting and promoting the following *Standards of Practice for Physical Therapy*. These Standards are the profession's statement of conditions and performances that are essential for provision of high-quality physical therapy. The Standards provide a foundation for assessment of physical therapy practice.

The Criteria for the Standards, promulgated by APTA's Board of Directors, are italicized beneath the Standards to which they apply.

I. Legal/Ethical Considerations

A. Legal Considerations
The physical therapist complies with all the legal requirements of jurisdictions regulating the practice of physical therapy.

The physical therapist assistant complies with all the legal requirements of jurisdictions regulating the work of the assistant.

B. Ethical Considerations
The physical therapist practices according to the *Code of Ethics* of the American Physical Therapy Association.

The physical therapist assistant complies with the *Standards of Ethical Conduct for the Physical Therapist Assistant* of the American Physical Therapy Association.

II. Administration of the Physical Therapy Service

A. Statement of Mission, Purposes, and Goals
The physical therapy service has a statement of mission, purposes, and goals that reflects the needs and interests of the patients/clients served, the physical therapy personnel affiliated with the service, and the community.

The statement of mission, purposes, and goals:
- *Defines the scope and limitations of the physical therapy service.*
- *Identifies the goals and objectives of the service.*
- *Is reviewed annually.*

B. Organizational Plan
The physical therapy service has a written organizational plan.

The organizational plan:
- *Describes relationships among components with the physical therapy service and, where the service is part of a larger organization, between the service and other components of that organization.*
- *Ensures that the service is directed by a physical therapist.*
- *Defines supervisory structures within the service.*
- *Reflects current personnel functions.*

C. Policies and Procedures
The physical therapy service has written policies and procedures that reflect the operation of the service and that are consistent with the mission, purposes, and goals of the service.

The written policies and procedures:
- *Are reviewed regularly and revised as necessary.*
- *Meet the requirements of federal and state law and external agencies.*
- *Apply to, but are not limited to:*
  - *Clinical education*
  - *Clinical research*
  - *Interdisciplinary collaboration*
  - *Criteria for access to care*
  - *Criteria for initiation and continuation of care*
  - *Criteria for referral to other appropriate health care providers*
  - *Criteria for termination of care*
  - *Equipment maintenance*
  - *Environmental safety*
  - *Fiscal management*
  - *Infection control*
  - *Job/position descriptions*
  - *Competency assessment*
  - *Medical emergencies*
  - *Care of patients/clients, including guidelines*
  - *Rights of patients/clients*
  - *Personnel-related policies*
  - *Improvement of quality of care and performance of services*
  - *Documentation*
  - *Staff orientation*

D. Administration
A physical therapist is responsible for the direction of the physical therapy service.

The physical therapist responsible for the direction of the physical therapy service:
- *Ensures compliance with local, state, and federal requirements.*
- *Ensures compliance with current APTA documents, including Standards of Practice for Physical Therapy and the Criteria, Guide to Physical Therapist Practice, Code of Ethics, Guide for Professional Conduct, Standards of Ethical Conduct for the Physical Therapist Assistant, and Guide for Conduct of the Affiliate Member.*
- *Ensures that services are consistent with the mission, purposes, and goals of the physical therapy service.*
- *Ensures that services are provided in accordance with established policies and procedures.*
- *Reviews and updates policies and procedures.*
- *Provides for training of physical therapy support personnel that ensures continued competence for their job description.*
- *Provides for continuous in-service training on safety issues and for periodic safety inspection of equipment by qualified individuals.*

E. Fiscal Management
The director of the physical therapy service, in consultation with physical therapy staff and appropriate administrative personnel, participates in planning for, and allocation of, resources. Fiscal planning and management of the service are based on sound accounting principles.

The fiscal management plan:
- *Includes a budget that provides for optimal use of resources.*
- *Ensures accurate recording and reporting of financial information.*
- *Ensures compliance with legal requirements.*
- *Allows for cost-effective utilization of resources.*
- *Uses a fee schedule that is consistent with the cost of physical therapy services and that is*

Figure 2–1. Standards of Practice for Physical Therapy is a policy document approved by the House of Delegates of the APTA. (From Standards of Practice for Physical Therapy, HOD 06-00-11-22. Alexandria, VA, American Physical Therapy Association, 2000.)

within customary norms of fairness and reasonableness.

F. Improvement of Quality of Care and Performance

The physical therapy service has a written plan for continuous improvement of quality of care and performance of services.

The improvement plan:
- *Provides evidence of ongoing review and evaluation of the physical therapy service.*
- *Provides a mechanism for documenting improvement in quality of care and performance.*
- *Is consistent with requirements of external agencies, as applicable.*

G. Staffing

The physical therapy personnel affiliated with the physical therapy service have demonstrated competence and are sufficient to achieve the mission, purposes, and goals of the service.

The physical therapy service:
- *Meets all legal requirements regarding licensure and certification of appropriate personnel.*
- *Ensures that the level of expertise within the service is appropriate to the needs of the patients/clients served.*
- *Provides appropriate professional and support personnel to meet the needs of the patient/client population.*

H. Staff Development

The physical therapy service has a written plan that provides for appropriate and ongoing staff development.

The staff development plan:
- *Includes self-assessment, individual goal setting, and organizational needs in directing continuing education and learning activities.*
- *Includes strategies for lifelong learning and professional and career development.*
- *Includes mechanisms to foster mentorship activities.*

I. Physical Setting

The physical setting is designed to provide a safe and accessible environment that facilitates fulfillment of the mission, purposes, and goals of the physical therapy service. The equipment is safe and sufficient to achieve the purposes and goals of physical therapy.

The physical setting:
- *Meets all applicable legal requirements for health and safety.*
- *Meets space needs appropriate*

for the number and type of patients/clients served.

The equipment:
- *Meets all applicable legal requirements for health and safety.*
- *Is inspected routinely.*

J. Collaboration

The physical therapy service collaborates with all appropriate disciplines.

The collaboration when appropriate:
- *Uses an interdisciplinary team approach to the care of patients/clients.*
- *Provides interdisciplinary instruction of patients/clients and families.*
- *Ensures interdisciplinary professional development and continuing education.*

III. Provision of Services

A. Informed Consent

The physical therapist has sole responsibility for providing information to the patient and for obtaining informed consent in accordance with jurisdictional law before initiating intervention.

In obtaining the informed consent of the patient/client, the physical therapist:
- *Clearly describes the proposed intervention, and delineates the expected benefits and material (decisional) risks as known with the proposed intervention.*
- *Compares known benefits and risks with and without the proposed intervention, and explains reasonable alternatives to the intervention.*

Patient/client informed consent obtained by the physical therapist:
- *Requires consent of a competent adult.*
- *Requires consent of a parent/legal guardian as the surrogate decision-maker when the adult patient is not competent or when the patient is a minor.*
- *Requires the patient/client or legal guardian to acknowledge understanding of the intervention and to give consent before intervention is initiated.*

B. Initial Examination/Evaluation/Diagnosis/Prognosis

The physical therapist performs an initial examination and evaluation to establish a diagnosis and prognosis prior to intervention.

The physical therapist examination:
- *Is documented, dated, and appropriately authenticated by the physical therapist who performed it.*
- *Identifies the physical therapy needs of the patient/client.*
- *Incorporates appropriate tests and measures to facilitate outcome measurement.*
- *Produces data that are sufficient to allow evaluation, diagnosis, prognosis, and the establishment of a plan of care.*
- *May result in recommendations for additional services to meet the needs of the patient/client.*

C. Plan of Care

The physical therapist establishes a plan of care for the patient/client based on the examination, evaluation, diagnosis, prognosis, anticipated goals, and expected outcomes of the planned interventions for identified impairments, functional limitations, and disabilities.

The physical therapist involves the patient/client and appropriate others in the planning, implementation, and assessment of the intervention program.

The physical therapist, in consultation with appropriate disciplines, plans for discharge of the patient/client, taking into consideration achievement of anticipated goals and expected outcomes, and provides for appropriate follow-up or referral.

The plan of care:
- *Is based on the examination, evaluation, diagnosis, and prognosis.*
- *Identifies anticipated goals and expected outcomes.*
- *Describes the proposed intervention, including frequency and duration.*
- *Includes documentation which is dated and appropriately authenticated by the physical therapist who established the plan of care.*

D. Intervention

The physical therapist provides, or directs and supervises, the physical therapy intervention consistent with the results of the examination, evaluation, diagnosis, prognosis, and plan of care.

The intervention:
- *Is based on the examination, evaluation, diagnosis, prognosis, and plan of care.*

Figure 2–1 *Continued*

Illustration continued on following page

- *Is provided under the ongoing direction and supervision of the physical therapist.*
- *Is provided in such a way that directed and supervised responsibilities are commensurate with the qualifications and the legal limitations of the physical therapist assistant.*
- *Is altered in accordance with changes in response or status.*
- *Is provided at a level that is consistent with current physical therapy practice.*
- *Is interdisciplinary when necessary to meet the needs of the patient/client.*
- *Documentation of the intervention is consistent with the Guidelines for Physical Therapy Documentation.*
- *Is dated and appropriately authenticated by the physical therapist or, when permissible by law, by the physical therapist assistant, or both.*

E. Reexamination
The physical therapist reexamines the patient/client as necessary during an episode of care to evaluate progress or change in patient/client status and modifies the plan of care accordingly or discontinues physical therapy services.

The physical therapist reexamination:
- *Is documented, dated, and appropriately authenticated by the physical therapist who performs it.*
- *Includes modifications to the plan of care.*

F. Discharge/Discontinuation of Intervention
The physical therapist discharges the patient/client from physical therapy services when the anticipated goals or expected outcomes for the patient/client have been achieved.

The physical therapist discontinues intervention when the patient/client is unable to continue to progress toward goals or when the physical therapist determines that the patient/client will no longer benefit from physical therapy.

Discharge documentation:
- *Includes the status of the patient/client at discharge and the goals and functional outcomes attained.*
- *Is dated and appropriately authenticated by the physical therapist who performed the discharge.*
- *Includes, when a patient/client is discharged prior to attainment of goals and functional outcomes, the status of the patient/client and the rationale for discontinuation.*

G. Communication/Coordination/Documentation
The physical therapist communicates, coordinates, and documents all aspects of patient/client management, including the results of the initial examination and evaluation, diagnosis, prognosis, plan of care, interventions, response to interventions, changes in patient/client status relative to the interventions, reexamination, and discharge/discontinuation of intervention.

Physical therapist documentation:
- *Is dated and appropriately authenticated by the physical therapist who performed the examination and established the plan of care.*
- *Is dated and appropriately authenticated by the physical therapist who performed the intervention or, when allowable by law or regulations, by the physical therapist assistant who performed specific components of the intervention as selected by the supervising physical therapist.*
- *Is dated and appropriately authenticated by the physical therapist who performed the reexamination and includes modifications to the plan of care.*

Figure 2–1 *Continued*

Glossary

Client—An individual who is not necessarily sick or injured but who can benefit from a physical therapist's consultation, professional advice, or services. A client also is a business, a school system, or other entity to whom physical therapists offer services.

Diagnosis—Both the process and the end result of the evaluation of information obtained from the patient examination. The physical therapist organizes the evaluation information into defined clusters, syndromes, or categories to determine the most appropriate intervention strategies for each patient.

Evaluation—A dynamic process in which the physical therapist makes clinical judgments based on data gathered during the examination.

Examination—The process of obtaining a history, performing relevant systems reviews, and selecting and administering specific tests and measures.

Intervention—The purposeful and skilled interaction of the physical therapist with the patient or client and, when appropriate, with other individuals involved with care, using various methods and techniques to produce changes in the condition of the patient or client. Intervention has three components: direct intervention; instruction of the patient or client and of the family; and coordination, communication, and documentation.

Patient—An individual who is receiving direct intervention for an impairment, functional limitation, disability, or change in physical function and health status resulting from injury, disease, or other causes; an individual receiving health care services.

Physical therapist patient/client management model—The model on which physical therapists base management of the patient throughout the episode of care, including the following elements: examination, evaluation and reevaluation, diagnosis, prognosis, and intervention leading to the outcome.

Plan of care—Statements that specify the anticipated long-term and short-term goals and the desired outcomes, predicted level of optimal improvement, specific interventions to be used, duration and frequency of the intervention required to reach the outcomes/goals, and the criteria for discharge.

Prognosis—The determination of the level of optimal improvement that might be attained by the patient/client and the amount of time needed to reach the level.

Treatment—The sum of all interventions provided by the physical therapist to a patient/client during an episode of care.

- *Is dated and appropriately authenticated by the physical therapist who performed the discharge, and includes the status of the patient/client and the goals and outcomes achieved.*
- *Includes, when a patient/client is discharged prior to achievement of goals and outcomes, the status of the patient/client and the rationale for discontinuation.*

IV. Education

The physical therapist is responsible for individual professional development. The physical therapist assistant is responsible for individual career development.

The physical therapist participates in the education of physical therapy students, physical therapist assistant students, and students in other health professions.

The physical therapist educates and provides consultation to consumers and the general public regarding the purposes and benefits of physical therapy.

The physical therapist educates and provides consultation to consumers and the general public regarding the roles of the physical therapist and the physical therapist assistant.

The physical therapist:
- *Educates and provides consultation to consumers and the general public regarding the roles of the physical therapist, the physical therapist assistant, and other support personnel.*

V. Research

The physical therapist applies research findings to practice and encourages, participates in, and promotes activities that establish the outcomes patient/client management provided by the physical therapist.

The physical therapist supports collaborative research.

The physical therapist:
- *Ensures that their knowledge of research literature related to practice is current.*
- *Ensures that the rights of study subjects are protected, and the integrity of research is maintained.*

- *Participates in the research process as appropriate to individual education, experience, and expertise.*
- *Educates physical therapists, physical therapist assistants, students, other health professionals, and the general public about the outcomes of physical therapist practice.*

VI. Community Responsibility

The physical therapist demonstrates community responsibility by participating in community and community agency activities, educating the public, formulating public policy, or providing pro bono physical therapy services.

The physical therapist:
- *Participates in community and community agency activities.*
- *Educates the public, including prevention education and health promotion.*
- *Helps formulate public policy.*
- *Provides pro bono physical therapy services.*

Adapted by the House of Delegates, June 1980

Amended June 2000, June 1999, June 1996, June 1991, June 1985

Figure 2–1 *Continued*

professionals, physical therapists collaborate with such practitioners as podiatrists, chiropractors, massage therapists, acupuncturists, and osteopaths. In addition, the therapist may communicate with other individuals, such as educators and insurers, for the ultimate benefit of the patient/client.

Prevention and Wellness

Fortunately, the general public has become more aware of healthy lifestyle habits and has engaged in activities and behavior that promote healthy living. By preventing or limiting dysfunction, individuals have more positive work and recreation experiences. In addition, the need and cost of health care are reduced.

Physical therapists, by virtue of their extensive education in normal body structure and function, are well qualified to provide services that prevent or limit dysfunction. These services may be categorized as screening or prevention activities.[6] In **screening**, the physical therapist determines whether further services are needed from a physical therapist or other health care professional. A common example is posture analysis in school-aged children to determine whether scoliosis may be present. In **prevention** activities, the physical therapist provides services designed to avoid the occurrence of pain and dysfunction or limit or reduce those that exist. These programs generally include several components: (1) history questionnaire, (2) medical screening and evaluation, (3) consultation, (4) exercise performance, and (5) reassessment.[8] The history questionnaire provides information about general health and related habits. A comprehensive medical and physical evaluation is necessary to establish a baseline and design a program. Consultation is provided individually or in a group to describe the results of the evaluation and compare them with norms. The results of the evaluation are used to design exercise programs, which may be conducted at home, at work, or at a health-related facility. Reassessment is done periodically to ensure program effectiveness and serve as a motivating factor.

Recently, the business and health care industries have been collaborating to establish health promotion programs to prevent injury and disease and thereby reduce health care costs while increasing productivity. Physical therapists are directly involved in these activities and may serve as consultants to establish programs or as health care providers to deliver services either on site or in a health-related facility. In these cases, the physical therapist may conduct an analysis of **ergonomics** at the work site and perform a **functional capacity evaluation**. Ergonomics is described as the relationship between the worker, the worker's tasks, and the work environment, whereas a functional capacity evaluation involves an examination of the physical abilities of the worker to perform the required tasks.[9] The therapist may then design a **work-conditioning program** or **work-hardening program**. In both cases, the goal is to return the individual to work. The work-conditioning program focuses more on the physical dysfunction, whereas the work-hardening program includes these aspects, in addition to behavioral and vocational management.[13]

Patient/Client Management Model

The *Guide to Physical Therapist Practice* has been instrumental in defining and describing what physical therapists do. Part of this achievement is due to promotion of the patient/client management model.[6] This model presents five components that reflect the process of gathering information, designing a plan of care, and implementing that plan to result in optimal outcomes for the patient/client. Before initiating services through this model, however, the therapist must obtain **informed consent** in accordance with the Standards of Practice for Physical Therapy (see Fig. 2–1).[14] The information provided should include (1) a clear description of the proposed intervention, expected benefits and known risks, and (2) a comparison of the benefits and risks with and without intervention, and an explanation of reasonable alternatives.[7] The physical therapist should provide adequate opportunity to answer any questions that the patient may have. The patient/client, parent, or legal guardian must confirm an understanding of the intervention and provide consent before interventions are begun.

Examination. After obtaining informed consent, the therapist may then move through the components of the patient/client management model (Fig. 2–2). The first component, **examination,** is the process of gathering information about the past and current status of the patient/client. It begins with a **history**

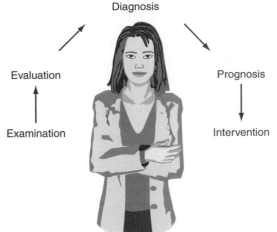

Diagnosis

Evaluation

Prognosis

Examination

Intervention

Figure **2–2.** The patient/client management model describes the sequence of events by physical therapists in the process of examination and intervention of individuals who receive care. (Adapted from Guide to Physical Therapist Practice. 2nd ed. Phys Ther 2001; 81:9–744.)

to describe the past and current nature of the condition or health status of the patient/client. Sources for this information include the patient/client, caregivers, other health professionals, and medical records. A **systems review** is then conducted to obtain general information about the overall medical and cognitive status of the patient/client. The final component of the examination, **tests and measures,** involves the selection and performance of specific procedures by the therapist to quantify the physical and functional status of the patient/client. An alphabetical list of these tests and measures is presented in Table 2–1. Figures 2–3 through 2–8 illustrate some examples of these tests and measures. Note that these activities involve observation, manual techniques, simple and complex equipment, and environmental analysis.

Evaluation. After the examination, the therapist performs an evaluation as the second component of the patient/client management model. As defined in the Standards of Tests and Measurements in Physical Therapy Practice, an **evaluation** is a *judgment* based on a measurement.[15] The standards further define **assessment** as the *measurement* or assigned value. Therefore, an evaluation is a process by which physical therapists make a clinical judgment based on an assessment.

Diagnosis. Evaluation is essential to establish a **diagnosis,** the next component of the model. The diagnosis is a categorization of the findings from the examination through a defined process. Establishing a diagnosis is performed in accordance with a policy adopted by the House of Delegates of the APTA (Box 2–1).[5] This policy recognizes the professional and autonomous judgment of the physical therapist and stipulates the responsibility of referral to other practitioners when warranted.

Prognosis. At this point in the model, attention shifts to the future to establish a **prognosis,** or a prediction of the level of improvement and time necessary to reach that level. The therapist also designs a **plan of care** that incorporates the

Table 2–1
Tests and Measures Used in a Physical Therapy Examination

TEST/MEASURE	DESCRIPTION
Aerobic capacity and endurance	Ability to use the body's O_2 uptake and delivery system
Anthropometric characteristics	Body measurements and fat composition
Arousal, attention, and cognition	Degree of responsiveness and awareness
Assistive and adaptive devices	Equipment to aid in performing tasks
Cranial and peripheral nerve integrity	Assessment of sensory and motor functions of cranial and peripheral nerves
Environmental, home, and work barriers	Analysis of physical restrictions to functioning in the environment
Ergonomics and body mechanics	Analyses of work tasks and postural adjustment to perform tasks
Gait, locomotion, and balance	Analyses of walking, moving from place to place, and equilibrium
Integumentary integrity	Health of the skin
Joint integrity and mobility	Assessment of joint structure and impact on passive movement
Motor function	Control of voluntary movement
Muscle performance	Analysis of muscle strength, power, and endurance
Neuromotor development and sensory integration	Evolution of movement skills and integration of information from the environment
Orthotic, protective, and supportive devices	Determination of need for fit of devices to support weak joints
Pain	Analysis of intensity, quality, and frequency of pain
Posture	Analysis of body alignment and positioning
Prosthetic requirements	Selection, fit, and use of prostheses
Range of motion	Amount of movement at a joint
Reflex integrity	Assessment of developmental, normal, and pathological reflexes
Self-care and home management	Analysis of activities necessary for independent living at home
Sensory integrity	Assessment of peripheral and central sensory processing, awareness of movement, and position
Ventilation and respiration/gas exchange	Assessment of movement of air into and out of the lungs, exchange of gases, and transport of blood to perform activities of daily living and exercises
Work, community, and leisure integration or reintegration	Analyses to determine whether the patient/client can assume a role in community or work

Data from Guide to Physical Therapist Practice. 2nd ed. Phys Ther 2001;81:9–744.

2

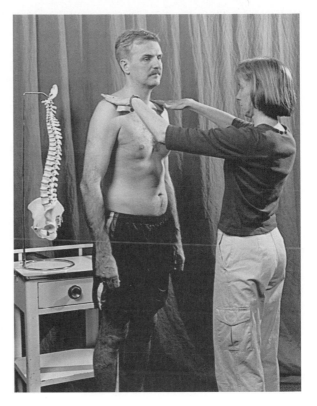

Figure 2–3. Observation is an essential component of a physical therapy examination. In this case, the therapist examines the cervical posture of the patient. Compare with Figure 2–9. (Courtesy of Dewey Neild.)

expectations of the patient/client. It identifies short- and long-term goals (alleviation of impairments), outcomes (results of interventions), interventions (type and frequency), and discharge criteria. The **goals** should be measurable, involve the patient/client or family member, and be linked to the impairments, functional limitations, and disabilities.[7] Only after these data-gathering and analysis activities have been completed can interventions begin.

Intervention. The last component of the model, **intervention,** occurs when the therapist and physical therapist assistant conduct procedures with the patient/client to achieve the desired outcomes. This component is subdivided into three activities, each of which is described further in the following paragraphs.

Coordination, Communication, and Documentation. These activities are essential to ensure that all personnel involved in care of the patient/client are well informed about the status of the individual by consistently exchanging information both verbally and in writing. This process requires effective communication in the verbal, written, and nonverbal arenas. Each deserves further description.

Verbal communication is a significant component of physical therapy service. The physical therapist must communicate orally with a variety of individuals, including the patient, family member, referral source, and additional practitioners providing care for the patient. Frequently, verbal and written commu-

Figure 2–4. Manual techniques such as manual muscle testing are also critical in physical examination. In this figure the therapist is performing a muscle test on the patient's shoulder musculature. (Courtesy of Dewey Neild.)

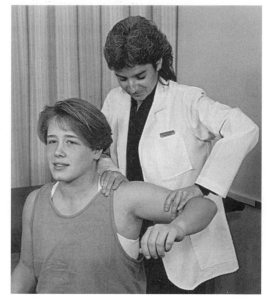

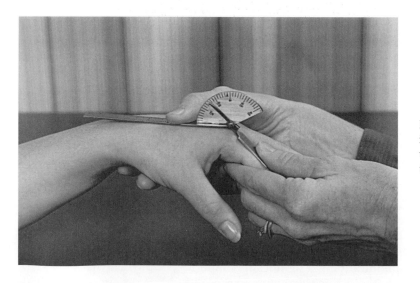

Figure 2–5. Passive range of motion in the joints of the fingers is measured with a simple finger goniometer. (Courtesy of Dewey Neild.)

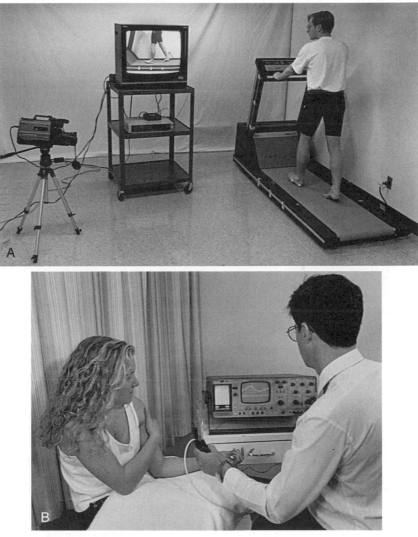

Figure 2–6. The equipment used by physical therapists for examinations can be complex. *A,* In motion analysis of the lower extremity, the patient is videotaped with markers at the joint axes while walking on a treadmill. The videotape is analyzed by computer technology to provide an objective measure of performance. *B,* Electrodiagnostic equipment is used to measure the conduction velocity of nerves. (Courtesy of Dewey Neild.)

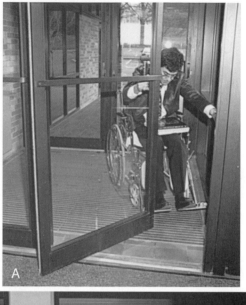

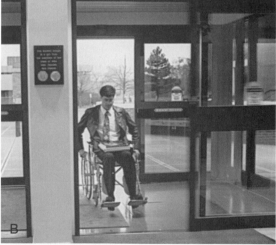

Figure 2–7. Architectural barriers in the environment, such as doorways that are difficult to manage in a wheelchair, are also examined by the physical therapist. *A,* Managing manual doorways can be difficult for individuals in wheelchairs. *B,* Automatic doorways provide excellent accessibility for individuals who use a wheelchair or assistive device. (Courtesy of Dewey Neild.)

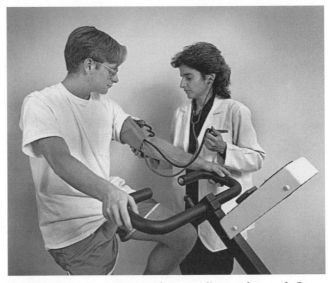

Figure 2–8. Physical therapists can conduct cardiovascular and fitness tests with a stationary bicycle. (Courtesy of Dewcy Neild.)

nication combines to provide a persuasive argument on behalf of the patient. Physical therapists must be skilled in these areas to describe their course of action.

Effective written communication is essential in the delivery of physical therapy services. Permanent records must be established to provide a baseline for future reference. They must be clear, concise, and accurate. Documentation is required by certain federal and state regulations and all insurance carriers. Fortunately, the APTA has constructed a set of *Guidelines for Physical Therapy Documentation* to assist physical therapists in this area.[7]

Written communication can follow many formats. Documentation regarding evaluation and treatment could be written as a narrative. This design allows maximum flexibility but is completely unstructured. Standardized forms are also frequently used to provide an efficient method to record information. They are helpful, but the structure of the form occasionally does not apply to the particular patient/client situation.

A third format, the **SOAP note,** combines the best attributes of the narrative and standardized form. It is taken from the problem-oriented medical record system introduced by Weed in 1969.[16] It is structured, yet adaptable and widely used among health care practitioners. The four components are (1) S for subjective (what the patient/client/family member describes), (2) O for objective (what the physical therapist observes or measures), (3) A for assessment (clinical judgment based on examination; includes goals), and (4) P for plan (plan of care). The abbreviations provide an effective and efficient method to outline and document information regarding the patient. It should be noted that use of the term "assessment" in this context is not the same as the

Box 2–1

Diagnosis by Physical Therapists

Physical therapists shall establish a diagnosis for each patient.

Prior to making a patient management decision, physical therapists shall utilize the diagnostic process in order to establish a diagnosis for the specific conditions in need of the physical therapist's attention.

A diagnosis is a label encompassing a cluster of signs and symptoms commonly associated with a disorder or syndrome or category of impairment, functional limitation, or disability. It is the decision reached as a result of the diagnostic process, which is the evaluation of information obtained from the patient examination. The purpose of the diagnosis is to guide the physical therapist in determining the most appropriate intervention strategy for each patient. In the event that the diagnostic process does not yield an identifiable cluster, disorder, syndrome, or category, intervention may be directed toward the alleviation of symptoms and remediation of impairment, functional limitation, or disability.

The diagnostic process includes the following: obtaining relevant history, performing systems review, selecting and administering specific tests and measures, and organizing and interpreting all data.

In performing the diagnostic process, physical therapists may need to obtain additional information (including diagnostic labels) from other health professionals. In addition, as the diagnostic process continues, physical therapists may identify findings that should be shared with other health professionals, including referral sources, to ensure optimal patient care. When the patient is referred with a previously established diagnosis, the physical therapist should determine that clinical findings are consistent with that diagnosis. If the diagnostic process reveals findings that are outside the scope of the physical therapist's knowledge, experience, or expertise, the physical therapist should then refer the patient to an appropriate practitioner.

From Diagnosis by Physical Therapists, HOD 06-97-06-19. Alexandria, VA, American Physical Therapy Association, 1997.

definition in the Standards of Tests and Measurements in Physical Therapy Practice, but more like the term "evaluation" in the same document.[15]

Another mode of communication that is occasionally overlooked is the nonverbal mode. It is important to note that facial expressions, body posture, and gestures often convey honest emotions (fear, pain, pleasure) that may be suppressed. In fact, Mehrabian reported that 55% of the impact of messages comes from facial expression, whereas only 38% comes from the vocal component and 7% from the verbal.[10] Physical therapists and physical therapist assistants must always be sensitive to the nonverbal signals displayed by themselves and their patients/clients.

Patient/Client-Related Instruction. This activity refers to education and training of the individual and caregivers regarding the plan of care and environmental transitions. Instruction may include audiovisual aids, demonstrations, and home programs and always incorporates the learning abilities and styles of the patient/client or caregiver.

Direct Intervention. Direct intervention is the major therapeutic interaction between the therapist/assistant and patient/client. A list of these interventions, in preferred order of use, is presented in Table 2–2. Figures 2–9 through 2–15 illustrate some examples of these direct interventions, which include manual techniques ("high-touch") and equipment ("high-tech"). At this point, a physical therapist assistant would be involved in a substantial component of the care as delegated by the physical therapist (see Chapter 3). Further descriptions of principles of direct interventions are found in Part II of this text.

Throughout the course of the patient/client management model, the physical therapist may periodically conduct re-examinations to determine the effect of the plan of care. If goals and outcomes are not being achieved, the plan, goals, and outcomes may be modified or the patient/client may be referred to other practitioners for services.

Ultimately, the patient/client will be discharged from physical therapy services. Normally, discharge occurs when the goals and outcomes have been achieved, but discharge may also occur because the patient/client terminates the services or the therapist believes that further intervention will not improve the status of the individual. In any case, the physical therapist must plan for this event and document reasons for discharge, status of the patient/client at that time, and any follow-up care that may be necessary.

OTHER PROFESSIONAL ROLES

Consultation

Physical therapists frequently provide consultation that is either patient centered or client centered. Patient-centered consultation refers to service provided by the physical therapist in making recommendations concerning the current or proposed physical therapy plan of care. It usually involves an examination but not intervention.

Client-centered consultation refers to the expert opinion or advice provided by the physical therapist regarding situations that do not directly involve patient care. These consultation services are provided to clients. Examples include court testimony, architectural recommendations, academic and clinical program evaluation, and suggestions for health care policies.

Education

Physical therapists and physical therapist assistants are constantly providing education to a variety of audiences because instruction is an inherent part of any patient care activity in physical therapy. Patients and sometimes family members are taught exercises or techniques to enhance function. Such instruction requires knowledge and skills that must be conveyed by the physical therapist or physical therapist assistant.

Text continued on page 41

Table 2–2
Direct Interventions Used in Physical Therapy

DIRECT INTERVENTION	DESCRIPTION
Therapeutic exercise	Activities to improve physical function and health status; performed actively, passively, or against resistance
Functional training in self-care and home management	Activities to improve function in activities of daily living and independence in home environment
Functional training in work, community, and leisure integration or reintegration	Activities to integrate or return the patient/client to work
Manual therapy techniques	Skilled hand techniques on soft tissues and joints
Prescription, application, and, as appropriate, fabrication of devices and equipment	Selection (or fabrication), fit, and training in the use of devices and equipment to improve function
Airway clearance techniques	Activities to improve airway protection, ventilation, and respiration
Integumentary repair and protective techniques	Activities to improve wound healing and scar management
Electrotherapeutic modalities	Use of electricity to decrease pain, swelling, and unwanted muscular activity; maintain strength; and improve functional training and wound healing
Physical agents and mechanical modalities	Use of thermal, acoustic, or radiant energy and mechanical equipment to decrease pain and swelling and improve skin condition and joint movement

Data from Guide to Physical Therapist Practice. 2nd ed. Phys Ther 2001;81:9–744.

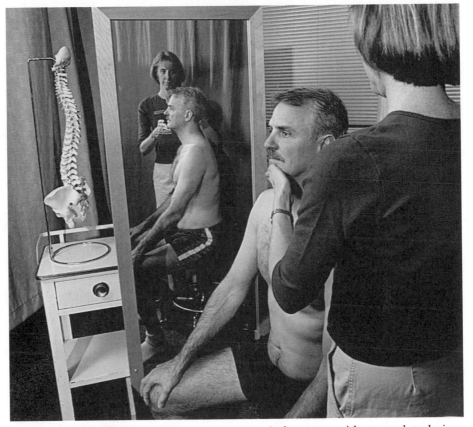

Figure 2–9. The physical therapist corrects cervical posture with manual techniques and instruction. Compare with Figure 2–3. (Courtesy of Dewey Neild.)

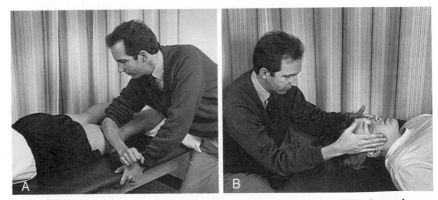

Figure 2–10. Myofascial release techniques are effective, rigorous, and gentle manual stretching techniques for soft tissue. Examples shown are in the posterior of the thigh (hamstring muscle) (*A*) and the temporomandibular joint region (*B*). (Courtesy of Dewey Neild.)

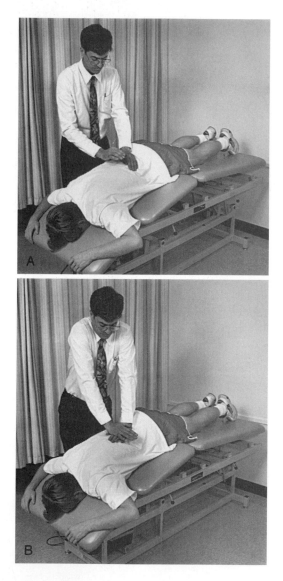

Figure 2–11. Postural drainage involves positioning, percussion, and coughing techniques to remove fluid from specific parts of the lungs. *A*, A cupping technique is applied to the lower ribs in a head-down position to loosen mucus in the lower lobes of the lungs (cupping done bilaterally). *B*, With outstretched arms, the therapist shakes the thoracic cage while the patient exhales to encourage coughing to remove fluid from the lungs. (Courtesy of Dewey Neild.)

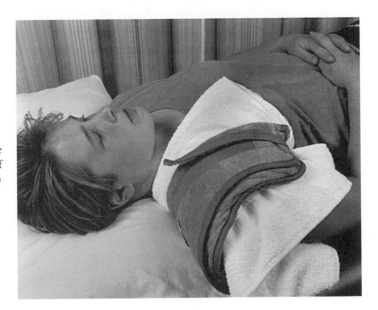

Figure 2–12. Hot packs applied to the shoulder region provide an effective form of superficial heat. (Courtesy of Dewey Neild.)

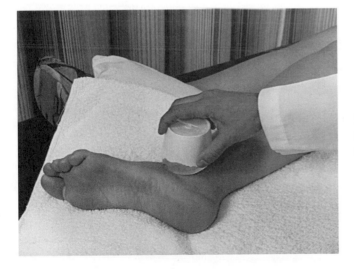

Figure 2–13. An ice massage is administered to the ankle to decrease pain and swelling. (Courtesy of Dewey Neild.)

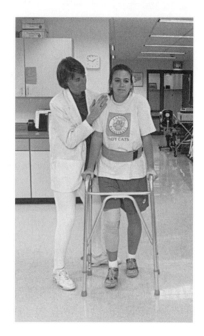

Figure 2–14. A walker is an example of an assistive device used to improve a person's functional abilities, such as ambulation. (Courtesy of Dewey Neild.)

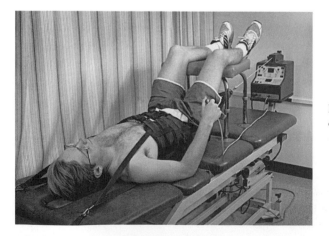

Figure 2–15. Mechanical traction units are used to open disk spaces between vertebrae and reduce pain. (Courtesy of Dewey Neild.)

2

Instruction also occurs in the clinical facility when students are supervised during internships. Demonstration, supervision, and feedback are important to practice and perfect skills.

Physical therapists and physical therapist assistants are also involved in academic education, either in the formal academic setting or in a continuing education program or presentation.

Critical Inquiry

Critical inquiry in physical therapy is essential for viability of the profession. Physical therapists and physical therapist assistants must be "healthy skeptics" and constantly ask "why." We must be able to respond to practitioners and those who pay for our services when questioned about the choice and efficacy of our direct interventions. Unfortunately, we do not have sufficient answers to these questions. Our practice must be based on sound evidence that comes from well-designed research (evidence-based practice). Sound practice is an inherent responsibility of every physical therapist and physical therapist assistant and is based on the selection of appropriate direct interventions, complete documentation, and outcomes assessment.

Research is the key to answer the critical questions proposed by the "healthy skeptics" within our profession and those outside the profession who challenge our practices. Experimental and case studies are common research methods to answer a research question or describe a technique or outcome. These studies are neither necessarily costly nor complex and are usually generated by astute clinical observation and questioning. While this type of research may require little more than good documentation and statistical comparison of two different direct interventions, it may involve substantial time, equipment, and cost. The Foundation for Physical Therapy supports this activity with grants and scholarships. Since its inception in 1979, it has provided nearly $6.5 million in awards and, in 1997, funded a $600,000 3 year grant to the University of Pittsburgh for a Clinical Research Center on Work-Related Low Back Injury. Activity at this comprehensive level, as well as at the individual level described earlier, is necessary to validate the direct interventions used by physical therapists and physical therapist assistants. (See Chapters 4 and 6 for more information on this foundation and evidence-based practice.)

Administration

Physical therapists and physical therapist assistants may move into a variety of administrative positions. Generally, the promotion ladder in clinical facilities involves more administrative responsibilities at the expense of patient care activities. An individual could also shift out of the patient care environment entirely and assume an executive position within a health care or related organization. In any case, administrative responsibilities include planning, communicating, delegating, managing, directing, supervising, budgeting, and evaluating. These activities are particularly important when the physical therapist is an owner or partner in an independent practice.

Somewhat related to this role is that of the physical therapist as a case manager. In this scenario, one individual is responsible for managing the health care of the patient/client with regard to the diagnosis. This manager may be a physician, nurse, or other designated health professional, including physical therapists.[4] Inherent in this model is an agreement by the provider to accept a predetermined fee for the services required for the diagnosis.[11] The case manager has the responsibility and authority to manage the necessary services in a cost-effective manner to achieve the desired outcomes of the plan of care. This area is relatively new for physical therapists, but one that is important for our profession to gain more control of reimbursement for necessary services by negotiating appropriate case fees and providing services that are efficient and effective.

EMPLOYMENT CHARACTERISTICS

The job market in physical therapy has changed recently in response to the impact of managed care and limited reimbursement from private and governmental payers. While the need for physical therapy services has not diminished, reimbursement for these services has. Employment opportunities have shifted relative to the coverage provided by third-party payers. To provide current and accurate data on these changes, the APTA is conducting an ongoing analysis of its members as they renew their membership. Numbers in these analyses range from 36,000 to 44,000 respondents. These data are reported several times each year, and data from the most recent analysis (February 2000) of the APTA Membership Database are presented in the following sections.[2] When available, data from earlier, less extensive membership surveys are included to demonstrate trends.[1]

Demographics

Gender. Females continue to predominate in the profession of physical therapy. They accounted for 68% of the respondents, with males accounting for 32%. This distribution increased from 71% in 1978 to 75% in 1987, and a slight decline is now seen in the proportion of females to males.

Age. The mean age of the respondents was 40 years. Since 1978, a modest and progressive increase in this figure has been noted (35 years); however, the members of this profession remain relatively young.

Education. The highest earned academic degree of the respondents is displayed in Figure 2–16. The baccalaureate degree continues to predominate at 56.1%; however, the percentage of respondents with this degree has declined steadily from 81% in 1978. In contrast, the percentage of respondents with a master's degree has steadily increased from 15.2% in 1978 to 40.4% in 2000. This increase is indicative of the transition to postbaccalaureate professional education at the master's and doctoral levels.

Employment Facility

A review of Figure 2–17 reveals that the highest percentage of respondents, 28.4%, are employed in a private office. This figure has remained relatively

2

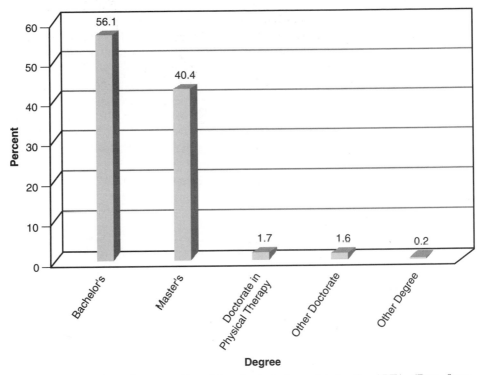

Figure 2–16. Highest degree achieved by physical therapists in the APTA. (Data from American Physical Therapy Association Membership Database. Alexandria, VA, American Physical Therapy Association, 2000.)

unchanged since 1993; however, previously, the hospital was the most common facility of employment. Regardless of the type of employment facility, the majority of respondents, 78%, held full-time positions.

Summary ——— The roles and activities of a physical therapist have begun an evolutionary change in response to the recent growth of managed care and health care cost containment. Despite these changes, diversity and opportunity remain widespread in physical therapy. Direct patient/client care continues to be the primary activity of physical therapists. Such care involves examination, evaluation, diagnosis, prognosis, and intervention as outlined in the patient/client management model. Physical therapists also provide services to prevent pain and dysfunction and promote wellness. Other roles include consultation, education, critical inquiry, and administration. Regardless of the area of activity, physical therapists must collaborate with other health care providers and communicate effectively in the verbal, written, and nonverbal modes.

In terms of demographics, the majority of physical therapists are female and relatively young. The baccalaureate degree predominates as the highest degree, but the number of therapists with a master's or doctoral degree continues to increase. The most common employment facility is a private office.

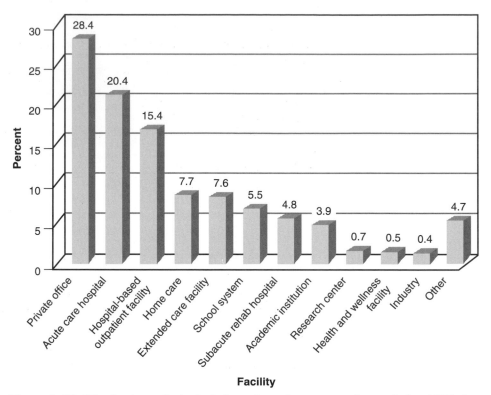

Figure 2–17. Distribution of physical therapists who are members of the APTA by facility of employment. (Data from American Physical Therapy Association Membership Database. Alexandria, VA, American Physical Therapy Association, 2000.)

These characteristics indicate that the profession is continuing to evolve and succeed. Such attributes contribute to the popularity of the profession and the enthusiasm of many individuals for pursuing a career as a physical therapist or physical therapist assistant.

References

1. American Physical Therapy Association 1987 Active Membership Profile Survey. Alexandria, VA, American Physical Therapy Association, 1987.
2. American Physical Therapy Association Membership Database. Alexandria, VA, American Physical Therapy Association, 2000.
3. Burch E: Direct access. *In* Matthews J (ed): Practice Issues in Physical Therapy. Thorofare, NJ, Slack, 1989.
4. Curtis KA: The Physical Therapist's Guide to Health Care. Thorofare, NJ, Slack, 1999.
5. Diagnosis by Physical Therapists, HOD 06-97-06-19. Alexandria, VA, American Physical Therapy Association, 1997.
6. Guide to Physical Therapist Practice. 2nd ed. Phys Ther 2001;81:9–744.
7. Guidelines for Physical Therapy Documentation, BOD 03-00-22-54. Alexandria, VA, American Physical Therapy Association, 2000.
8. Huhn RH, Volski RV: Primary prevention programs for business and industry. Phys Ther 1985;65:1840–1844.

9. Key GL: Industrial physical therapy. *In* Gould JA III (ed): Orthopaedic and Sports Physical Therapy, ed 2. St Louis, CV Mosby, 1990.
10. Mehrabian A: Silent Messages. Belmont, CA, Wadsworth, 1971.
11. Nosse LJ, Friberg DG, Kovacek PR: Managerial and Supervisory Principles for Physical Therapists. Baltimore, Williams & Wilkins, 1999.
12. Pritchett P: The Employee Handbook of New Work Habits for a Radically Changing World. Dallas, Pritchett & Associates, 1994.
13. Resource Guide: Industrial Physical Therapy. Alexandria, VA, American Physical Therapy Association, 1992.
14. Standards of Practice for Physical Therapy, HOD 06-00-11-12. Alexandria, VA, American Physical Therapy Association, 2000.
15. Task force on standards for measurements in physical therapy. Standards for tests and measurements in physical therapy practice. Phys Ther 1991;71:589–622.
16. Weed LL: Medical Records, Medical Education and Patient Care. Chicago, Year Book, 1970.

2

Suggested Readings

Davis CM: Patient Practitioner Interaction, ed 3. Thorofare, NJ, Slack, 1998.

Addresses the affective domain of behavior and includes content on self-awareness and communicating with others in the context of health care.

Gould JA III (ed): Orthopaedic and Sports Physical Therapy, ed 2. St Louis, Mosby–Year Book, 1990.

A comprehensive review of examination and direct intervention techniques in orthopaedic and sports physical therapy arranged by technique and body region.

Hayes W: Manual for Physical Agents, ed 5. E Norwalk, CT, Appleton & Lange, 2000.

A concise presentation on physical agents, including description, purpose and effects, advantages, disadvantages, indications, contraindications, precautions, instructions, and frequency.

Hecox B, Mehretab TA, Weisberg J: Physical Agents: A Comprehensive Text for Physical Therapists. E Norwalk, CT, Appleton & Lange, 1994.

Includes a thorough description of the physical agents used in physical therapy and their mechanisms of action and physiological effects.

Irwin S, Tecklin JS (eds): Cardiopulmonary Physical Therapy, ed 3. St Louis, Mosby–Year Book, 1995.

Presents the physiology, examination, and treatment of cardiac and pulmonary disorders seen by physical therapists.

Minor MA, Minor SD: Patient Care Skills, ed 4. Stamford, CT, Appleton & Lange, 1999.

Presents a comprehensive review of patient handling techniques (e.g., transfers, ambulation). Photos and a section on the Americans with Disabilities Act supplement the text.

Myers RS: Saunders Manual of Physical Therapy Practice, Philadelphia, WB Saunders, 1995.

Comprehensive resource text written for experienced practicing physical therapy practitioners.

Pauls JA, Reed KL: Quick Reference to Physical Therapy. Gaithersburg, MD, Aspen, 1996.

Synopsis of diseases, disorders, and dysfunctions referenced in the physical therapy literature. Extensive references are included.

Purtillo R: Health Professional and Patient Interaction, ed 4. Philadelphia, WB Saunders, 1990.

Focuses on the psychosocial aspects of interpersonal communication between the practitioner and patient.

Scully RM, Barnes ML: Physical Therapy. Philadelphia, JB Lippincott, 1989.

A comprehensive text on the profession and practice of physical therapy for advanced-level students or practitioners.

Umphred DA (ed): Neurological Rehabilitation, ed 3. St Louis, Mosby–Year Book, 1995.

Includes the theoretical foundations, evaluation, and treatment techniques of neurological disorders seen by physical therapists.

Walter J: Physical Therapy Management: An Integrated Science. St Louis, Mosby–Year Book, 1993.

Presents current issues and strategies relating to management in physical therapy. Chapter topics include an overview of health care systems, laws and regulations, ethics, organizational behavior, marketing, and fiscal management. Case studies are used to illustrate managerial concepts.

REVIEW QUESTIONS

1. Why is the phrase "direct access" preferred over "practice without referral"?

2. You go to a physical therapist for an injury sustained while skiing. Describe what you should expect at the first meeting before intervention begins.

3. Describe the steps in an initial examination.

4. What is included in a plan of care?

5. Discuss how you would decide which documentation format might best suit a physical therapist's needs in any given situation. Show the advantages and disadvantages of each.

6. What is the difference between patient-centered and client-centered consultation?

*W*hat matters is not the letters that come after your name, but what
you can do.
Nancy Watts, PT, FAPTA

The Physical
Therapist
Assistant

Cheryl A. Carpenter

KEY TERMS

active member
Affiliate Assembly
affiliate member
Affiliate Special Interest Group
career ladder
National Assembly of Physical Therapist
Assistants (National Assembly)
physical therapist assistant (PTA)
physical therapy aide
Representative Body of the National Assembly
(RBNA)
Student Assembly

OBJECTIVES   After reading this chapter, the reader will be able to

- Identify historical milestones in the development of the role of the physical therapist assistant
- Differentiate between the role of the physical therapist and the physical therapist assistant in the practice setting
- Define physical therapist assistant educational competencies in the areas of examination, measurement, and intervention.
- Identify the rights and privileges of affiliate members in the American Physical Therapy Association (APTA) and the National Assembly of Physical Therapist Assistants.

> The dilemma with which physical therapy is faced is that there are not enough physical therapists to perform the essential physical therapy services, and it is apparent from identifiable trends that there will not be enough physical therapists for this purpose in the foreseeable future. Yet the need for physical therapy services is constantly growing and will accelerate in coming years.[18]

This comment was made by Catherine Worthingham as a member of a panel discussion on nonprofessional personnel in physical therapy at the 1964 Annual Conference of the APTA. The shortage of physical therapy personnel identified in that address was exacerbated by the continued increased demand for services. This shortage identified the need for a new kind of health care team member—one who had knowledge of the life sciences, first aid, and physical therapy techniques and, most important, one who could problem-solve to make patient care decisions. This void was filled by the creation of a formally educated physical therapist assistant (PTA).

DEFINITION   A **physical therapist assistant** is defined as a health care provider who assists the physical therapist (PT) in the provision of physical therapy and has graduated from an accredited PTA associate degree program (Box 3–1).[7] The function of a PTA is to assist the PT in the delivery of physical therapy services in compliance with federal and state regulations regarding the practice of physical therapy. While in all jurisdictions the PTA carries out tasks delegated by the PT, the degree of supervision and autonomy varies by state.

Box 3–1

Definition of the Physical Therapist Assistant

The physical therapist assistant is a technically educated health care provider who assists the physical therapist in the provision of physical therapy. The physical therapist assistant is a graduate of a physical therapist assistant associate degree program accredited by the Commission on Accreditation in Physical Therapy Education (CAPTE).

From Direction and Supervision of the Physical Therapist Assistant, HOD 06-00-16-27. Alexandria, VA, American Physical Therapy Association, 2000.

ORIGIN AND HISTORY

The role of the PT and the use of support personnel have been influenced by events that occurred over the last few decades. The Hill-Burton Act of 1946 and the subsequent amendment in 1954 provided specific funds for the construction of nursing homes, diagnostic and treatment centers, rehabilitation facilities, and chronic disease hospitals.[11] The provision for rehabilitation facilities created a new need for physical therapy.

Changes in human resource needs resulted in a shift from the exclusive use of PTs to the use of support personnel for efficient and cost-effective delivery models of patient care. The anticipated growth of the profession prompted the 1949 APTA House of Delegates to adopt the first resolution concerning the use of nonprofessional personnel.

During the 1960s, efforts were made to ensure the continued provision of health care in response to the increased demand. The number of employees in the health services industry in 1960 was 2.6 million, a 54% increase over 1950. In 1965, the 89th Congress enacted laws that created Medicare and Medicaid. These laws began to officially recognize the need for innovative trends in health care. It was believed that the establishment and growth of new health care programs would create a need for supportive personnel. Medicare and Medicaid identified categories of these personnel and their relationships to primary care providers.[3]

Several agencies began to investigate the creation of supportive personnel in physical therapy, including the American Association of Junior Colleges; the U.S. Department of Labor; the U.S. Department of Health, Education, and Welfare; vocational schools; proprietary agencies; physician groups; nursing homes; and state health departments.

Changes in the roles and responsibilities of support personnel resulted in a shift in the site of preparation from the work setting (hospital) to the educational setting (campus).[4] The APTA recognized problems regarding shortages in support personnel and unregulated education programs. Concern was expressed over the development of training programs without the benefit of physical therapy leadership and input.[12] A task force was established in 1964 to investigate the role of support personnel for the professional PT and the criteria for PTA education programs. In 1967, the task force submitted to the APTA House of Delegates a proposal for guidelines for use of the PTA.

On July 5th of that same year, after deliberation the House of Delegates adopted a policy statement regarding standards for PTA education programs, essentially giving birth to the PTA. The policy statement recommended the following: "(1) that APTA was to establish the standards for the program, which also meant an attendant process of some form of accreditation; (2) that a supervisory relationship should exist between the physical therapist and the physical therapist assistant; (3) that the functions of the assistant be identified; (4) that mandatory licensure or registration, incorporated into existing physical therapy laws, should be encouraged; and (5) that a category of membership be established in APTA for the physical therapist assistant."[17]

A subsequent policy further defined the PTA education program as a 2-year college program located in an accredited educational institution. For approval,

3

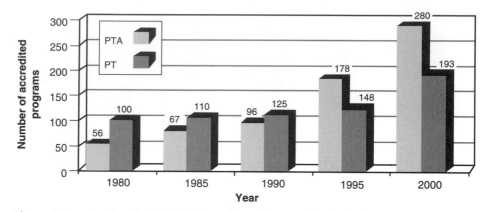

Figure 3–1. Growth of physical therapist assistant and physical therapist education programs. (From Department of Accreditation, American Physical Therapy Association.)

the education program had to provide information to the APTA Board of Directors, which evaluated the program against the standards and curriculum guidelines published by the APTA,[6] similar to the current accreditation process followed by existing PTA programs. Two PTA education programs were created in 1967. Two years later, these institutions graduated the first 15 PTAs. The growth as well as development of new PTA education programs was and remains phenomenal. Figure 3–1 indicates that the number of PTA education programs now substantially exceeds the number of PT education programs.

CURRICULUM AND ACCREDITATION STANDARDS

The curricula for all 2-year associate degree PTA education programs are designed to meet the accreditation standards outlined by CAPTE, the same agency that accredits education programs for the PT.

In comparing the accreditation criteria for the PTA and the PT, many similarities exist. The curricula for both these health care providers must consist of a combination of didactic and clinical learning experiences that are reflective of contemporary practice.[8, 9] This similarity is indicative of their complementary and interactive roles in clinical practice. A comparison of the similarities and differences in their education programs provides a basis for understanding the tasks appropriate for delegation, supervision, and autonomy in clinical practice.

Educational similarities begin in their core curricula. Both PTA and PT students must complete courses such as anatomy, physiology, biology, kinesiology, and general education courses that lead to the students' respective degrees awarded by the college or university. The difference in the PT's education is the depth of theory and practice provided during mandatory advanced courses such as anatomy, physiology, neuroanatomy, physics, research, pathophysiology, neurology, and pharmacology.

Courses in the professional portions of the curricula are also similar in content areas. In regard to assessment and measurement techniques, specific areas must be included in accordance with accreditation criteria (Box 3–2;

Box 3–2

Assessment and Measurement Techniques in Physical Therapist Assistant Curriculum

Architectural Barriers and Environmental Modifications
Endurance
Flexibility/Range of Motion and Muscle Length
Functional Activities
Gait and Balance
Pain
Posture
Righting and Equilibrium Reactions
Segmental Length, Girth, and Volume
Skin and Sensation
Strength
Vital Signs

Reprinted from *Evaluative Criteria for Accreditation of Education Programs for the Preparation of Physical Therapist Assistants* with the permission of the American Physical Therapy Association. Alexandria, VA, American Physical Therapy Association, 1998.

compare with Table 2–1).[9] Likewise, intervention techniques in specific areas must also be addressed (Box 3–3; compare with Table 2–2).[9] Figure 3–2 illustrates a PTA performing an assessment and an intervention.

Clinical education is also a requirement in both curricula. Programs must provide the PTA or PT student with clinical rotations in a variety of settings and with different patient populations. Students have the opportunity to work with numerous medical diagnoses in acute care, rehabilitation, outpatient, and school settings while supervised by a clinical instructor. Graduate PTAs may supervise PTA students, with additional direction provided by the center coordinator of clinical education or PT at the facility. Graduate PTs serve as clinical instructors to both PTA and PT students.

Often, PTA and PT students are involved in clinical affiliations at the same location, which provides an opportunity for students to communicate with each other regarding similarities in the physical therapy education programs. Delegation of tasks and the responsibility for patient follow-up could be simulated with guidance of the respective clinical instructors.

In addition to specific content areas, the accreditation criteria emphasize that PTA program graduates practice in an ethical, legal, safe, caring, and effective manner. The graduate must understand principles of authority and responsibility, planning and time management, the supervisory process, performance evaluations, policies and procedures, fiscal considerations for physical therapy, and quality assurance and must be able to plan for future professional development to maintain practice consistent with acceptable standards. PTA graduates must demonstrate the ability to modify intervention techniques as

Box 3–3

Intervention Techniques in Physical Therapist Assistant Curriculum

Activities of Daily Living and Functional Training
Assistive/Adaptive Devices
Balance and Gait Training
Biofeedback
Developmental Activities
Electric Current
Electromagnetic Radiations
External Compression
Hydrotherapy
Orthoses and Prostheses
Patient and Family Education
Postural Training and Body Mechanics
Pulmonary Hygiene Techniques
Therapeutic Exercise
Therapeutic Massage
Thermal Agents
Topical Application (including those for iontophoresis)
Traction
Ultrasound
Universal Precautions/Infection Control
Wound Care

Reprinted from *Evaluative Criteria for Accreditation of Education Programs for the Preparation of Physical Therapist Assistants* with the permission of the American Physical Therapy Association. Alexandria, VA, American Physical Therapy Association, 1998.

indicated in the plan of care designed by the PT or as necessitated by acute changes in the client's physiological state. The PTA graduate must also be able to read and interpret professional literature and critically analyze new concepts.

The PTA must also be proficient in communication. The graduate must be able to interact with patients and families in a manner that provides the desired psychosocial support; teach other health providers, patients, and families to perform selected intervention procedures; participate in discharge planning and follow-up; document relevant aspects of patient treatment; and promote effective interpersonal relationships. Skill development in these areas requires knowledge and training in written, oral, and nonverbal communication.

UTILIZATION

Physical Therapist Assistant

When describing the utilization of a PTA, it is often helpful to acknowledge and discard some of the myths that surround the topic, including the following: (1) it is essential for PTs to perform all physical therapy techniques with patients, (2) the assistant should administer only physical agents to patients,

3

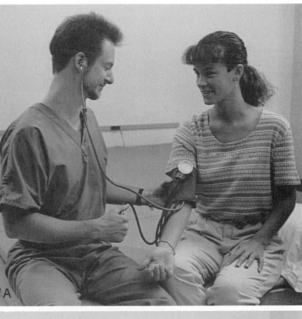

Figure 3–2. A physical therapist assistant performing an assessment (blood pressure measurement) (*A*) and an intervention (balance and strengthening exercises) (*B*).

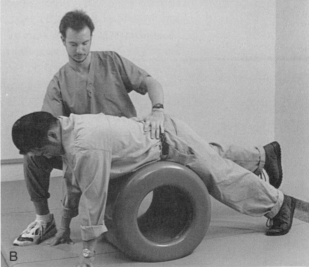

(3) the assistant requires step-by-step instructions, (4) the PTA is someone to whom the PT delegates noncompliant patients, and (5) the assistant is trying to take over the job of the PT. This section will dispel these myths and provide an accurate description of the roles of the PTA and PT.

While many similarities exist, differences in roles appear soon after initial employment. In a study conducted on utilization of PTAs, Gossett reported, "Where simultaneous or near-simultaneous employment did occur, the new assistant graduate and the new physical therapy graduate appeared to function similarly, initially. The new physical therapist, however, soon was expected to accept more responsibility in the areas of departmental supervision, patient evaluations, and performance of more complex treatment procedures."[10]

The area of evaluation serves as a clear example of role distinction. It is the responsibility of the PT to perform the patient's physical therapy evaluation. This act requires interpreting the results of the examination and using the results as a guide to set realistic goals and design an appropriate plan of care. This process requires understanding and judgment based on the theoretical premises of life sciences that have been provided in the physical therapy curriculum.

Many aspects of the plan of care may be delegated to the PTA. Delegation of patient intervention after the initial evaluation requires supervision and ongoing communication. The exchange of information is crucial to physical therapy practice.

These and related responsibilities are delineated in the APTA policy titled *Direction and Supervision of the Physical Therapist Assistant* (HOD 06-00-16-27), which states in part, "Direction and supervision are essential in the provision of quality physical therapy services. The degree of direction and supervision necessary for assuring quality physical therapy services is dependent upon many factors, including the education, experience, and responsibilities of the parties involved, as well as the organizational structure in which the physical therapy services are provided" (Box 3–4).[7]

The factors of education, experience, and responsibilities deserve further analysis. *Education* has been previously reviewed in the Curriculum and Accreditation Standards section. Competency in such areas as therapeutic exercise, goniometry, manual muscle testing, and application of physical agents is a requirement of a PTA graduate.

The degree of delegation and supervision is also dependent on *experience*. PTAs and PTs continue to expand their knowledge base and skills after graduation. Continuing education courses, staff development seminars, and individual in-services by colleagues take place on an ongoing basis. For example, a PTA may attend an ergonomic seating seminar. Expertise in this area may lend itself to performance of ergonomic assessments for the patient population that the PTA is treating. The PT may have included ergonomic instruction as part of the plan of care to be performed based on patient need and, if delegated to the PTA, based on the assistant's ability. If the PT did not delegate this component of care to the PTA, the PT could decide to (1) conduct the

Box 3–4

Direction and Supervision of the Physical Therapist Assistant

3

Physical therapists have a responsibility to deliver services in ways that protect the public safety and maximize the availability of their services. They do this through direct delivery of services in conjunction with responsible utilization of physical therapist assistants who assist with specific components of intervention. The physical therapist assistant is the only individual permitted to assist a physical therapist in selected interventions under the direction and supervision of a physical therapist.

Direction and supervision are essential in the provision of quality physical therapy services. The degree of direction and supervision necessary for assuring quality physical therapy services is dependent upon many factors, including the education, experiences, and responsibilities of the parties involved, as well as the organizational structure in which the physical therapy services are provided.

Regardless of the setting in which the service is given, the following responsibilities must be borne solely by the physical therapist:

1. Interpretation of referrals when available.
2. Initial examination, evaluation, diagnosis, and prognosis.
3. Development or modification of a plan of care which is based on the initial examination or reexamination and which includes the physical therapy anticipated goals and expected outcomes.
4. Determination of when the expertise and decision-making capability of the physical therapist requires the physical therapist to personally render physical therapy interventions and when it may be appropriate to utilize the physical therapist assistant that provides for the delivery of service that is safe, effective and efficient.
5. Reexamination of the patient in light of the patient's anticipated goals and revision of the plan of care when indicated.
6. Establishment of the discharge plan and documentation of discharge summary/status.
7. Oversight of all documentation for services rendered to each patient.

From Direction and Supervision of the Physical Therapist Assistant, HOD 06-00-16-27. Alexandria, VA, American Physical Therapy Association, 2000.

assessment personally or (2) refer the patient for ergonomic assessment elsewhere.

The third factor affecting delegation is *responsibilities*. Part of the APTA policy cited earlier (HOD 06-00-16-17) addresses the responsibilities of the PT. While the PT may delegate all, some, or none of the intervention tasks to the PTA, the ultimate responsibility for the physical therapy services provided to the patient, including evaluations (initial, interim, and final), rests with the PT.

Figure 3–3 depicts the delegation of responsibilities and interaction between the PT and PTA as a decision tree.

Supervision is an inherent component of delegation, and although certain tasks may be delegated to a PTA, as noted earlier, the PT remains ultimately responsible for the patient. Supervision must be provided by the PT, and the PTA should be able to request supervision as needed.

This relationship is frequently regulated by PTA/PT ratios. Although PTA/PT ratios are not defined specifically in APTA policies, these ratios may be established in a state physical therapy practice act. When establishing these ratios, the supervising PT, the PTA, and the facility management should be

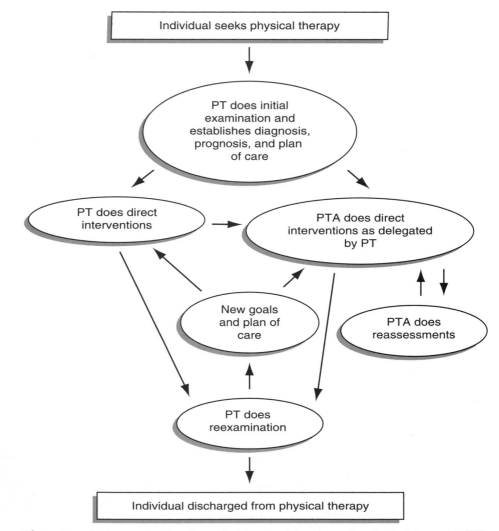

Figure 3–3. Pathways of delegation (decision tree) involving the physical therapist (PT) and physical therapist assistant (PTA).

involved. The ratio should take into account the *experience* of the PT and PTA, the *impairment* of the patients, the *patient caseload* per therapist/assistant, and the *accessibility* of the PT by telecommunication. The APTA policy on direction and supervision of the PTA also addresses this issue (Box 3–5).[7]

For example, consider a therapist who is consulting at three clinical facilities in a rural area with one PTA in each facility. The patient load is approximately 15 to 18 patients a day for each PTA. The level of impairment varies from a few patients in intensive care units to patients in the acute care sections of the facilities. In addition, the therapist needs to evaluate approximately 4 to 5 patients per day among the three facilities. The PT carries a beeper and is accessible at all times. Supervision is provided in accordance with the state practice act, which defines it as being available at all times through telecommunication, with weekly on-site visits.

In this scenario, the therapist is responsible for 45 to 54 patients with varying levels of impairment seen by the PTAs and for 4 to 5 patient evaluations per day. As noted from this example, special consideration should be given to establish appropriate PTA/PT ratios.

Delegation in physical therapy cannot rely on myths. Facts to consider are that (1) PTAs are competent to perform many aspects of patient care delegated, including assessment and intervention techniques; (2) PTAs are competent to carry out a plan of care based on well-formulated goals with general instruction from the PT; (3) PTAs do not initially evaluate patients, nor do they diagnose or make a prognosis; (4) PTAs continue to gain expertise through continuing education and work-related experience; and (5) PTAs are routinely performing the kinds of procedures that were once believed to be beyond a PTA's comprehension, just as PTs are diagnosing conditions and performing advanced examinations once deemed to be beyond the scope of the practice of physical therapy.[2]

As the physical therapy profession progresses, the personnel within it will be required to adapt to the changes. Traditionally considered support personnel, PTAs are now recognized as paraprofessionals. Although correct use of the title physical thera*pist* assistant implies that ultimate responsibility for physical therapy services rests with the PT, partnership is a key ingredient to success in the changing environment of physical therapy.

Physical Therapy Aide

As the role and utilization of the PTA continue to evolve, confusion remains regarding the role and utilization of the **physical therapy aide**. In part, this uncertainty is due to the variety of state laws that regulate or are silent on the physical therapy aide. To provide clarity and consistency, the APTA adopted a position in 2000 to address the definition and utilization of the physical therapy aide (Box 3–6).[16] The position indicates that the scope of support services is very limited and that direct personal supervision must be continuous throughout each session. In some jurisdictions, supervision may be provided by the PTA.

Box 3–5

Utilization of the Physical Therapist Assistant

The physical therapist is directly responsible for the actions of the physical therapist assistant. The physical therapist assistant may perform physical therapy interventions that have been selected by the supervising physical therapist. Where permitted by law, the physical therapist assistant may also carry out routine operational functions. The ability of the physical therapist assistant to perform the selected interventions shall be assessed on an ongoing basis by the supervising physical therapist. The physical therapist assistant may modify an intervention in accordance with changes in patient/client status within the scope of the established plan of care.

The physical therapist assistant must work under the direction and supervision of the physical therapist. In all practice settings the performance of selected interventions by the physical therapist assistant must be consistent with safe and legal physical therapy practice and shall be predicated on the following factors: complexity and acuity of the patient/client's needs; proximity and accessibility to the physical therapist; supervision available in the event of emergencies or critical events; and type of setting in which the service is provided.

When supervising the physical therapist assistant in any off-site setting, the following requirements must be observed:

1. A physical therapist must be accessible by telecommunications to the physical therapist assistant at all times while the physical therapist assistant is treating patients/clients.
2. There must be regularly scheduled and documented conferences with the physical therapist assistant regarding patients/clients, the frequency of which is determined by the needs of the patient/client and the needs of the physical therapist assistant.
3. In those situations in which a physical therapist assistant is involved in the care of a patient/client, a supervisory visit by the physical therapist will be made:
   a. Upon the physical therapist assistant's request for a re-examination, when a change in treatment plan of care is needed, prior to any planned discharge, and in response to a change in the patient/client's medical status.
   b. At least once a month, or at a higher frequency when established by the physical therapist, in accordance with the needs of the patient.
   c. A supervisory visit should include:
      1. An on-site re-examination of the patient/client.
      2. On-site review of the plan of care with appropriate revision or termination.
      3. Evaluation of need and recommendation for utilization of outside resources.

From Direction and Supervision of the Physical Therapist Assistant, HOD 06-00-16-27. Alexandria, VA, American Physical Therapy Association, 2000.

Box 3–6

Position on the Provision of Physical Therapy Interventions and Related Tasks

Physical therapy aides are any support personnel who perform designated tasks related to the operation of the physical therapy service. Tasks are those activities that do not require the clinical decision making of the physical therapist or the clinical problem solving of the physical therapist assistant. Tasks related to patient/client management must be assigned to the physical therapy aide by the physical therapist, or where allowable by law, the physical therapist assistant, and may only be performed by the aide under direct personal supervision of the physical therapist, or where allowable by law, the physical therapist assistant. Direct personal supervision requires that the physical therapist, or where allowable by law, the physical therapist assistant, be physically present and immediately available to direct and supervise tasks that are related to patient/client management. The direction and supervision is continuous throughout the time these tasks are performed. The physical therapist or physical therapist assistant must have direct contact with the patient/client during each session. Telecommunication does not meet the requirement of direct personal supervision.

From Position on the Provision of Physical Therapy Interventions and Related Tasks, HOD 06-00-17-28. Alexandria, VA, American Physical Therapy Association, 2000.

STATE REGULATION

Physical therapy practice is regulated in all 50 states by practice acts (see Chapter 5). These practice acts define not only physical therapy but also the qualifications required for use of the title and practice. As an example, each PT must be licensed by the state in which practice is being conducted. The purpose of licensure is to provide standards and protect the public from harm.

These acts also address the PTA. Variations in practice acts across the United States give rise to some of the confusion regarding utilization of the PTA. For instance, PTAs are regulated in 42 states and U.S. territories by licensure, registration, or certification.[15] Where these statutes exist, the PTA is most often defined as a graduate of an accredited PTA program. Although some states do not regulate PTAs, supervisory requirements may be delineated in the physical therapy rules and regulations for support personnel. Many state regulations specify that the PT may delegate aspects of physical therapy care to appropriately trained individuals. This policy directly affects the manner in which the PTA is used and supervised.

These interstate variations result in a broad range of responsibilities and considerable confusion. For example, a state might mandate that the PT be available at all times via telecommunication while the PTA is providing patient care. This requirement would allow a PT to be off-site when a PTA is treating a patient as long as the PT is available by telecommunication. In contrast, if the practice act defines supervision as on-site, the PT must be within the same facility while a PTA is providing patient care.

The state physical therapy practice act provides the legal basis for physical therapy practice. It is imperative that the PT and PTA be familiar with the rules and regulations that pertain to their roles and practice in physical therapy.

EMPLOYMENT CHARACTERISTICS

Demographic characteristics and information regarding the current primary employment position of PTs were described in Chapter 2. Similar data were obtained from renewal applications by PTAs. The following two subsections are based on data from this APTA Membership Database compiled in 2000.[1]

Demographics

Gender. Females accounted for 80.2% of the respondents. This degree of dominance exceeded that for active members (PTs) of the APTA, which was 68.3%.

Age. The mean age of the respondents was 37.5 years, which indicates a younger population than PTs, whose mean age was 40.4 years. This difference may be explained by the fact that the PTA position is relatively new in comparison to the PT position.

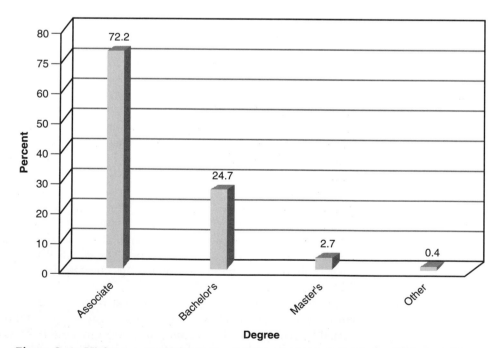

Figure 3–4. Highest earned academic degree of physical therapist assistants. (From American Physical Therapy Association Membership Database. Alexandria, VA, American Physical Therapy Association, 2000.)

Education. The associate degree was the highest earned academic degree of 72.2% of the respondents (Fig. 3–4), which reflects the degree requirement. A substantial number, 24.7%, hold a bachelor's degree.

Employment Facility

3

For PTAs, the primary employment patterns were similar to those for PTs, except for extended care facilities (Fig. 3–5). On a percentage basis, twice as many PTAs (15.1%) were employed in an extended care facility as PTs (7.6%). This difference in employment indicates the important role that PTAs perform in tasks delegated by PTs in these facilities. It also provides a context for studying the levels of responsibility of the PT and adequate supervision (see the preceding Utilization section). The current transition to a cost containment environment may play a role in economic decisions regarding the relative staffing mix of PTAs and PTs in these settings. Regardless of the employment setting, the majority of respondents held full-time salaried positions (71.0%).

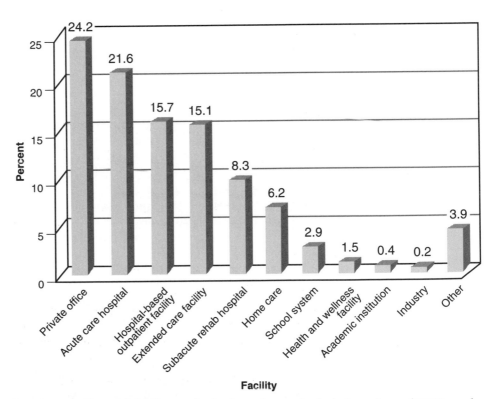

Figure 3–5. Type of facility or institution where physical therapist assistants work. Compare with Figure 2–17 for physical therapists. (Data from American Physical Therapy Association Membership Database. Alexandria, VA, American Physical Therapy Association, 2000.)

Career Development

When choosing a career, students consider the field of physical therapy for a variety of reasons. The most common reason is that they want to work with patients. When considering a career as a PTA versus a PT, many factors must be taken into account, some of which are finances, family, location of the education program, and future career goals.

In the job market, demand will vary at times in accordance with society's need for the service. The need for physical therapy personnel has resulted in a steady job market for the PTA. According to the U.S. Bureau of Labor Statistics, PTA is considered to be among the fastest-growing occupations through the year 2006.[14] Licensed PTAs can enhance the cost-effective provision of physical therapy services.

The variety of positions in physical therapy departments provides many opportunities for advancement. Like the PT, a PTA may have previous work experience in such areas as public relations, business, or education. Further analysis reveals individual characteristics such as organizational skills, in-depth knowledge of reimbursement and documentation guidelines, and/or strategic planning skills. All these characteristics can be used in a physical therapy department in a variety of capacities such as utilization coordinator, center coordinator of clinical education, or in-service coordinator. To make the greatest use of talented employees, most departments do make a concerted effort to use any special skills.

The issue of retention was studied by the APTA in 1988 by conducting a survey of PTAs and PTs in hospital settings. The results revealed that PTAs remained employed at a facility for an average of 5 to 6 years, whereas PTs remained employed at a facility for an average of 1 to 2 years.[5] PTA respondents who had resigned from acute care settings cited low salary, limited opportunity for advancement, and a "nonflexible administration" as reasons for their decision to resign.

The results of this survey prompted some facilities to begin designing **career ladders** for the PTA similar to career ladders for the PT. Eligibility requirements are based on years of experience and tenure at the facility. Duties describing the three position levels (PTA I, II, III) are categorized as clinical, administrative, teaching, educational, and professional. These career ladders are described in Table 3–1.

Another form of career development for a PTA is to return to an education program to pursue an advanced degree. For example, a degree in business may augment the assistant's ability to be involved in the administrative component of a physical therapy practice.

A PTA may make the choice to pursue a degree as a PT. The reasons cited are often greater autonomy, greater responsibility for patient care, and an increase in pay. If a PTA makes the choice to pursue a degree as a PT, it is especially important to note that the coursework previously completed may not be acceptable in the physical therapy program. Many physical therapy programs allow the PTA to test out of certain courses, but such is not always the case.

RIGHTS AND PRIVILEGES IN THE APTA

The development of PTA education programs and the definition of utilization of support personnel eventually led to discussion regarding the formation of a class of membership in the APTA for the PTA. Heated debates over the nonprofessional assistant joining the APTA ensued.

In his 1969 presidential address, Eugene Michels, PT, stated, "I am aware of the reasons given against the extension of voting privileges. Those reasons are insufficient and unconvincing. Some say that students and assistants will not know enough about the issues to vote intelligently. That argument is unsound

3

Table 3–1
Career Development for the Physical Therapist Assistant

DUTIES	PHYSICAL THERAPIST ASSISTANT LEVEL I (New Graduate)
Clinical	Assists physical therapist in overall assessment of patient Assists in implementation of patient treatment
Administrative	Knowledgeable regarding department policy and procedures Organizes own schedule Carries a standard caseload Provides appropriate and accurate documentation Participates in quality improvement programs Participates in department administration
Teaching	Teaches appropriate techniques to patients and families Provides in-services to staff Provides educational opportunities to physical therapy students
Educational	Attends continuing education programs Attends facility meetings and orientations Attends departmental in-services Reads professional literature and remains current on physical therapy techniques Possesses current CPR certification
Professional	Demonstrates appropriate verbal communication skills Follows appropriate administrative policy Demonstrates professional behavior Actively participates in administrative meetings Demonstrates a willingness to participate in departmental functions

Table continued on following page

Table 3–1
Career Development for the Physical
Therapist Assistant *Continued*

DUTIES	PHYSICAL THERAPIST ASSISTANT LEVEL II (2 yr of Experience, Same Job Description as that of PTA I and Additional Duties Listed Below)
Clinical	Performs and interprets the results of selected measurement procedures in consultation with the physical therapist Makes modification in patient treatment based on information for less frequent diagnoses Knowledgeable about community services and makes recommendations to the team
Administrative	Familiar with policies and procedures and recommends changes as needed Cognizant of patient care priorities and facility responsibilities and adapts accordingly Participates on facility committees
Teaching	Provides facility and community in-services Provides educational opportunities to PTA students of at least 1 full-time affiliation per year
Educational	Attends 3 continuing education programs per year Participates in 1 or more patient or community educational programs per year
Professional	Demonstrates appropriate professional conduct Supportive of management response to staff

for two reasons. First, give students and assistants half a chance, and you will soon find out what they do know. Second, every active and life member who currently holds a vote does not know what the issues are. Others fear the consequences of being out-voted by the combined power of students and assistants. If that should ever happen, and it is conceivable, the answers to the following two questions deflate that fear: (1) If it does happen, whose fault will it be? and (2) If it does happen, is it necessarily bad? I find it incredible that we place so little trust in others who, we assume, are perfectly content to place their full trust in us. What a familiar ring that has!''[13]

The 1973 APTA House of Delegates approved a proposal that provided an affiliate membership category for PTAs. PTAs have been affiliate members of the APTA since that action. The rights and privileges of an **affiliate member** (PTA) were different from those of an **active member** (PT). The affiliate member was entitled to (1) attend all meetings; (2) speak and make motions; (3) hold committee appointments, including chairman, but not any office at

Table 3–1
Career Development for the Physical Therapist Assistant Continued

3

DUTIES	PHYSICAL THERAPIST ASSISTANT LEVEL III (4 yr of Experience, Same Job Description as that of PTA II and Additional Duties Listed Below)
Clinical	Able to interpret and follow the plan of care established by the physical therapist for less frequent diagnoses Assists those at the PTA I and PTA II level with the interpretation of subjective and objective evaluation information Assesses the available community services and makes recommendations to the team May initiate patient care conferences after consulting with the evaluating physical therapist
Administrative	Participates in updating policies and procedures with an awareness of standards of accrediting agencies Provides mentoring of those at the PTA I and PTA II level Investigates and initiates equipment repair and potential replacement
Teaching	Participates in orientation of new staff Provides educational opportunities to PTA students of at least 2 full-time affiliations per year
Educational	Attends 4 continuing education programs per year Participates in APTA activities
Professional	Provides insight to management regarding staff concerns

APTA, American Physical Therapy Association; CPR, cardiopulmonary resuscitation; PTA, physical therapist assistant.
From Carpenter C: PTA career ladders. PT—Magazine of Physical Therapy 1993;1(1):56–61. Reprinted from PT—Magazine with the permission of the American Physical Therapy Association.

the national or component level; (4) serve as a chapter affiliate delegate; (5) assert a one-half vote; and (6) receive the official journal of the APTA.

In 1983, the House of Delegates adopted a proposal to support the formation of an Affiliate Special Interest Group to manage the concerns of the affiliate and provide more opportunities within the APTA for interaction. After this action, affiliate leaders began to formalize the **Affiliate Special Interest Group,** later known as ASIG, to identify concerns of affiliate members across the country. Regions were identified and assigned to people within the ASIG, and a chairperson was elected. This person served as the liaison with the APTA

Board of Directors. The continued support of PTAs throughout the country made apparent the need for a formalized group within the APTA specifically for the PTA.

The issues surrounding categories of membership continued to plague the association. In even-numbered years, when amendments to the bylaws were proposed, topics from the past continued to be presented and defeated. The APTA Board of Directors responded by creating an organizational task force, which studied the issue for 2 years and presented its findings to the 1989 House of Delegates.

Among the proposals was the formation of an assembly. The purpose of an assembly is to provide a means by which members of the same class may meet, confer, and promote the interests of the respective membership class. This proposal was adopted in 1989, along with formation of the first assembly, called the Affiliate Assembly.

The **Affiliate Assembly** was an officially recognized component of the APTA. The officers were PTAs elected by their peers. The assembly officers were the affiliate's formal liaisons with the APTA officers and staff. Their mission was to promote the role of the PTA within the association in keeping with the goals and objects of the association.

One year after the Affiliate Assembly was created, the House of Delegates approved the **Student Assembly** (1990). The Student Assembly is composed of PT and PTA students. This networking ability will continue to provide a forum in which PTA and PT students can better understand their roles and responsibilities in physical therapy practice.

In 1992, a motion was proposed to the House of Delegates to allow PTAs to hold office at the component level (chapter and section) with the exception of the office of president. This motion was passed in 1992 and amended in 1994 to further delineate that the PTA was ineligible to hold an office that was in direct succession to the presidency of the component.

This motion provided additional rights and privileges to the affiliate member. The adoption of such proposals further builds on the mission of the APTA to meet the needs and interests of its membership. Over the past 5 years, great strides have been made in the inclusion of PTAs as affiliate members of the APTA to assume a role in the leadership of physical therapy.

In 1998, a controversial action was taken by the House of Delegates when that body passed RC-1. RC-1 created what is now called the **National Assembly of Physical Therapist Assistants**, or simply the National Assembly. In addition to officers, the National Assembly has regional directors who serve geographical locations. Although this action excluded the affiliate as a voting member of the House of Delegates, it provided for the creation of a separate deliberative body unique to the PTA. Consequently, the **Representative Body of the National Assembly (RBNA)** was created and had its first meeting in 1999. Its structure is similar to that of the House of Delegates and consists of affiliate representatives from all chapters. The issues put forth in the RBNA deal solely with issues that affect PTAs. Issues passed by the RBNA are sent to the House of Delegates for final approval. Two National Assembly delegates attend the House of Delegates and may speak, debate, and make and second motions, but they may not vote.

In addition, three National Assembly board consultants attend sessions of the House to answer questions posed by the speaker of the House of Delegates.

TRENDS

Trends in health care will continue to influence the way in which PTs and PTAs are professionally prepared and function in the provision of service. PTA education programs will continue to expand their curricula to meet the needs of practice. The increased curriculum demands may result in a reconsideration of the degree awarded.

Continued growth in academic and clinical programs will result in greater utilization of the PTA, with an increased number hired by PTA education programs as instructors, academic coordinators of clinical education, and program directors. PTAs in the clinic will continue to be directly involved in the supervision of PTA students during their clinical rotations, where their advanced clinical expertise can be put to maximum use and allow them to be positive role models.

Clinical research is another area in which PTAs will play a greater role. To a large extent, the credibility of physical therapy will depend on continued research related to physical therapy outcome studies and provision of effective and efficient models of patient care. Such studies are continually needed to prove the worth of physical therapy services and thus ensure reimbursement for services rendered by all levels of physical therapy professionals.

The diversity of physical therapy services and society's need for these services from prevention to the provision of care for the aging population will create new demands for physical therapy practitioners. PTAs can provide the opportunity for PTs to spend additional time performing patient evaluation, diagnosis, prognosis, re-evaluation, and research, which is not to say that the PTA can replace the therapist in patient care. Certain patient impairment levels will continue to demand the presence of a PT.

PTAs will also continue to advance their skills and knowledge and become involved in departmental activities such as community education to facilitate health and wellness. Advanced clinical skills will lead to PTA specialization and an expanded need for PTA continuing education courses.

It should be no surprise, in view of all this growth, that the APTA affiliate membership will continue to grow, with reliance on the National Assembly to serve as a voice of the affiliate. We should also expect to see affiliate members forming groups at the state level to address regional concerns, addressing issues of member rights and privileges at future meetings of the RBNA, and serving more frequently as component officers and committee chairs. Eventually, the APTA will be faced with the issue of elected affiliate representation on the APTA Board of Directors.

Case Studies

The following case studies illustrate just two examples of the various roles that the PTA can take in the practice setting.

Physical Therapist Assistant I (Novice)

Jackie, a PT working in a private practice setting, recently hired Don, a new graduate PTA. Before assigning patients, Jackie spoke with Don regarding his course work and the physical therapy experience he had during his clinical rotations.

Shortly after this conversation, Jackie reviews with Don the diagnosis, plan of care, and precautions for a new patient with the diagnosis of a frozen shoulder (adhesive capsulitis). After the patient's third treatment, Jackie questions Don on the patient's progress. Don reports that the treatment has consisted of the exercise program Jackie had suggested but that the patient continues to have difficulty moving his arm in the correct patterns.

Jackie asks Don to suggest an exercise that may work better. He mentions that the patient tends to compensate with his body during pulley activities. He also adds that the corrections made to the patient's position have not worked very well. Instead, he would like to try diagonal movement patterns with verbal cueing. Jackie suggests positioning the patient supine (lying face up) and using some of the diagonal patterns with verbal and physical cueing. Don agrees that positioning the patient supine would provide better trunk stability and decrease the compensatory patterns of the trunk. Then, Jackie makes plans to work with Don and the patient during the next exercise session to problem-solve together.

Physical Therapist Assistant III (Senior)

Eric, a PT in a rural community hospital, has been working with the same PTA, Cindy, for 6 years. After a patient evaluation, Eric confers with Cindy regarding a patient with the diagnosis of a cerebrovascular accident (stroke). He asks Cindy to review the evaluation and address any questions with him before beginning treatment in the afternoon. He requests that Cindy see the patient twice daily.

Cindy reviews the evaluation and notes that the short-term goals of treatment are for the patient to sit unsupported for 5 minutes and transfer three of five times with standby assistance. Eric's long-term goal is for this patient to ambulate with an appropriate assistive device (e.g., cane, walker). Cindy also notes the patient's previous history of a myocardial infarction and coronary artery disease. Cindy determines that she will need to monitor blood pressure and pulse throughout the patient's treatment. Treatment sessions will be limited by the patient's endurance.

Later, Cindy walks into the patient's room, where she finds him sitting in a wheelchair at bedside. She introduces herself as a PTA on staff at the hospital. She reminds the patient of the PT who examined him in the morning and further explains that the PT has assigned her to work with the patient on movement activities. She explains that she will be taking the patient's blood pressure and pulse throughout the treatment sessions.

After informing the nurse, Cindy wheels the patient around the corner to the physical therapy gym. She transfers him to the mat and assesses his transfer and sitting balance. She uses some of the neurodevelopmental techniques that she learned at the fall conference to decrease the patient's sacral sitting posture. She then incorporates upper extremity activities of weight bearing and crossing the body midline. She monitors the patient's pulse and blood pressure during treatment. At the completion of the session, Cindy transports the patient back to his room and informs the nurse that she did so. After she returns to the physical therapy department, she sees Eric. She tells him that the patient did well during the first session and tolerated 20 minutes of treatment before becoming tired. She provides Eric with information regarding the patient's blood pressure and pulse responses during treatment. The PT concurs with the treatment approach.

After a week of treatment, the patient is able to sit unsupported for 5 minutes and transfers from sitting to standing with standby assistance. Cindy has reported this progress to Eric. After re-examining the patient together, they establish new short-term goals for the patient to stand with standby assistance for 5 minutes in the parallel bars, ambulate in the parallel bars for 5 to 10 ft with minimal to moderate assistance, perform dynamic sitting activities with extended reach, and maintain the appropriate posture three of five times without loss of balance.

The next day, Cindy speaks with the social worker and is advised that the patient has reached his insurance limit for skilled physical therapy services and will be leaving the hospital for an extended care facility. She reports this information to Eric and provides him with data on the patient's functional status, manual muscle test grades, and balance/endurance status. Eric re-evaluates the patient with the input from Cindy and develops a discharge summary that includes the necessary equipment and a plan of care for the personnel at the extended care facility to follow. Eric writes the final discharge note based on the patient's last physical therapy treatment while Cindy orders the necessary equipment for the patient to take with him.

Summary _____   Many turning points have occurred in the growth and development of the profession of PTA. The APTA responded positively to an early need by creating the position of PTA in 1967. As a result, the profession has reaped the benefits of extending its influence and thereby expanding the provision of services to more people.

As PTs became involved in conducting more complicated evaluations and establishing diagnoses, utilization of the PTA was advanced to include assessment and measurement activities and selected interventions as delegated by the PT. Education programs for the PTA proliferated and now exceed the number of educational programs for the PT. The APTA membership responded to affiliate needs by creating the Affiliate Assembly and finally the National Assembly of Physical Therapist Assistants.

Physical therapy services continue to evolve in variety and mechanism of provision. Greater understanding regarding the personnel who provide these services will result in more effective and efficient health care. This evolution will result in a profession that is empowered and prepared to face the challenges of tomorrow.

References

1. American Physical Therapy Association Membership Database. Alexandria, VA, American Physical Therapy Association, 2000.
2. Bashi HL, Domholdt E: Use of support personnel for physical therapy treatment. Phys Ther 1993;73:421–429.

3. Blood H: Supportive personnel in the health-care system. Phys Ther 1970;50:173–180.
4. Blood H: Report of the Ad Hoc Committee to study the utilization and training of nonprofessional assistants. Phys Ther 1967;47(11, Part 2):31–39.
5. Carpenter C: PTA career ladders. PT—Magazine of Physical Therapy 1993;1(1):56–61.
6. Collopy S, Schenck J, Wood W: Report of a three-year study on the physical therapist assistant. Phys Ther 1972;52:1300–1307.
7. Direction and Supervision of the Physical Therapist Assistant, HOD 06-00-16-27. Alexandria, VA, American Physical Therapy Association, 2000.
8. Evaluative Criteria for Accreditation of Education Programs for the Preparation of Physical Therapists. Alexandria, VA, American Physical Therapy Association, 1996.
9. Evaluative Criteria for Accreditation of Education Programs for the Preparation of Physical Therapist Assistants. Alexandria, VA, American Physical Therapy Association, 1998.
10. Gossett R: Assistant utilization: A pilot study. Phys Ther 1973;53:502–506.
11. Hill Burton State Plan Data: A National Summary. Washington, DC, U.S. Department of Health, Education and Welfare, January 1962.
12. Hislop H: Man power versus mind power. Phys Ther 1963;43:711.
13. Michels E: The 1969 Presidential Address. Phys Ther 1969;49:1191–1200.
14. 1998–1999 Occupational Outlook Handbook. Washington, DC, Bureau of Labor Statistics, 1999.
15. 1999 State Licensure Reference Guide. Alexandria, VA, Federation of State Boards of Physical Therapy, 1999.
16. Position on the Provision of Physical Therapy Interventions and Related Tasks, HOD 06-00-17-38. Alexandria, VA, American Physical Therapy Association, 2000.
17. White B: Physical therapy assistants: Implications for the future. Phys Ther 1970;50:674–679.
18. Worthingham CA: Nonprofessional personnel in physical therapy. Phys Ther 1965;45:112–115.

Suggested Readings

Brister S: Mosby's Comprehensive Physical Therapist Assistant Board Review. St Louis, Mosby–Year Book, 1996.

This manual was written and "field-tested" for PTA students in their second year of study who are preparing for the required board certification examination. It is designed to assist students in the review process by helping them examine their knowledge base and by pointing out areas of weakness. Includes 200 illustrations, study questions for every chapter, a comprehensive glossary, and two practice examinations.

Canan B: What changes are predicted for the physical therapist assistant in the 1980s? Phys Ther 1980;60:312.

Guest commentary on the role of the PT and the assistant as a health care team.

Carpenter C: Physical therapist assistant issues in the 1980s and 1990s. *In* Mathew JS (ed): Practice Issues in Physical Therapy: Current Patterns and Future Directions. Thorofare, NJ, Slack, 1989.

Overview of PTA origin, education, licensure, specialization, advancement opportunities, and APTA membership.

Larson CW, Davis ER: Following up the physical therapist assistant graduate: A curriculum evaluation process. Phys Ther 1975;55:601–606.

Survey analysis of frequency and independence in performance of 111 tasks by PTA graduates of St. Mary's Junior College to ascertain how well they had been prepared for the demands of their jobs and discover what revisions in the program curriculum might be appropriate.

Lovelace-Chandler V, Lovelace-Chandler B: Employment of physical therapist assistants in a residential state school. Phys Ther 1979;59:1243–1246.
Provides an analysis of PTA educational preparation and ethical guidelines to aid in the determination of appropriate utilization within a given facility.

Lupi-Williams F, James S, Murphy P: The PTA role and function. Clin Manage Phys Ther 1983;3(3):35–40.
A three-part overview of the education, utilization in general practice, and a job description of the PTA in a school setting.

Robinson A, McCall M, DePalma MT, et al: Physical therapists' perceptions of the roles of the physical therapist assistant. Phys Ther 1994;74:571–582.
A longitudinal study that investigated PTs' perception of the roles of the PTA through surveys conducted in 1986 and 1992.

Schunk C, Lippert L, Reeves B: PTA practice: In reality. Clin Manage Phys Ther 1992;12(6):88–92.
A survey of licensed PTAs in the state of Oregon conducted by the Affiliate Affairs Committee of the Oregon Physical Therapy Association regarding how PTAs practice, supervision standards, and what PTAs believe about their utilization.

Woods: PTA twentieth anniversary. PT—Magazine of Physical Therapy 1993; 1(4):34–45.
Describes the evolution of the PTA in relation to the APTA and the profession.

3

REVIEW QUESTIONS

1. Contrast competencies in a PTA curriculum with those in a PT curriculum.

2. Identify common myths regarding the role and utilization of PTAs. Can you combat these myths with "myth-breaking" facts about PTA competence?

3. Describe the scope of PTA competency in the practice setting.

4. What is the difference between a PTA and a physical therapy aide?

5. Discuss the wide-ranging supervision requirements for using physical therapy aides.

6. How might such skills as in-depth knowledge of reimbursement and documentation guidelines and/or strategic planning skills be used in the physical therapy setting?

7. Distinguish the roles of the following organizations: Affiliate Special Interest Group, National Assembly, Student Assembly.

Approximately 70 percent of Americans are members of at least one association; 25 percent belong to four or more. Although the role of associations varies, these organizational entities offer forums for communication and collaboration, develop ethical standards for the individuals or groups they represent, educate members and the public, and provide a vehicle for change in society.
APTA Environmental Statement

American Physical Therapy Association

Michael A. Pagliarulo

MISSION AND GOALS
ORGANIZATIONAL STRUCTURE
  Membership
  Districts
  Chapters
  Sections
  Assemblies
  House of Delegates
  Representative Body of the National
    Assembly of Physical Therapist Assistants
  Board of Directors
  Staff

ASSOCIATED ORGANIZATIONS
  American Board of Physical Therapy
    Specialties
  Commission on Accreditation in
    Physical Therapy Education
  Federation of State Boards of Physical
    Therapy
  Foundation for Physical Therapy
  Trialliance
  World Confederation of Physical
    Therapy

OTHER RELATED ORGANIZATIONS
   American Academy of Physical Therapists
   United Societies of Physiotherapists, Inc.
BENEFITS OF BELONGING
SUMMARY

KEY TERMS

American Board of Physical Therapy
Specialties (ABPTS)
American Physical Therapy Association (APTA)
annual conference and exposition
assembly
Board of Directors (BOD)

chapter
Combined Sections Meeting
Commission on Accreditation in Physical
Therapy Education (CAPTE)
components
district
Federation of State Boards of Physical Therapy
(FSBPT)
Foundation for Physical Therapy
House of Delegates (HOD)
section
special interest group (SIG)
Trialliance
World Confederation of Physical Therapy

OBJECTIVES   After reading this chapter, the reader will be able to

- Describe the structure and function of the American Physical Therapy Association
- Distinguish between sections and assemblies within the association
- Identify and describe organizations that are associated and related to the association
- Describe the benefits of belonging to the association

The definition of physical therapy presented in Chapter 1 demonstrated that this field is a profession because it possesses all the qualities or criteria of a profession. One of these criteria is a representative organization. This chapter focuses on the **American Physical Therapy Association (APTA)**, which is the national organization that represents physical therapy. The organization's mission, structure, and benefits are described here. We already saw a historical account of the association in Chapter 1. Affiliated and related organizations representing physical therapy interests are included at the end of this chapter.

MISSION AND GOALS   The APTA is a national member-driven organization that represents the profession of physical therapy (Fig. 4–1). It is composed of more than 70,000 physical therapists, physical therapist assistants, and students throughout the United States and abroad. Membership is strictly voluntary.

   In 1993, the House of Delegates (HOD) of the APTA adopted a mission statement and related policy. The statement[1] (Box 4–1) and policy[6] (Box 4–2) demonstrate the profession's interest in serving the public and its members through practice, education, and research.

   Goals for the APTA are established annually by the Board of Directors

APTA

American Physical Therapy Association

Figure 4–1. Logo for the American Physical Therapy Association. (Reprinted with permission from the American Physical Therapy Association.)

(BOD). They are then reviewed and approved by the HOD. The goals for 2000 were approved by the HOD in June 1999 and are presented in Box 4–3.[5] These goals direct the activities and funding priorities for the new year and reiterate the grounding in education, research, and practice.

ORGANIZATIONAL STRUCTURE

The organizational structure of the APTA is depicted in Figure 4–2. This structure provides a three-tiered approach (local, state, and national) to serve the members and the public. Three units at the state and national levels—chapters, sections, and assemblies—are the **components** of the APTA. Policymaking bodies, with their respective committees and task forces, and staff complete the general plan of this organization. Each level is described in this section, beginning with the primary unit, the membership.

Membership

As stated earlier, membership in the APTA is voluntary; however, it is estimated that approximately two thirds of licensed physical therapists in the United States are members. This extensive membership provides strength and diversity to the organization.

The primary membership categories of the APTA are active (physical therapist), affiliate (physical therapist assistant), and their respective student categories, student and student affiliate. Other categories include life (retired), honorary (not a member in any other category and has made outstanding contributions to the association or health of the public), and Catherine Worthingham Fellow of the APTA (active member for at least 15 years who has made notable contributions to the profession; may use the initials FAPTA). All active and life members are automatically members of the American College of Physical Therapists, whereas all affiliate and life affiliate members are automatically members of the National Assembly of Physical Therapist Assistants. Requirements for membership include graduation from (or enrollment in) an education program approved (or seeking candidacy) by a recognized accrediting agency. In addition, the applicant must sign a pledge indicating compliance

Box 4–1

Mission of the American Physical Therapy Association

The mission of the American Physical Therapy Association (APTA), the principal membership organization representing and promoting the profession of physical therapy, is to further the profession's role in the prevention, diagnosis, and treatment of movement dysfunctions and the enhancement of the physical health and functional abilities of members of the public.

From APTA Mission Statement, HOD 06-93-05-05. Alexandria, VA, American Physical Therapy Association, 1993.

Box 4–2

Policy on the American Physical Therapy Association Mission Statement

To fulfill the American Physical Therapy Association's Mission to meet the needs and interests of its members and to promote physical therapy as a vital professional career, the Association shall:

- Promote physical therapy care and services through the establishment, maintenance, and promotion of ethical principles and quality standards for practice, education, and research;
- Influence policy in the public and private sectors;
- Enable physical therapy practitioners to improve their skills, knowledge, and operations in the interest of furthering the profession;
- Develop and improve the art and science of physical therapy, including practice, education, and research;
- Facilitate a common understanding and appreciation for the diversity of the profession, the membership, and the communities we serve; and
- Maintain a stable and diverse financial base from which to fund the programs, services, and operations that support this mission.

From Policy on APTA Mission Statement, HOD 06-93-06-07. Alexandria, VA, American Physical Therapy Association, 1993.

Box 4–3

Goals that Represent the 2001 Priorities of the APTA

4

Goal I. Participate actively in shaping the current and emerging health care environment to promote the development of high-quality, cost-effective health care services and to further the recognition of and support for the profession of physical therapy and the role of physical therapists.

Goal II. Stimulate innovation in the practice of physical therapy that supports physical therapists and physical therapist assistants.

Goal III. Quantify and interpret the demand for, the need for, and the access to physical therapist services.

Goal IV. Stimulate innovation in physical therapy education and professional development at all levels to ensure currency with the changing environments in health care and education and with student and professional needs.

Goal V. Stimulate research to further the science of physical therapy, to influence current and emerging health care trends, and to advance the profession.

Goal VI. Increase APTA's responsiveness to the needs of current and future members.

These goals are based on the priorities that have been adopted annually by the House of Delegates since 1988 to provide direction to the APTA Board of Directors and have been established based on practice, research, and education being the highest priorities of the Association. The Board is committed to these goals as the foundation from which to lead the Association. The Association's awareness of cultural diversity, its commitment to expanding minority representation and participation in physical therapy, and its commitment to equal opportunity for all members permeate these goals. The goals are not ranked and do not represent any priority order.

From Goals that Represent the 2001 Priorities of the Association, HOD 06-00-11-03. Alexandria, VA, American Physical Therapy Association, 2000.

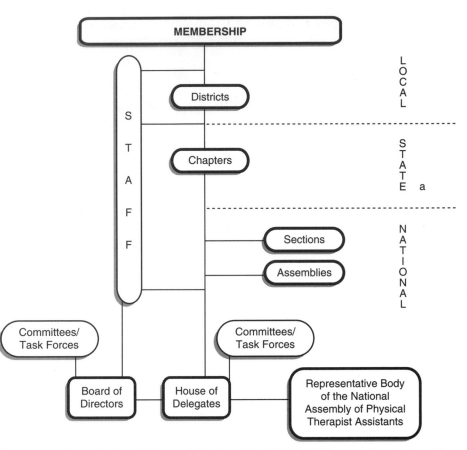

Figure 4–2. Organizational chart of the American Physical Therapy Association. Note how the membership drives this organization. Staff members provide support at all levels, including membership, local, state, and national. a, Washington, DC, and Puerto Rico are also chapters.

with the Code of Ethics (active and related categories) or Standards of Ethical Conduct for the Physical Therapist Assistant (affiliate and related categories) and pay dues.

Service to the membership has always been one of the main purposes of the APTA. Likewise, members have had a sense of pride and commitment to the organization. In fact, during the formative years of the profession, membership in this organization was considered the standard for competence. This proud heritage remains today; however, membership is not required to demonstrate competence.

Districts

Figure 4–2 indicates that a **district** is the most local organizational unit in the structure of the APTA. Districts do not exist in all jurisdictions, such as small states. Membership is automatic where they do exist and may be based on location of residence or employment as provided in the bylaws of the APTA.

Districts are more common in locations with high population densities or large geographical areas and frequently consist of one or more counties. This arrangement provides a mechanism for convenient meetings and participation. It also provides a basis for representation in a body that conducts business at the next level of organization, the chapter.

Chapters

In accordance with the standing rules of the APTA, a **chapter** "must coincide with or be confined within the legally constituted boundaries of a state, territory, or commonwealth of the United States or the District of Columbia."[7] In 2001, the APTA consists of 52 chapters, one for each state, the District of Columbia, and Puerto Rico. Membership in a chapter is *automatic* and based on location of residence, employment, education, or greatest active participation (in the last case, only in an immediately adjacent chapter). In contrast to districts, which are not permitted to assess dues, each chapter requires dues for active and affiliate members and, in a few cases, student categories.

Chapters are an important component of the APTA. They provide a mechanism for participation at a state level and proportionate representation at the national level (see House of Delegates later). Participation is facilitated through authorized special interest groups (SIGs) and assemblies to address the needs of recognized subsidiary groups. They also provide an important voice for members at the state level of government. This capacity is essential to maintain statewide legislation and regulations appropriate to the profession and practice of physical therapy.

Sections

A **section** is organized at the national level exclusively. In accordance with the bylaws of the APTA, sections provide an opportunity for members with similar areas of interest to "meet, confer, and promote the interests of the respective sections."[2] Membership in 1 or more of the 19 sections listed in Table 4–1 is voluntary; however, one must be a member of the APTA to join a section.[2, 3] Students are permitted and encouraged to join.

In addition to the publications listed in Table 4–1, section members share information at an annual **Combined Sections Meeting** in early February. This meeting provides a mechanism for educational and business sessions. Section leadership can then accurately represent the members at other APTA and government arenas.

A specialty area within a section may form a **special interest group**. Bylaws authorize SIGs within a chapter, section, and assembly, but they are most common in sections. This capability provides an opportunity for members in one of these components to further organize into smaller areas of common interest. For example, the Section for Education has four SIGs, two for aca-

4

Table 4–1
Sections of the American Physical Therapy Association

SECTION	AREA(S) OF INTEREST	PUBLICATION(S)
Acute Care/Hospital Clinical Practice	PTs practicing in acute care/hospital setting SIG: Rehab/Long-Term Care	*Acute Care Perspectives*
Administration	Business, leadership, and management	*The Resource*
Aquatic Physical Therapy	Administrative and clinical needs of members to define and enhance the scope of practice	*Journal of Aquatic Physical Therapy* *Waterlines Newsletter*
Cardiopulmonary	Heart and lung dysfunction caused by disease, injury, or birth defects	*Cardiopulmonary Physical Therapy Journal*
Clinical Electrophysiology	Electrotherapy, electrophysiological evaluation, physical agents, and wound management SIGs: Electrotherapeutics, Electrophysiological Testing, Wound Care	*Clinical Electrophysiology Newsletter*
Education	Education of PTs and PTAs SIGs: PTA Educators, Academic Administrators, Academic Faculty, Clinical Educators	*Journal of Physical Therapy Education* *The Bulletin*
Geriatrics	Clinical excellence of PTs and PTAs working with older adults	*Issues on Aging* *GeriNotes*
Hand Rehabilitation	Hand and upper extremity rehabilitation	*Hand Prints*
Health Policy, Legislation, and Regulation	Health policy, legislation, and regulations affecting the practice of physical therapy SIGs: Cross-Cultural and International; Advocates for the Disabled and Access	*Policy Watch*
Home Health	Practice in home or community setting	*Quarterly Report*
Neurology	Neurological Injury and Disease SIGs: Brain Injury, Degenerative Diseases, Spinal Cord Injury, and Vestibular Rehabilitation	*Neurology Report* *Neuro Notes*
Oncology	Physical therapy for individuals with cancer SIG: HIV and AIDS	*Oncology Rehabilitation*
Orthopaedic	Management of patients with musculoskeletal disorders SIGs: Occupational Health, Foot and Ankle, Performing Arts, Pain Management, and Animal Physical Therapy	*Journal of Orthopaedic and Sports Physical Therapy* *Orthopaedic Physical Therapy Practice*

Table 4–1

Sections of the American Physical Therapy Association *Continued*

SECTION	AREA(S) OF INTEREST	PUBLICATION(S)
Pediatrics	Excellence in pediatric practice and research	*Pediatric Physical Therapy* *Section on Pediatrics Newsletter*
Private Practice	Successful management of a physical therapy practice	*Membership Directory* *IMPACT* *NetIMPACT* "Doing Business" in *Advance for Directors in Rehabilitation*
Research	Clinical and basic scientific research	*Section on Research Newsletter* *Michels Research Forum Proceedings*
Sports Physical Therapy	Rehabilitation, prevention, recognition, and treatment of injuries in athletes SIGs: Athletes with Disabilities, Sports, Pediatrics, Residency, Knee, and Shoulder	*The Journal of Orthopaedic and Sports Physical Therapy* *Sports Section Newsletter*
Veterans Affairs	High-quality physical therapy in VA Medical Centers	*VAntage PoinT*
Women's Health	Women's health and wellness across the life span	*Journal of the Section on Women's Health* *Highlights in Women's Health*

AIDS, acquired immunodeficiency syndrome; HIV, human immunodeficiency virus; PT, physical therapist; PTA, physical therapist assistant; SIG, special interest group.

Data from Enhancing Your Membership: Sections. Alexandria, VA, American Physical Therapy Association, 1999.

demic administrators (physical therapist and physical therapist assistant education programs) and one each for clinical education and academic faculty. Participation in any SIG is voluntary.

Assemblies

An **assembly** is similar to a section in that it provides a mechanism for members with common interests to meet, confer, and promote their objectives. The differences are that assemblies are composed of members of the same class (category) and may exist at the state and national levels. One exception to the class limitation applies to student and student affiliate members, who may combine into one assembly.

Only two assemblies currently exist: the Student Assembly and the National

Assembly of Physical Therapist Assistants (National Assembly). Each provides an important vehicle for communication and a voice for its members. Membership in each assembly is automatic for APTA members in specific categories—the Student Assembly for students and student affiliates and the National Assembly for affiliates and life affiliates. (For more information on the origin and function of the National Assembly, see Chapter 3.)

House of Delegates

The **House of Delegates** is the highest policymaking body of the APTA. Officers, directors, and members of the Nominating Committee are elected by the HOD. Its general powers, noted in Box 4–4,[2] are derived from the bylaws of the APTA.

The HOD is composed of delegates from all chapters, sections, assemblies, as well as members of the BOD. Representation is proportionate; however, the complex formula for determining the size of the HOD ensures that the total number of delegates will always be slightly above 400. In addition, each chapter has at least 2 delegates, each section 1 delegate, and each assembly 2 delegates. Delegates from sections and assemblies and members of the BOD may speak and make motions, but they do not have the right to vote.

In accordance with the bylaws, the annual session of the APTA is the HOD meeting. This session occurs in June, spans 3 days, and is held in conjunction with an **annual conference and exposition.** The conference (known as "PT XXXX," which represents the year) continues for another 2 to 3 days and includes an extensive program of presentations and activities.

Ad hoc committees and task forces, in addition to standing committees, may be created by the HOD to address issues that it deems important. When these groups are created, definite charges and time lines are stipulated in the motion that created the unit.

Box 4–4

General Powers of the House of Delegates

The House of Delegates of the American Physical Therapy Association has all legislative and elective powers and authority to determine policies of the Association, including the power to:

A. Amend and repeal these Bylaws;
B. Amend, suspend, or rescind the Standing Rules;
C. Adopt ethical principles and standards to govern the conduct of members of the Association in their roles as physical therapists or physical therapist assistants; and
D. Modify or reverse a decision of the Board of Directors.

Reprinted from Bylaws of the American Physical Therapy Association. Phys Ther 2000;80:1026–1035, with permission of the American Physical Therapy Association.

Representative Body of the National Assembly of Physical Therapist Assistants

The Representative Body of the National Assembly (RBNA) is similar to the HOD in that it is a representative and policymaking body for its constituents, in this case, the physical therapist assistant. It is composed of one representative from each chapter and the BOD of the National Assembly. Representatives from both groups may speak and make motions, but only chapter representatives may vote. In addition, three members of the association BOD serve as consultants to respond to inquiries.

An annual meeting is held before the HOD convenes so that pertinent issues can be brought to the latter body by the two delegates from the National Assembly, one of whom is the president of that body and the other is elected by the RBNA. The RBNA had its inaugural meeting in 1999.

4

Board of Directors

Six officers of the APTA and nine directors constitute the **Board of Directors.** The officers are the president, vice president, secretary, treasurer, speaker of the HOD, and vice speaker of the HOD. The duty of the BOD is to carry out the mandates and policies established by the HOD. Full meetings generally occur in November and March.

The BOD and HOD must work closely together for effective operation of the APTA. While the HOD establishes the policies and positions of the APTA, the BOD, elected by the HOD, communicates these issues to internal and external personnel or agencies. This communication of issues is an important representative function of the BOD.

Similar to the HOD, the BOD may create ad hoc committees and task forces to carry out its business. These units will also have specific charges and time lines. In addition, the BOD may establish councils to respond to unique service needs of the APTA.

Staff

The organizational chart in Figure 4–2 indicates that APTA staff serve the organization at multiple levels. During any business hour, a member (or non-member) can call the APTA headquarters in Alexandria, Virginia, on its toll-free number, (800) 999-APTA (2782), and speak to any of its more than 150 staff members. Staff may also be contacted through links from the APTA website (*http://www.apta.org*). This direct benefit is important to access information and services. Staff also provide support for activities of the chapters, sections, and assemblies and for operation of the HOD, BOD, RBNA, and all committees and task forces.

Key staff members also provide important representative functions to outside agencies, similar to duties of the BOD. This role is particularly true for the chief executive officer and senior vice presidents. These individuals are respon-sible for the following divisions: Executive; Communications; Education; Finance and Administration; Governance, Components, and Meetings; and Practice and Research.

ASSOCIATED ORGANIZATIONS

In addition to the components identified in Figure 4–2, several other organizations have a mission and set of goals that complement those of the APTA. Some of these agencies function completely independently of the APTA, whereas for others, the link is more than philosophical. In all cases, the association is mutually beneficial. These organizations are briefly described in the following sections and labeled in Figure 4–3.

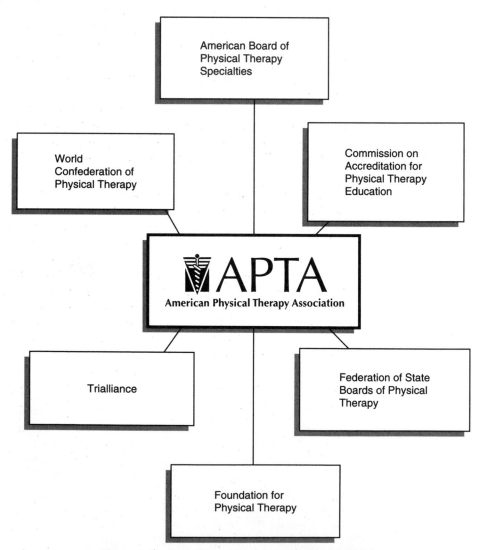

Figure 4–3. Organizations associated with the APTA.

American Board of Physical Therapy Specialties

The **American Board of Physical Therapy Specialties (ABPTS)** was created by the HOD in 1978 to provide a formal mechanism to recognize physical therapists with advanced knowledge, skills, and experience in a special area of practice. A specialization program was established to achieve board certification and enhance the quality of care in the specialty area. Participation in the program is voluntary; however, physical therapists shall not present themselves as "board-certified clinical specialists" unless they have successfully completed the certification process.

Each specialty area must be approved by the HOD; however, criteria for each area are established by the ABPTS. Seven specialty areas have been approved and are listed in Table 4–2.

To be recognized as a "board-certified clinical specialist," a physical therapist must pass a written examination and present the following qualifications: (1) licensure to practice physical therapy in one of the chapters of the APTA and (2) evidence of at least 2000 hours of clinical practice in the specialty area, at least 25% of which must have been done within the 3 years preceding the examination. The first three specialists were recognized in 1985 in the area of cardiopulmonary physical therapy. Currently, over 2000 clinical specialists have been certified. For more information on the ABPTS, visit the APTA website.

Commission on Accreditation in Physical Therapy Education

The **Commission on Accreditation in Physical Therapy Education (CAPTE)** is responsible for evaluating and accrediting professional (entry-level) physical therapy and physical therapist assistant education programs. It is recognized by the U.S. Department of Education and Council for Higher Education Accreditation. CAPTE is composed of 26 members from the educational community, the physical therapy profession, and the public. (See Chapter 1 for a historical account of accreditation in physical therapy.)

Table 4–2
Approved Specialty Areas in Physical Therapy

SPECIALTY AREA	YEAR APPROVED
Cardiopulmonary Physical Therapy	1981
Clinical Electrophysiology	1982
Geriatrics	1989
Neurology	1982
Orthopaedics	1981
Pediatrics	1981
Sports Physical Therapy	1981

The relationship between the APTA and CAPTE is integrated, yet they are technically independent. A Department of Accreditation within the APTA manages the accreditation program. However, CAPTE reviews the data and determines the accreditation status of each education program. Moreover, CAPTE establishes the evaluative criteria for the accreditation decisions. For more information on CAPTE, visit the APTA website.

Federation of State Boards of Physical Therapy

The **Federation of State Boards of Physical Therapy (FSBPT)** is an independent agency that has been instrumental in coordinating activity among all of the state boards that regulate physical therapy. It exists to protect the health, safety, and welfare of the public by promoting uniformity in regulations pertaining to physical therapy in each state. Areas of attention include the licensing examination and state practice acts for physical therapy. Regarding the examinations, the FSBPT develops, maintains, and administers the national licensing examination for physical therapists and physical therapist assistants. It has been involved in revising the examination and standardizing passing criteria among the states. Concerning state practice acts, the FSBPT has created a model practice act for physical therapy to be used in these laws. This model is an attempt to standardize language and legal references to the practice of physical therapy. For more information on the FSBPT, visit its website (*http://www.fsbpt.org*) or call (800) 881-1430.

Foundation for Physical Therapy

The **Foundation for Physical Therapy** was established in 1979 by an action of the APTA HOD. It was created to promote and provide financial support for scientific research, clinical research, and health services research in physical therapy. Because it is an independent entity, its governing body is separate from the APTA and consists of clinicians, researchers, and business leaders. Awards are distributed in the areas of research grants, scholarships for doctoral degree education, and postdoctoral fellowships. Special projects are also funded. For example, in 1999 the Foundation issued a call for proposals for three $40,000 research grants on the effectiveness of physical therapist practice in preventing work-related injuries and reducing frailty in older adults. Through these comprehensive programs, the Foundation promotes clinically focused research to improve the practice and cost-effectiveness of physical therapy. For more information on the foundation, visit the APTA website or call (800) 875-1378.

Trialliance

The **Trialliance** was formed in 1988 and consists of the APTA, the American Occupational Therapy Association, and the American Speech-Language and Hearing Association. This organization meets three times per year to discuss issues of mutual concern. Current issues focus on legislation and regulations that address reimbursement. This unified voice provides greater strength when interacting with governmental and private agencies.

World Confederation of Physical Therapy

The **World Confederation of Physical Therapy** represents physical therapy on a global level. Member organizations are from 82 nations around the world, including the APTA. In addition to annual business meetings, an international congress is held every 4 years to provide a forum to share information and collaborate on mutual goals. For more information, contact the secretariat of the World Confederation of Physical Therapy at 46–48 Grosvenor Gardens, London, SW1W OEB, United Kingdom.

4

OTHER RELATED ORGANIZATIONS

American Academy of Physical Therapists

This organization was founded in 1989 to address the professional needs and concerns of black Americans and other minorities in regard to the profession and practice of physical therapy. Its mission includes encouraging minority students to pursue careers in the allied health professions. The academy also promotes clinical research related to the health of minorities. Business and education programs are conducted at its annual conferences. For more information, visit its website (*http://www.aaptanet.org*) or call (888) 292-AAPT.

United Societies of Physiotherapists, Inc.

The United Societies of Physiotherapists is another organization that consists of and represents physical therapists. Membership qualifications are not limited to one group; however, most of the members are engaged in private practice. The purpose is to improve the professional status of "licensed physiotherapists," create fair reimbursement rates and methods, and maintain the highest level of competency in physical therapy services. It is composed of independent physical therapy associations in several states and at-large members, who send representatives to an executive board. The United Societies of Physiotherapists retains a legislative representative and legal counsel and has been active in legislative efforts regarding the practice of physical therapy.

BENEFITS OF BELONGING

Benefits of belonging to the APTA are both intangible and tangible. The intangible benefits relate to the commitment to high-quality service that the organization provides to its members and public. As the recognized voice for this profession in the United States, it is appropriate for physical therapists, physical therapist assistants, and students to join the APTA. Through the organizational structure described previously, members are represented in a wide variety of public and governmental areas. No other organization will advocate for the best interests of physical therapists, physical therapist assistants, or the patients and clients whom they serve.

The tangible benefits of belonging to the APTA are identified in Table 4–3 and briefly described here.[4] Legislative efforts are provided through lobbying,

Table 4–3
Benefits of Belonging to the APTA

BENEFIT	EXAMPLES
Legislative efforts	Medicare reimbursement
	Preservation of the ban on physician self-referral
	Protecting spinal manipulation
Information	*Physical Therapy*
	PT—Magazine of Physical Therapy
	PT Bulletin Online
	Website (*http://www.apta.org*)
	Staff consultation on practice, reimbursement, and research
Continuing education	Annual Conference and seminars
	Combined Sections Meeting
	Home study courses
Professional development	Networking and education through districts, chapters, sections, and assemblies
Practice and research	Fostering clinical competency through policies, guidelines, and core documents
	Advising agencies about professional standards
	Conducting and attending meetings with federal funding agencies on need for research funding
Reimbursement	Input into CPT coding
	Workshops on reimbursement and managed care
Insurance and member benefits	Professional liability insurance plan
	Visa and Mastercard
	Investment and retirement planning program
	Long-term disability plan

CPT, Current Procedural Terminology.
Data from Extend Your Reach: Benefits of Belonging Checklist. Alexandria, VA, American Physical Therapy Association.

direct contact with government officials, and a strong infrastructure to represent the members. In this era of rapidly changing health care management and reimbursement, this membership benefit is critical for success of the profession. Information is made available through World Wide Web access to the APTA, phone contact with staff (see the earlier section on staff), and publications. The website contains a great deal of current and reference information; however, some of it is restricted to members only. Continuing education offerings, including annual events and home study courses, are available to members at considerable discount from nonmember prices. Professional development occurs through interaction at the local, state, and national levels, which is available through district, chapter, section, and assembly events. Practice and research activities include promoting clinical competency through guidelines and policies, advising government agencies and insurance companies of practice standards, and defending the need for research funding to appropriate sources. Services in the area of reimbursement, perhaps the most significant issue currently confronting the profession, include input into Current Procedural Terminology (CPT) coding changes, workshops for both members and payers, and coordinated legislative efforts on behalf of physical therapists, physical therapist assistants, and students. Finally, insurance and other financial benefits include low-cost group programs and investment/retirement planning.

Special incentives are provided for student membership. Fees for membership and participation in activities are generally 10% to 25% of the cost for an active member. In addition, a 3-year dues increment to convert from student to active member after graduation (from one-third to two-thirds to full dues) eases the financial transition to the higher dues level.

Summary ———— This chapter described the purposes, infrastructure, benefits, and organizations related to the APTA. Purposes of the APTA include serving the public and its members to enhance the profession and practice of physical therapy. Its governing bodies are organized into three levels: local (districts), state (chapters), and national (HOD and BOD). Opportunities for participation in areas of special interest exist in sections and assemblies. Staff members are readily available to support the organization at all levels and interact with external agencies. Other related organizations in the United States and across the globe further promote physical therapy, and the APTA participates in these organizations through either direct membership or interaction. Benefits of belonging include outcomes that are intangible (professional commitment) and tangible (legislative efforts, information, continuing education, professional development, practice and research support, reimbursement actions, and low-cost insurance). Through its purpose, organization, and activities, the APTA provides widespread opportunities and strong representation for the profession and practice of physical therapy.

References

1. APTA Mission Statement, HOD 06-93-05-05. Alexandria, VA, American Physical Therapy Association, 1993.

2. Bylaws of the American Physical Therapy Association. Phys Ther 2000;80:1026–1035.
3. Enhancing Your Membership: Sections. Alexandria, VA, American Physical Therapy Association, 1999.
4. Extend Your Reach: Benefits of Belonging Checklist. Alexandria, VA, American Physical Therapy Association.
5. Goals that Represent the 2001 Priorities of the Association, HOD 06-00-11-03. Alexandria, VA, American Physical Therapy Association, 2000.
6. Policy on APTA Mission Statement, HOD 06-93-06-07. Alexandria, VA, American Physical Therapy Association, 1993.
7. Standing rules of the American Physical Therapy Association. Phys Ther 2000;80:1023–1025.

REVIEW QUESTIONS

1. Select at least three components of the APTA mission statement and apply them to Figure 4–2 by indicating at what level of APTA each goal should be most logically tackled. (There may be more than one answer.)

2. Apply the goals listed in Box 4–3 to the various levels of the APTA's organizational structure (Fig. 4–2) and compare them with your applications in question 1 and with the definitions of the various APTA components given in this chapter.

3. What is the difference between an assembly, section, and SIG? How do they differ in function and membership?

4. Write to one of the physical therapy organizations besides the APTA to discern differences in scope and function. What advantage do they offer over membership in the APTA alone?

*N*o civilization . . . would ever have been possible without a framework of stability, to provide the wherein for the flux of change. Foremost among the stabilizing factors, more enduring than customs, manners, and traditions, are the legal systems that regulate our life in the world and our daily affairs with each other.
Hannah Arendt

Laws, Regulations, and Policies

Laurie A. Walsh

KEY TERMS

certification
civil law
Code of Ethics
common law
contract
criminal law
law
licensure
malpractice
negligence
policy
practice act

professional misconduct
registration
regulation
risk management

Standards of Ethical Conduct for the Physical
Therapist Assistant
statute
vicarious liability

OBJECTIVES   After reading this chapter, the reader will be able to

- Distinguish between laws, regulations, and policies and how they are made
- Understand basic concepts regarding how various laws, regulations, and policies affect physical therapy practice
- Identify resources that physical therapists and physical therapist assistants may use to find out more about laws, regulations, and policies affecting physical therapy practice
- Identify ways in which individuals and groups can effect change in the regulation of physical therapy practice
- Understand the basic issues involved in the various ways that physical therapists and physical therapist assistants can be held legally liable for the care that they provide and the consequences of liability

The primary purpose of laws, regulations, and policies governing the practice of physical therapy is to protect the public by (1) trying to ensure that providers are competent and (2) where services are paid for by government programs, to ensure that taxpayer dollars are being spent appropriately. Laws, regulations, and policies serve to create, in legal terms, a scope of practice for physical therapy and to distinguish it from other professions. In accepting government regulation, physical therapists (PTs) and physical therapist assistants (PTAs) receive a double-edged sword: providers receive rights and protection under regulation, but they must also accept responsibilities and limits imposed by regulation.

A detailed examination of the legal regulation of physical therapy practice is beyond the scope of this chapter, and the reader is referred elsewhere for more detail. As you read this chapter, the following basic principles should be kept in mind:

1. Many of the laws, regulations, and policies affecting physical therapy practice vary from state to state and from program to program. This chapter will focus on general principles, so readers should look to individual state laws, program regulations, and the like for specific information.
2. Various aspects of practice may be governed by both state and federal law. When they come into conflict, federal law generally prevails.
3. Some laws, regulations, and policies govern what services PTs and PTAs may legally provide, whereas others may address how these services are reimbursed. The fact that reimbursement may be denied does not necessarily mean that the services cannot be legally provided, only that the therapist must look elsewhere for reimbursement.

STATUTORY, REGULATORY, AND COMMON LAW

Law is "a body of rules of action or conduct prescribed by the controlling authority and hav[ing] binding legal force."[1] The law of a jurisdiction may be composed of laws created by legislatures, decrees handed down by courts, or regulations created by government agencies. Laws may address offenses against society or the private wrongs that one individual commits against another. This section will address the various components of the law and how they affect the practice of physical therapy. This section will also discuss distinctions between three major topic areas in law: criminal law, civil law, and contract law.

Statutes

Statutes are a type of law that is "enacted and established by the will of the legislative department of government."[1] Statutes affecting the practice of physical therapy may be enacted at the federal level by Congress or at the state level by the various state legislatures. Provisions of federal and state statutes can be enforced through the state and federal court systems.

Federal Statutes. These laws address areas that the federal government is constitutionally permitted to regulate, such as interstate commerce and taxation. Federal statutes apply consistently to all citizens across state lines and, when they conflict with related state laws, supersede state law. A number of federal statutes may have an impact on the provision of physical therapy services. For example, the Americans with Disabilities Act (ADA) requires that goods and services (including health care) available to the public be made accessible to persons with disabilities. The Individuals with Disabilities Education Act requires that special education and related services (including physical therapy) be provided at public expense to students with disabilities when needed for students to benefit from an education program (see Chapter 11). The Social Security Act contains, among other provisions, the foundation for the Medicare program, a federally subsidized health insurance program for people 65 years and older. Medicaid, jointly funded by the state and federal governments, is a program designed to provide health care services to the poor. Physical therapy is among the health care services reimbursed under Medicare and Medicaid.

The consequences for violating federal laws vary. Violations of the ADA may result in fines or injunctions (in this case, court orders requiring defendants to make their businesses more accessible to persons with disabilities). Fraudulent billing of federal benefit programs, such as Medicare, is vigorously prosecuted. One example involved a physical therapist who pled guilty to billing the federal government and private insurance companies $1 million for therapy services that were never provided.[12] The therapist was criminally prosecuted, ordered to repay $125,000, and sentenced to 27 months in a federal penitentiary.

State Statutes. State statutes are enacted in areas that states are constitutionally permitted to regulate, such as education, professional licensing, and insurance. When no superseding federal law exists, each state is entitled to tailor its laws

5

to meet the needs of its citizens. Consequently, laws in these areas vary from state to state.

State statutes can affect the practice of physical therapy in a number of ways, such as through regulation of the insurance industry, availability of state health care funding for the poor, and state health department requirements. The single most important statute, however, is the state practice act. The **practice act** is the legal foundation for the scope and protection of physical therapy practice. Among the areas covered by the practice act are the state definition of physical therapy practice, identification of providers who may be legally provide physical therapy services, identification of tasks that may be delegated and to which persons they may be delegated, and supervisory requirements. Physical therapy providers are legally permitted to practice only when they comply with their state's practice act, and it is assumed that they are knowledgeable about the provisions of the practice act. The practice act is the final word regarding what is legal physical therapy practice in a given state; it supersedes the provisions of other state practice acts and the guidelines of private organizations, such as the American Physical Therapy Association (APTA). The consequences of violating state practice acts are often stated in the act or accompanying regulations. In some states, such as New York, the unlawful practice of physical therapy is a criminal offense.[21]

One may obtain a copy of a state practice act in many ways. The state physical therapy licensing board may have copies available, and many state legislatures now have official websites with all state laws, including practice acts, available on-line. State practice acts may also be accessed at the APTA website (*http://www.apta.org*) through the Government Affairs Department/PT Advocacy. (*Note:* While this information is currently available to the public, some information on the website is accessible only to APTA members.)

With respect to efforts to obtain more consistent physical therapy regulation, the reader is also advised to be aware of the Model Practice Act for Physical Therapy (MPA). The MPA is not a statute and does not have the force of law, but it is intended as an "integrated model for the regulation of physical therapy practice" and a guide to assist in the modification of state practice acts.[20] The MPA was developed by the Federation of State Boards of Physical Therapy, a private organization consisting of members of physical therapy licensing boards from all 50 states and the federal territories. The federation is also responsible for developing national licensing examinations for the PT and PTA. More information about the Federation can be obtained from their website (*http://www.fsbpt.org*), which also contains basic information about the licensing examinations and a directory of all state licensing boards.

Although a great deal of overlap is seen among practice acts, they also have significant differences. Given that physical therapy providers are legally responsible for knowing their own practice acts, providers must educate themselves and cannot assume that what is legal therapy practice in another state is also legal in their own state. One example is direct access to physical therapy services, which permits a patient to obtain services without first obtaining a referral from another provider, usually a physician. As of this writing, 47 states permit evaluation without referral and 33 states permit some form of intervention without referral.[6] States vary in terms of the amount of experience that a therapist must have before being allowed to provide direct access and may impose time limits on the number of days that service may be provided before a referral must be obtained.

The manner in which physical therapy providers are regulated also varies from state to state. All 50 states license physical therapists. A license, however, cannot automatically be transferred from one state to another. If a provider moves to another state, that person must apply for a new license according to that state's requirements and procedures. **Licensure** creates a scope of practice, authorizes the individual to practice in a given state, and legally protects the professional title "physical therapist"; only licensed individuals may refer to themselves as such. All states require graduation from an accredited program and a passing score on the licensing examination to be licensed, but exact procedures, forms, costs, and other requirements vary from state to state.[18]

The PTA is also recognized under the practice acts of 43 states and may be licensed, certified, or registered. Functionally, **certification**, like licensure, legally protects the title of the PTA; however, unlike licensure, it does not create a separate scope of practice or a monopoly to provide a particular service.[14] **Registration** is the least rigorous form of governmental regulation and requires only that registrants periodically provide the state with updated information on their name, address, and qualifications and pay a registration fee. Individuals who are licensed or certified are generally required to periodically reregister as well.

The reader should not confuse state certification with certification by private organizations. The APTA, for example, has a program to certify practitioners as specialists in particular areas of practice. The Neurodevelopmental Treatment Association, as well as other organizations, has programs to certify practitioners. These private forms of certification establish that an individual has met the standards of these organizations in terms of competency in a certain therapeutic approach or specialty area.[14] Unlike state certification, they do not create a legally enforceable professional title.

Regulations

Unlike statutes, regulations are developed not by the legislature but by governmental agencies. Administrative agencies exist at all levels of government and serve to regulate industries and government benefit programs, such as Medicare and Medicaid. Such agencies are created by statutes for the purpose of regulating a particular industry or program. Agencies are overseen by the legislative branch and can perform only those duties delegated by the legislature.[15] Unlike legislators, appointees to agencies generally have specific expertise and experience in the industry or program being regulated.

Having been delegated authority in a specific area by the legislature, agencies have the authority to develop regulations and enforce them within a specific industry or program. A **regulation** is a rule controlling the practices of individuals or organizations under the authority of the agency.[15] For example, regulations may support, clarify, or give further definition to terms in the statutes that created the agency, or they may set forth procedures for programs created by statute. A practice act, for example, may require that a PTA be supervised on site by a PT. The legislature may then delegate to an appropriate state agency the responsibility for developing a regulation defining what constitutes appropriate supervision. Consequently, one must be familiar with both the statutes and regulations of a given jurisdiction to have full knowledge of the law.

Federal Regulations. Federal agencies regulate a wide variety of industries and benefit programs. One example of a federal agency with great impact on the provision of physical therapy services is the Health Care Financing Administration (HCFA), part of the federal cabinet Department of Health and Human Services. Among HCFA's responsibilities is regulation of the Medicare and Medicaid programs. While it is beyond the scope of this chapter to discuss the Medicare program and the role of the HCFA in detail, HCFA regulations determine to what extent therapists may participate as providers within the Medicare program and how much and for what services they will be reimbursed.[16] Radical changes have occurred during the 1990s regarding reimbursement within the various aspects of Medicare, and reimbursement for physical therapy services in many areas has been dramatically reduced.[19] The APTA has struggled on the behalf of consumers and the profession to restore adequate levels of reimbursement (see Chapter 6).

Failure to abide by Medicare regulations may result in denial of reimbursement for services rendered. Federal statutes and regulations also prohibit fraudulent billing; consequently, when evidence of fraud is uncovered, fines and criminal prosecution may follow, as noted earlier in this chapter. In the absence of fraud, however, denial of reimbursement does not mean that services were illegally provided, only that they are not covered by the Medicare program, and providers must seek reimbursement elsewhere.

The APTA updates members frequently regarding the activities of the HCFA and other government agencies through publications such as *PT Bulletin* and *PT—Magazine of Physical Therapy.* The Government Affairs Department/PT Advocacy section of the APTA website also maintains current information and links to government websites. Information specific to the HCFA may be accessed on the World Wide Web (*http://www.hcfa.gov*).

State Regulations. State agencies also regulate a variety of industries and programs. Among the most important for the practice of physical therapy is the state physical therapy board. The composition and functions of physical therapy boards are set by each state's law. While they cannot change the practice acts adopted by state legislatures, state boards serve many important functions. They advise the legislature or other governmental bodies to clarify the scope of practice, as well as provide advice to state-licensed practitioners seeking guidance on practice issues in that state. They also assist in administering the licensing procedures and are generally consulted by prosecutors in professional misconduct cases. More information on the role of a state board can be obtained directly from the licensing board of an individual state.

Professional misconduct is often regulated by a state disciplinary agency and is a topic that deserves further discussion. **Professional misconduct** involves actions by licensed professionals that demonstrate an inability to competently perform the duties of a licensed professional. Actions that constitute professional misconduct are defined in the practice act or accompanying regulations and may include physical/sexual abuse of a patient, patient abandonment (discharge of a patient while services are still needed), improper delegation or supervision of treatment activities, provision of unnecessary treatment, fraud, incompetence, and practicing while intoxicated, among other activities. Complaints of unprofessional conduct are typically prosecuted by administrative bodies set up for that purpose by the states rather than being prosecuted in courts of law. The state physical therapy board is usually consulted regarding the proceedings. A finding that a PT or PTA has committed professional misconduct may result in that individual's being reprimanded, fined, required to obtain remedial professional education, or placed on probation or having the license suspended or revoked.[11]

5

Creating Statutes and Regulations

Given the profound effect that statutes and regulations can have on the practice of physical therapy (and the consequences of violations), it is necessary that therapists and assistants remain aware of and be in compliance with the applicable laws and regulations. When laws and regulations unnecessarily limit the provision of services to the public, therapists and assistants must work to educate lawmakers. First, however, physical therapy providers must educate themselves on how laws and regulations are made and where they can have an impact on the final outcome.

How Laws Are Made. Enacting or amending statutes is often a lengthy process involving negotiation and compromise. It varies somewhat from state to state and between state and federal governments. In general, however, the process involves introducing a proposed statute (or bill) in one house of the legislature, where it will be referred to at least one committee assigned to address all bills pertaining to a certain topic (e.g., Finance, Education, Appropriations).[10] Committees will gather additional information on the bill and debate and amend it. If passed, the committee's version of the bill is referred to the entire house (or "floor") for debate. If passed by one house of the legislature, the bill is then forwarded to the other house to undergo the same process. Only when passed by both legislative houses in identical form is a bill then forwarded to the executive branch (president or governor) to be signed into law or vetoed. While the process of enacting statutes is lengthy and complicated, the many steps involved give interested parties, such as physical therapy providers, ample opportunity to contact their legislators to make sure that the interest of the profession and the public is represented. The process of persuading lawmakers, or lobbying, is essential to ensure the well-being of the public and the health of the profession. The APTA is actively involved at both the state and national levels to ensure that the profession's interests are represented. Therapists and assistants must become aware of pending legislation that may affect the practice of physical therapy and become involved in lobbying efforts, such as writing to their legislators at various points in the process.

The APTA keeps members updated on current legislative issues through publications such as *PT Bulletin* and *PT—Magazine of Physical Therapy* and through the Government Affairs Department/PT Advocacy on the APTA website. State chapters also keep members apprised through newsletters, and a number of chapters now have websites that may carry legislative information. Again, the national APTA website contains links to state chapters that have websites. State and federal governments also have a number of official publications on pending and recent legislation. For example, the *Congressional Record* publishes a daily record of House and Senate proceedings. The Library of Congress has extensive federal legislative information available on-line through its service THOMAS (*http://thomas.loc.gov*). Among the information available at this site is the most recent *Congressional Record*, bill texts, committee reports, and summaries of the legislative process.

How Regulations Are Made. Procedures have also been established for promulgating regulations, which may vary from state to state. In general, though, an agency must first publish a proposed regulation and give interested parties time to comment on it. This "comment period" gives physical therapy providers an opportunity to educate regulatory bodies on the issues and influence the form that the final rule takes.[22] At the federal level, proposed and final regulations are published daily in the *Federal Register* and can be accessed via a link at the APTA website under the Government Affairs Department/PT Advocacy.

Common Law

The courts serve a number of functions in our legal system, including clarifying and interpreting statutes. The court system serves as an additional source of law: **common law** is law that has been created by court decisions, written by judges, and handed down.[16] Areas of common law evolve as new court decisions are added to the existing body of law in that area and may modify or overrule previous decisions. Certain areas of the law, such as negligence, are governed primarily through common law, although some states have developed statutory definitions of professional negligence.[4] Negligence and malpractice will be discussed further under the section on civil law.

CRIMINAL LAW VERSUS CIVIL LAW

The reader should also understand that within the law are different areas, or topics. One important distinction is the difference between criminal and civil law. Legal matters may be handled differently, depending on this distinction, and the penalties imposed for a finding of liability also differ.

Criminal Law

Criminal law involves prosecution in a court of law for acts "done in violation of those duties which an individual owes to the community."[1] Thus, crimes are considered to be infractions committed against society, and the state prosecutes these actions on behalf of the public. Criminal laws are generally found today as state and federal statutes rather than common law.[1] The consequences of being tried and convicted or pleading guilty to a crime may involve fines, probation, and/or imprisonment and will vary depending on the type of crime committed and the law of the particular jurisdiction involved (state or federal). Criminal prosecution will not directly affect a provider's license but may result in referral to a state professional disciplinary agency to initiate such an action. Earlier in this chapter, an example was given of a therapist prosecuted criminally for insurance fraud. Other possible sources of criminal liability may involve sexual abuse of patients or, depending on the state law, unlawful practice of a profession.

Civil Law

Unlike criminal law, **civil law** is concerned with private wrongs and remedies.[16] Civil actions are also prosecuted in courts of law, but in these cases, one private citizen brings a lawsuit against another to seek compensation for injuries received. Unlike criminal cases, persons found liable in civil cases cannot be punished by the state with fines or incarceration; the only remedy available for civil liability is for the defendant to pay money damages to the plaintiff (the person who brings the lawsuit) to compensate that person for injuries that can be shown to be caused by the defendant's actions. A civil lawsuit also cannot affect a person's license, but it may, depending on the nature of the wrong, result in a complaint to the state disciplinary agency to initiate a separate action for professional misconduct. Physical therapy providers may be named in civil lawsuits for a variety of reasons, including defamation (saying or writing something untrue that harms another person's reputation) or breach of contract. The most common grounds for civil actions involving physical therapy providers, however, involve claims of negligence or malpractice.

Negligence and Malpractice. **Negligence** is defined as the failure to act as a reasonably prudent person: doing (or failing to do) something that a reasonably prudent person would have done (or would not have done) under similar circumstances.[1] An example of negligence in a physical therapy clinic would be failure to mop up water that had been tracked onto the clinic floor, with someone subsequently slipping and getting injured. A reasonably prudent person would have recognized that the water posed a risk of injury and promptly cleaned it up. **Malpractice**, or professional negligence, is failure to do (or avoid doing) something that a reasonably prudent member of that profession would have done (or avoided doing), with subsequent injury to the patient.[1] An example of malpractice would be a therapist who excessively mobilizes a joint and thereby causes injury. A reasonably prudent person would not be expected to know whether or how much to mobilize a joint in a given patient. A therapist, as a professional, is held to a higher standard of care and is expected to exercise appropriate clinical judgment to avoid patient injury.

Delegation and Supervision: Vicarious Liability: It is essential that the reader understand that the legal duty to provide a professional standard of care—and the ultimate responsibility for patient care—always remains with the PT. The therapist may therefore be held liable for a patient's injury even if the therapist was not directly providing services at that time. This liability is due to the fact that a therapist's professional duty to the patient includes appropriate decision making regarding delegation and supervision of interventions. PTAs or students on affiliation can be held legally liable for their own negligent clinical judgments; however, the therapist may also be liable if tasks were negligently delegated or supervised. If a therapist determines that delegation is appropriate, the therapist should always advise the patient of the credentials of the person to whom tasks have been delegated to avoid misunderstandings.

Similarly, an employer may be held legally responsible for the negligence or malpractice of employees when it is committed within the scope of their employment duties, regardless of whether the employer was involved in rendering care at the time.[16] This form of liability, known as **vicarious liability**, is based on the fact that the employer can control the quality of care rendered by controlling the workplace (policies, hiring, etc.). Thus, a therapist who owns a private practice may be held liable for the injuries caused by one of the practice's PTs or PTAs while these employees are treating patients. In contrast, the employer would not be liable for any negligent acts (such as causing a car accident on the way to work through negligent driving) that employees may commit when not performing their professional duties.

Risk Management. **Risk management** involves a coordinated effort by an organization to "identify, assess, and minimize, where possible, the risk of suffering harm or loss to patients, visitors, staff and the organization."[9] To decrease the risk of lawsuits, PT providers are advised to constantly monitor the quality of the services that they provide to avoid or minimize the occurrence of activities that increase the risk of patient injuries and other incidents that may impose legal liability. Additionally, they are advised to carry professional liability insurance that would cover the cost of legal fees and settlements or judgments arising from civil liability.[8] Under ordinary circumstances, however, liability insurance will not cover legal fees for professional misconduct or criminal actions.

Contracts. A **contract** is "an agreement between two or more persons which creates mutual obligations to do or not do particular things."[1] Contractual obligations are a matter of civil law and can be enforced in court. It is beyond the scope of this chapter to fully discuss the various types of contracts that physical therapy providers may encounter, but a few of the more prominent ones will be mentioned here. For example, providers may sign employment contracts with their employers, although most providers are employed without having signed contracts.[16] Therapists may also contract independently to provide services for an agency or facility without becoming employees. Providers are advised to thoroughly review any contract before signing it, preferably with legal counsel. Should a provider breach an employment contract, the employer may seek to legally enforce it. While providers cannot be forced to stay at a job against their will, the employer may be entitled to monetary damages, as set forth in the contract. For example, some employers may offer tuition reimbursement or other inducements in return for one's agreement to work for the employer for a set period. If the provider breaches the agreement, the employer may be entitled to all or a percentage of the reimbursement provided, with interest.

In an increasingly managed care environment, therapists may also sign agreements with managed care organizations (MCOs) and other payers to become recognized providers for patients enrolled with or covered by those organizations.[9] It is not uncommon for an MCO to refuse to reimburse or to limit reimbursement for services rendered to enrollees if the provider has not signed an agreement with the MCO. If a provider does not abide by the agreement, the MCO can deny reimbursement or, if the breach is severe enough, drop the therapist as a recognized provider.

5

POLICIES

The APTA defines and applies a **policy** as "a decision which obligates actions or subsequent decisions on similar matters."[5] Procedures, on the other hand, describe the actions required to implement policies. Policies affecting physical therapy may be set by other private entities, such as employers and payers. Policies, unlike laws, cannot be legally enforced unless set forth in a contract. They do, however, represent the consensus of the members of an organization on a given issue. Consequently, policies related to physical therapy can influence the relationships between physical therapy providers and private organizations, or they can be used to provide some momentum to effect change within private and public organizations.

APTA *Policies*

As noted elsewhere in this text, the APTA is the primary professional organization representing the physical therapy profession in the United States. Through the activities of its Board of Directors and the House of Delegates, it establishes and annually reviews policies for its members. Policies of the APTA address a number of areas relating to practice, from documentation to the use of support personnel to national health care policy. Therapists and assistants are encouraged to become participative members of the APTA to ensure that their voices are heard and their efforts can be of assistance as policies affecting current and future practice are developed.

Information on a number of APTA policies can be obtained from the national organization website. The reader is reminded that because the APTA is a private organization, its policies are binding only on members. These policies, however, can have wide-ranging effects as they drive changes in practice, such as entry-level degree requirements (through accreditation activities), scope of practice (through lobbying efforts), and reimbursement issues (through lobbying and dialogue with payers).

Certain policies and interpretive guidelines, clustered as core documents, address practice standards and ethical conduct. One example is the "Standards of Practice for Physical Therapy," which was identified and described in Chapter 2 (see Fig. 2–1). Two documents that establish standards of ethical conduct for physical therapy providers are the **Code of Ethics** (for physical therapists, Box 5–1) and the **Standards of Ethical Conduct for the Physical Therapist Assistant** (Box 5–2).[2, 17] Companion documents, the "Guide for Professional Conduct" (for the Code of Conduct) and the "Guide for Conduct of the Affiliate Member" (for the Standards), interpret each item in the policies.[3] Violations of these policies by members can be prosecuted by the APTA.[13] A complaint must first be lodged with the state chapter president, who will refer it to the state chapter ethics committee for investigation. The member accused of the violations will be notified and given an opportunity to respond. After completing the investigation, the state chapter ethics committee will forward the matter to the Ethics and Judicial Committee of the national organization if the complaint is found to have any merit. The Ethics and Judicial Committee will then review the matter and impose sanctions ranging from reprimanding the member to expulsion from the organization. The APTA action can affect only membership; it has no jurisdiction to levy fines or affect the member's license to practice.

Payer Reimbursement Policies

A full description of reimbursement policies is beyond the scope of this chapter. Different insurance companies, MCOs, government benefit programs, and so forth have different policies regarding, among other topics, who can be a provider, what services will be reimbursed and for how much, documentation requirements, and procedures for claims review and appeals for claim denials. Physical therapy providers must become familiar with these various policies and adhere to them to be reimbursed for their services. Payer policies may be found in government regulations, provider agreements, and provider manuals.

Changes in reimbursement policies in recent years have created dilemmas for providers because of the temptation to allow reimbursement to drive

---

Box 5–1   **Code of Ethics**

Preamble

This Code of Ethics of the American Physical Therapy Association sets forth principles for the ethical practice of physical therapy. All physical therapists are responsible for maintaining and promoting ethical practice. To this end, the physical therapist shall act in the best interest of the patient/client. This Code of Ethics shall be binding on all physical therapists.

Principle 1

A physical therapist shall respect the rights and dignity of all individuals and shall provide compassionate care.

Principle 2

A physical therapist shall act in a trustworthy manner towards patients/ clients, and in all other aspects of physical therapy practice.

Principle 3

A physical therapist shall comply with laws and regulations governing physical therapy and shall strive to effect changes that benefit patients/clients.

Principle 4

A physical therapist shall exercise sound professional judgment.

Principle 5

A physical therapist shall achieve and maintain professional competence.

Principle 6

A physical therapist shall maintain and promote high standards for physical therapy practice, education and research.

Principle 7

A physical therapist shall seek only such remuneration as is deserved and reasonable for physical therapy services.

Principle 8

A physical therapist shall provide and make available accurate and relevant information to patients/clients about their care and to the public about physical therapy services.

Principle 9

A physical therapist shall protect the public and the profession from unethical, incompetent, and illegal acts.

Principle 10

A physical therapist shall endeavor to address the health needs of society.

Principle 11

A physical therapist shall respect the rights, knowledge, and skills of colleagues and other healthcare professionals.

From Code of Ethics, HOD 06-00-12-23. Alexandria, VA, American Physical Therapy Association, 2000.

Box 5–2

Standards of Ethical Conduct for the Physical Therapist Assistant

Preamble

This document of the American Physical Therapy Association sets forth standards for the ethical conduct of the physical therapist assistant. All physical therapist assistants are responsible for maintaining high standards of conduct while assisting physical therapists. The physical therapist assistant shall act in the best interest of the patient/client. These standards of conduct shall be binding on all physical therapist assistants.

Standard 1

A physical therapist assistant shall respect the rights and dignity of all individuals and shall provide compassionate care.

Standard 2

A physical therapist assistant shall act in a trustworthy manner towards patients/clients.

Standard 3

A physical therapist assistant shall provide selected physical therapy interventions only under the supervision and direction of a physical therapist.

Standard 4

A physical therapist assistant shall comply with laws and regulations governing physical therapy.

Standard 5

A physical therapist assistant shall achieve and maintain competence in the provision of selected physical therapy interventions.

Standard 6

A physical therapist assistant shall make judgments that are commensurate with their educational and legal qualifications as a physical therapist assistant.

Standard 7

A physical therapist assistant shall protect the public and the profession from unethical, incompetent, and illegal acts.

From Standards of Ethical Conduct for the Physical Therapist Assistant, HOD 06-00-13-24. Alexandria, VA, American Physical Therapy Association, 2000.

practice. Providers must be actively engaged in a dialogue with payers to educate them and ensure that reimbursement is adequate to meet patient needs. Providers must be able to successfully advocate on behalf of patients by using tools such as the *Guide to Physical Therapist Practice* and research demonstrating the effectiveness of physical therapy. Therapists must also become more involved in clinical research to increase the body of knowledge establishing the effectiveness of physical therapy interventions. (See Chapter 6 for further description of reimbursement, the *Guide,* and research.)

Employer Policies

Various employment settings also establish policies and procedures that are specific to that facility or organization. These policies and procedures address a wide variety of employment issues, including job descriptions, intervention protocols, record-keeping requirements, safety issues, and activities to ensure quality of care.[7] It should be noted that the "Standards of Practice for Physical Therapy" requires that physical therapy services have written policies and procedures to ensure the provision of high-quality physical therapy.[3]

Employer policies cannot be legally enforced unless contained in an employment contract. They can, however, be grounds for disciplinary actions or firing. In addition, inquiries regarding whether facility policies and procedures were followed are often made during legal actions for negligence or malpractice as part of the determination regarding whether the appropriate standard of care was met. As professionals, however, therapists should not blindly follow policies without question, but should be engaged in active dialogue with their employers to ensure that their policies promote ethical, legal, and effective patient care.

5

Case Study

You are a physical therapist operating an outpatient clinic that provides services for patients with a wide variety of needs. One of your patients is a 28-year-old construction worker who injured his knee in a work-related accident. He was referred to your clinic after surgery to repair the anterior cruciate ligament. You have completed your examination and evaluation, generated a diagnosis and prognosis, developed a plan of care, and delegated implementation of the intervention plan to an athletic trainer (ATC) who works for you in your clinic. The patient attends routine therapy visits over the next 2 weeks but then fails to show up for further visits. Calls to the patient are not returned and communication with his physician fails to explain the patient's apparent decision to terminate therapy. Several months later, legal papers are served at the clinic indicating that a lawsuit has been filed against you. The patient claims that the treatment received reinjured his knee. You discuss the case with the ATC, who after reviewing his notes can recall no incidents or complaints involving the patient. From conversations with the patient, the ATC had suspicions that the patient was not adhering to activity precautions appropriate for his stage of recovery. However, the ATC did not believe that these suspicions were strong enough to share with you or document in the patient's chart. You immediately contact your malpractice insurance carrier and forward all the legal papers and patient records.

An attorney for the insurance company contacts you to discuss the case. While noting that the patient needs to prove his case to win in court, she states that the failure to follow up on concerns regarding the patient's failure to adhere to precautions will hurt your case. Additionally, the attorney advises that she has confidentially contacted a representative of your state's Physical Therapy Board, who has advised her that your state law does not permit delegation of physical therapy interventions to ATCs. Given the problems with this case, she notifies you that she will be recommending that the insurance company settle the case.

QUESTIONS

1. Can the PT be held liable for the patient's injuries in this case? If so, on what grounds? What penalties can be imposed on the therapist for negligence/malpractice?

2. Assume that the PT's conduct also constitutes professional misconduct in this case. What penalties may be imposed on the basis of professional misconduct?

3. Were any policies implicated in this case? Identify possible areas of policy violations.

4. What actions could the PT have taken to minimize liability risks in this case? With whom could the PT have consulted?

Summary

Regulation of the physical therapy profession provides practitioners with both opportunities and limitations. Regulation occurs through the enactment of statutes by state and federal legislatures and through regulations developed by state and federal agencies under statutory delegation. Physical therapy providers must work with legislators and regulatory bodies to ensure that statutes and regulations accurately reflect the current state of practice. Court decisions clarify and interpret statutory language and, in the civil law arena, also shape practice through the imposition of liability for acts of malpractice. Policies adopted by private organizations, such as the APTA, can also affect the evolution of physical therapy practice. Examples cited in this chapter indicate how laws, regulations, and policies can have an impact on the practice of physical therapy. Knowledge of and adherence to the applicable laws, regulations, and policies are necessary for safe, legal, ethical, and reimbursable practice.

References

1. Black's Law Dictionary, ed 5. St Paul, MN, West Publishing, 1990.
2. Code of Ethics, HOD 06-00-12-23, Alexandria, VA, American Physical Therapy Association, 2000.

3. Core documents. Phys Ther 2000;80:78–86.

4. Cowdrey M, Drew M: Basic Law for the Allied Health Professions, ed 2. Boston, Jones & Bartlett, 1995.

5. Definitions, BOD 06-95-12-01. Alexandria, VA, American Physical Therapy Association, 1995.

6. Direct access to physical therapy services. Retrieved from *http://www.apta.org/Advocacy/state/State2*, American Physical Therapy Association, 2000.

7. Gaynor L: High quality, low risk. Clin Manage Phys Ther 1991;11(3):16–19.

8. Lewis K: Professional liability insurance: Are you covered? PT Magazine Physical Therapy 1994;2(7):49–54.

9. Nosse J, Friberg D, Kovacek P: Managerial and Supervisory Principles for Physical Therapists. Baltimore, Williams & Wilkins, 1999, p 248.

10. Olsen GG: Understanding and influencing the legislative process. *In* Mathews J (ed): Practice Issues in Physical Therapy. Thorofare, NJ, Slack, 1989.

11. Penalties for professional misconduct, New York State Education Law, Article 130, Subarticle 3, Section 6511. Retrieved from *http://www.assembly.state.ny.us/cgi-bin/claws?law= 30&art= 120*, New York State Assembly, 2000.

12. Physical therapist sentenced for billing fraud. PT Bull 1993;1(11):4.

13. Procedural Document on Disciplinary Action of the American Physical Therapy Association. Alexandria, VA, American Physical Therapy Association, 1996.

14. Reforming Health Care Workforce Regulation: Policy Considerations for the 21st Century. San Francisco, Pew Health Professions Commissions, 1995.

15. Schwartz B: Administrative Law: A Casebook, ed 3. Boston, Little, Brown, 1988.

16. Scott RW: Promoting Legal Awareness in Physical and Occupational Therapy. New York, CV Mosby, 1997.

17. Standards of Ethical Conduct for the Physical Therapist Assistant, HOD 06-00-13-24. Alexandria, VA, American Physical Therapy Association, 2000.

18. State Licensure Reference Guide. Alexandria, VA, American Physical Therapy Association, 1997.

19. The Balanced Budget Act: How it affects physical therapy. Retrieved from *http://www.apta.org/Advocacy/national/National*, American Physical Therapy Association, 2000.

20. The Model Practice Act for Physical Therapy. Alexandria, VA, Federation of State Boards of Physical Therapy, 1997.

21. Unauthorized practice a crime, New York State Education Law, Article 130, Subarticle 4, Section 6512. Retrieved from *http://www.assembly.state.ny.us/cgi-bin/claws?law= 30&art= 121*, New York State Assembly, 2000.

22. Wilbanks J. The regulatory branch and you. PT—Magazine of Physical Therapy 1995;3(7):18.

5

Websites Referenced

http://thomas.loc.gov
http://www.apta.org
http://www.fsbpt.org
http://www.hcfa.gov

Suggested Readings

House of Delegates Policies. Alexandria, VA, American Physical Therapy Association, 1999.

This document contains standards, policies, and positions adopted by the House of Delegates of the APTA and is updated annually. It governs the activities of the organization and its members. Also available on the World Wide Web to members only at www.apta.org/MembersOnly/governance/house_policy.html.

Law and Liability: Professional Issues Learning Series. Alexandria, VA, American Physical Therapy Association. 1999.

A two-part collection of articles from PT—Magazine of Physical Therapy and

Physical Therapy, *including such topics as licensure, liability insurance, malpractice, delegation and supervision, and legislation.*

Purtilo R: Ethical Dimensions in the Health Professions, ed 3. Philadelphia, WB Saunders, 1999.

The text assumes no formal previous study of ethics. It addresses basic concepts of morality and ethics, applies them to specific dilemmas in health care, and includes a process for ethical decision making. It makes extensive use of case studies and study questions.

Scott RW: Promoting Legal Awareness in Physical and Occupational Therapy, New York, CV Mosby, 1997.

The text is intended for use by, among others, clinicians, students, and educators as a basic overview of health care–related legal issues. It begins with an overview of health care law and ethics and then develops issues in specific areas of liability. It includes study cases and questions and a glossary.

REVIEW QUESTIONS

1. Suggest examples of decisions that would be considered (1) a statute, (2) a common law decision, (3) a regulation, and (4) a policy.

2. Explain the different purposes and effects of a practice act versus federal legislation. Cite examples.

3. Describe how state regulations for professional conduct differ from HCFA regulations.

4. Cite major differences between the "Code of Ethics" and the "Standards of Practice for Physical Therapy."

The time is now for us to face the current crisis so that we ensure that the horizon ahead of us is not a receding one. The current health crisis should result in the opening of even greater doors for our profession.
Marilyn Moffat, PT, FAPTA
1994 APTA Presidential Address

Current Issues

Susan E. Bennett

KEY TERMS

alliance

ambulatory center

Balanced Budget Act of 1997 (BBA)

continuous quality improvement/total quality management (CQI/TQM)

continuum of care

critical pathways

cross-training

customer satisfaction

Diagnostic Related Groups (DRGs)

doctor of physical therapy (DPT)

encroachment

Evaluative Criteria for Accreditation of Education Programs for the Preparation of Physical Therapists

Evaluative Criteria for Accreditation of Education Programs for the Preparation of Physical Therapist Assistants

evidence-based practice

gatekeeper

Health Care Financing Administration (HCFA)

health maintenance organization (HMO)

managed care

managed care network

Medicaid

Medicare

Minimum Data Set (MDS)

A Normative Model of Physical Therapist Assistant Education

A Normative Model of Physical Therapist Professional Education

patient-focused care (PFC)

physician-owned physical therapy service (POPTS)

postprofessional education

preferred provider

professional physical therapy education

Prospective Payment System (PPS)

OBJECTIVES   After reading this chapter, the reader will be able to describe

- The difference between professional and postprofessional education and the need for both in physical therapy
- The pros and cons of obtaining a doctor of physical therapy degree
- Three practice issues having an impact on the physical therapist assistant
- The results of the Vector Study
- The development of health care systems and the benefits of continuum of care
- In what setting the physical therapist may be a primary care provider
- How encroachment may have an impact on physical therapy
- The effects of the Balanced Budget Act of 1997 on the practice of physical therapy
- The importance of evidenced-based practice

The issues that affect the profession of physical therapy are very similar to those affecting other health care professions. All health care providers are concerned about changes in the delivery of health care that may impinge on their current practice environment. One of the biggest factors to have an impact on all of health care has been the **Balanced Budget Act of 1997 (BBA)**. This federal legislation was enacted to save the Medicare program from dissolution. Compliance with the BBA was accomplished through cost-cutting measures that have an impact on all providers of health care. Changes in Medicare reimbursement have also had an effect on where we practice and on referral sources, reimbursement from other insurance carriers, encroachment, and peer review. In addition, our profession has been changing to meet the demands of the patients we serve, patient access to our care, and the health care system in which we practice under the BBA.

This chapter will examine how issues in education, practice, and research are affecting the profession of physical therapy. The historical perspective will be presented, as appropriate, to demonstrate the longevity and evolution of some of these issues.

EDUCATION

Historical Overview

The extent of the educational preparation and degree required to practice physical therapy has been a topic of debate for some time. The physical therapist (PT) evolved from the reconstruction aides established during World War I (see Chapter 1). These reconstruction aides were trained in emergency courses but were phased out at the end of the war. "Standards for Schools of Physical Therapy," published in 1928, was the first recommended course of study for physical therapy. The American Physical Therapy Association (APTA), at that time called the American Physiotherapy Association, was closely involved in the development of these programs until 1936, when the American Medical Association (AMA) assumed responsibility for overseeing the educational preparation.[17] This change was initially perceived to be a positive step for the profession, but as it turned out, the AMA limited the input from PTs and never revised or updated the curricula until 1955.

The first discussion of academic degree requirements occurred in 1955, when it was determined that if physical therapy education was integrated with a bachelor's degree program, the graduates could receive a bachelor's degree in physical therapy. This action was formalized in 1960 by the APTA's House of Delegates and provided strong support to move the first professional degree in physical therapy from a certificate to a bachelor's degree. In 1977, the APTA was recognized as an independent accrediting agency, and in 1983 the APTA became the only recognized accrediting agency for PT and physical therapist assistant (PTA) education programs. The conflict created by the AMA's limiting the growth and independence of education programs for physical therapy was eliminated with the 1977 action.[17]

Professional-Level Education

More controversy was to follow, however, when the APTA House of Delegates adopted a policy in 1979 with amendments in 1980 ruling that "physical therapist professional education be that which results in the awarding of a postbaccalaureate degree" and "that all physical therapist professional education programs and all developing physical therapist professional educational programs shall comply with this policy by December 31, 1990."[5] Postbaccalaureate education moved academic preparation of the PT beyond the bachelor's degree and into the master's degree level. By January 1994, 55% of PT education programs were at or had received approval to move to the postbaccalaureate level. While this figure reflects a substantial transition to postbaccalaureate-level education, it also indicates that the policy adopted by the House of Delegates in 1979 could not supersede each state's requirements for education and licensure for PTs. Each state is responsible for establishing and regulating the education and practice of licensed professionals. A national organization, such as the APTA, cannot supersede any rules and regulations set by each state. Awarding of the bachelor's or master's degree remained a controversy for many years.

New terminology was adopted by the House of Delegates in June 1993 to

6

differentiate entry-level education for PTs from advanced preparation in physical therapy. **Professional physical therapy education** refers to all academic programs that prepare students for *entry* into the field of physical therapy regardless of the degree. **Postprofessional education** is *advanced* education (at either the master's or doctoral level) of a licensed PT.

In 1993, a policy was to be presented to the House of Delegates to investigate the **doctor of physical therapy (DPT)** as the professional degree. Students in this program, though receiving a doctoral degree, would be entry-level graduates in the field of physical therapy. Other doctoral programs have been proposed, but at the postprofessional level (an advanced degree for licensed PTs). This policy did not reach the House floor for discussion; however, it did generate much discussion outside the House of Delegates. As previously noted, the policy adopted in 1979 by the House of Delegates could not mandate a postbaccalaureate degree for physical therapy education, so it was believed that the DPT would meet the same fate. Even discussing a DPT as the professional degree seemed premature to many members of the House of Delegates, especially in view of the status of the postbaccalaureate degree.

Education Today

Two documents, *A Normative Model of Physical Therapist Professional Education*[15] and the *Evaluative Criteria for Accreditation of Education Programs for the Preparation of Physical Therapists*,[6] serve as guidelines and standards, respectively, for existing and developing professional-level programs in physical therapy. The Normative Model is a standardized framework for all PT education programs that serves to "translate practice expectations into educational outcomes, identify necessary content strategies, and describe possible strategies to achieve these outcomes based on a conceptual framework that places the curriculum in the context of its immediate settings and the extended environment."[15] The Evaluative Criteria describe the specific components that must be in place for accreditation of professional-level programs. These components include the organization of the department and institution that provides the resources to support the program, curriculum development and content, and the means by which the program is continually assessed. The recent revisions of the Evaluative Criteria were particularly significant because the document stipulated that accrediting activities for professional-level education programs would be limited to those that awarded postbaccalaureate degrees beginning January 1, 2002.

These two documents are reflective of the role that the PT plays in health care today. Programs that follow the Normative Model and meet the Evaluative Criteria graduate students who are ready to enter a health care system in which they may serve as primary care providers and in which patients may have access to physical therapy care without a physician's referral. The education programs commonly require a total of 90 or more credits in professional study to complete the requirements for practice as a PT. In many instances, students are now required to have a bachelor's degree before entering the professional program in physical therapy. At several academic institutions, the clinical education component of the professional program is a residency requirement, and in some regions, 1-year paid residencies have been established (similar to the medical model).

With the expanding autonomy of the PT in health care now and the extensive educational preparation required to practice, more PTs are supporting adoption of the DPT as the professional degree in physical therapy. The professional doctorate has been described as "the appropriate degree for preparation of practitioners who are competent to meet the broad societal need for physical therapy services now and in the future."[22] As of January 1, 2000, 8 DPT professional programs were accredited, with another 20 to 25 in transition.

With all the debate over the DPT as the professional degree for physical therapy, one might ask whether advanced degrees are needed at all. According to Rothstein in his May 1998 editorial in *Physical Therapy,* "The DPT prepares an individual for practice, not for a career as an academic. If we substitute the DPT for the PhD, the EdD, the ScD, and the like, we will have abandoned any hope of developing a mature academic enterprise, one that can supply clinicians with the research and scholarship they need to be better practitioners."[19] Sahrmann echoed the sentiment of Rothstein in the 29th Mary McMillan Lecture when she stated, "I believe the development of these postprofessional programs should be encouraged so that the practicing therapist will have the opportunity to be a scholar-clinician, as well as a diagnostician."[20] We have much to learn in our role as movement scientists, and a scientific foundation must be established from which we can justify the effectiveness of interventions that we provide.

Will the DPT become the *required* professional degree of our profession? Action taken by the 2000 House of Delegates clearly indicates that the DPT is the degree for the physical therapist of the future. That body endorsed a Vision Sentence that reads, "By 2020, physical therapy will be provided by physical therapists who are doctors of physical therapy, recognized by consumers and other healthcare professionals as the practitioners of choice to whom consumers have direct access for the diagnosis of, interventions for, and prevention of impairments, functional limitations, and disabilities related to movement, function, and health."[3]

What of the practicing PTs with a bachelor's or master's degree? Do they need to earn a DPT degree or do they receive the credentials based on years of competent practice? How will postprofessional education for physical therapy change if the DPT is the professional degree? These questions and the advent of the DPT have fostered widespread debate in academic and clinical arenas across the country as the profession continues to evolve.

Supply and Demand

It was not very long ago that graduates of PT and PTA programs could go anywhere in the country and find employment. In most instances, new graduates could be selective of which job offer to accept. However, within a short span of 4 to 5 years, the job market has changed dramatically. Is it because too many education programs are graduating PTs and PTAs? Is the need for physical therapy services dwindling even though the number of individuals 75 years and older continues to increase?

In 1997 the APTA commissioned Vector Research, Inc., to conduct a study examining the demand for physical therapy services for the years 1995, 2000, and 2005. The results of the study were surprising to many, in that the demand for PTs was projected to be met by 1998, with a mild surplus in 2000 and a large surplus of therapists projected by 2005.[23] Many blamed the surplus on the expansion of existing education programs and development of new programs driven by market demand and the extent of qualified applicants seeking admission to PT and PTA education programs. Others realized that the delivery of physical therapy was changing, as was the reimbursement for services provided. The old model of treating the patient three times a week for 2 to 3 months was no longer being reimbursed. Therapists and employers recognized that they had to do more with less (effects of managed care). The reimbursement rate for services provided was dwindling, and thus therapists were expected to see more patients each day to compensate for the diminished revenue.

The current surplus of PTs and PTAs is probably related to a combination of the effects of managed care and the expansion of education programs. The 1999 House of Delegates endorsed the position that "The American Physical Therapy Association recommends against the development of new entry-level physical therapist and physical therapist assistant education programs and the expansion of existing programs until June 30, 2002."[18] Will this recommendation create new jobs for future graduates? No, but it temporarily eases the proliferation of graduates in the context of the current job market. Does the surplus of PTs reinforce the need for education programs to prepare graduates who have time management skills, organization and administrative skills, business skills, program development in wellness and prevention, effective communication skills, and knowledge in marketing? Yes! Does a DPT degree versus a master's degree make the new graduate more marketable? These issues are part of the current debate.

Physical Therapist Assistant

Evolution of the educational requirement for the PTA has been less controversial. Chapter 3 provides a thorough description of the educational preparation of the PTA. The House of Delegates created the PTA position and originally defined the role of PTAs as technicians, although the position has evolved and today PTAs are referred to as paraprofessionals. In 1999, the House of Delegates adopted *A Normative Model of Physical Therapist Assistant Education,* which provides guidelines for the content of these education programs. The document *Evaluative Criteria for Accreditation of Education Programs for the Preparation of Physical Therapist Assistants* is used in the accreditation of PTA programs and is currently undergoing revision. The current controversy with PTA education involves three issues: the attendance and participation of PTAs at continuing education courses offered for PTs, opportunity for advanced recognition of clinical skills, and restricting interventions performed by the assistant. Some may also argue that adoption of the Normative Model for PTA education raises the issue of requiring a bachelor's degree program versus the current associate's degree preparation.

Many PTs believe that PTAs should be excluded from attending continuing education courses offered for PTs because the PTA academic preparation prepares them to serve in a supportive role. The PTA does not receive academic preparation equivalent to that of the PT in the theoretical basis for treatment or in sciences such as gross anatomy (detailed human anatomy), physics, or neuroscience. Without this academic preparation, PTAs may be unable to thoroughly understand the concepts provided in continuing education courses for PTs. With a mixed audience, the course instructor might add information to provide the PTAs with the necessary knowledge at the expense of the PTs in the audience. If the PTA learns and practices these examination and intervention skills in a continuing education course, would the expectation be that the PTA could perform those procedures in the clinic without the direction and supervision of the PT?

The problem is magnified by the limited number of continuing education courses specifically offered for the PTA. Many PTAs have developed the background knowledge needed to attend the continuing education courses offered for PTs through their work experience and interaction with PTs. The majority of continuing education courses provided continue to offer open enrollment, which means that this debate remains unsolved.

Assistants have argued that they are instructed in higher-level intervention skills both in their academic preparation and by the supervising therapist. An example is the intervention of mobilization and manipulation, which is part of the curriculum in several PTA education programs. The APTA is currently examining the role of the PTA in performing interventions that require constant re-examination and clinical decision making by the physical therapist (e.g., mobilizations, wound débridement with sharp instruments).

The APTA Board of Directors, in collaboration with the National Assembly of Physical Therapist Assistants, is also examining the feasibility and need for recognition of advanced achievement by PTAs. PTs have the opportunity to pursue board certification as clinical specialists. The National Assembly is interested in exploring the establishment of a similar recognition program for PTAs.

PRACTICE

Background

Health care reform and the distribution of reimbursement dollars have changed the practice of physical therapy. Historically, physical therapy evolved to meet the rehabilitative needs of soldiers from the war and children with polio. Most of these individuals needing physical therapy were treated in hospitals or long-term care facilities. As the profession has expanded, PTs can be found treating individuals across the life span who display a variety of problems that impair their ability to move and function. PTs evaluate and treat patients/clients in a variety of practice settings. In addition, PTs are adapting their practices to accommodate the rapidly changing health care system.

Managed Care

Escalating costs of health care resulted in the dramatic growth of **managed care** during the 1990s. In managed care, the insurance company contracts with health care providers to provide health care to consumers who subscribe to the insurance plan. Private practitioners in physical therapy may become what is known as **preferred providers** for insurance company X, which means that when a consumer insured by company X needs physical therapy, the insurance company will refer the consumer to its physical therapy preferred provider. The preferred provider is usually selected on the basis of quality of care and cost containment.

Of concern is the selection of health care providers in managed care settings. If a PT is a preferred provider in a managed care setting, that therapist may be dropped as a provider if the cost for services becomes too high, even if the quality of care remains excellent. This policy becomes a problem for consumers who want to have access to the best PT for their rehabilitation but are unable to do so because of the insurance company's refusal to pay the PT's rates. The eight top insurance companies own nearly half the health maintenance organizations (HMOs), so the selection problem can be found in the HMO as well.[1]

Of greater concern is the inability of all PTs in private practice to become members of a **managed care network.** A managed care network is a group of health care providers who form a professional cooperative relationship for the purpose of referring individuals to health care providers within the network. The intent of the network is to maintain quality standards of practice by all health care providers in the network. PTs in private practice may be denied the opportunity to become participating providers in managed care networks even though they meet the same quality standards established for the network. As health care reform continues to move toward managed care, private practices have closed because physicians are encouraged to refer patients to the health care system or managed care network in which they are affiliated. Referrals from physicians remain a large source of business for private practitioners.

Health Maintenance Organizations

The private practice environment in physical therapy has traditionally consisted of one or more PTs who own a practice and provide physical therapy services. In many of these private practices, other PTs are employed to provide care for the patients. The physical therapy private practice is an ambulatory setting; however, it is limited in that the only service provided is physical therapy. Many of the health care reform proposals were designed to use ambulatory settings that are multipurpose. A good example is the **health maintenance organization,** which provides all the health care services needed under one roof. In this arrangement, the insurance is prepaid, and you can have access to your physician, nurse practitioner/physician's assistant, and PT, as well as services of the pharmacy, radiologist, and laboratories, in one setting.

Health care reform has emphasized the use of HMOs because of greater accountability for quality care, peer review, and cost containment. Approximately 40 million members are enrolled in 550 HMOs across the country,[13] so a large percentage of the population uses health care providers who work in HMOs. For physicians, this change has not been a major problem because many HMOs contract with several physicians, especially in specialty areas. Physicians can contract with the HMO and practice in a managed care environment with the HMO while also maintaining their private practice. PTs, however, are not as highly sought after by the HMO as physicians are; consequently, to save cost, the HMO employs (rather than contracts with) PTs to provide care to their members. The majority of PTs working in this environment do not maintain a separate private practice, so their sole employment is with the HMO.

Ambulatory Centers

Health care reform and advances in medical technology have also caused a shift in the delivery of care to ambulatory settings. An **ambulatory center** is any facility in which health care is provided on an outpatient basis. The patient is able to walk into the facility, receive health care, and walk out of the facility the same day. Health care systems usually have several ambulatory centers in the different geographical regions that they serve. Outpatient clinics and HMOs are examples of ambulatory centers. Health care in this environment is less costly to the consumer and the insurance companies overall. Therefore, this type of setting is becoming more common. In fact, the APTA Membership Database for 2000 indicates that 43.8% of PTs were practicing in a private office or hospital-based outpatient facility, whereas only 15.4% of the therapists were practicing in an acute care hospital (see Fig. 2–17).[2]

Reimbursement

Who pays for health care? That was a question most of our patients or colleagues never considered until the health care reform of the 1990s. The answer is essential to understand because decreases in reimbursement have had a significant negative impact on the number of jobs and salaries for PTs.

Basically, payment comes from two sources. The first is the patient/client, and the second, frequently known as the third party, is a health insurance company or the government. With health care costs so high, much of the coverage comes from third-party payers.

Health care insurance companies offer managed care or indemnity plans that are paid for predominantly by the employer. One obtains health insurance through one's employer, who then pays a premium to the health insurance agency. The managed care option is the less expensive of the two and is

6

usually strongly recommended by the employer. Insurance companies have also promoted managed care arrangements to control the escalating cost of health care, to the point that currently the majority of individuals under 65 years of age are insured through some form of managed care.[7]

The increasing cost of health care over the past 30 years has also resulted in an increased charge for the services rendered. To stay in business and cover these costs, the health insurance agency increases the premiums to the employer, which in some cases has resulted in the small business owner's terminating health insurance coverage, leaving the employees uninsured.

The government also pays for health care. **Medicare**, the health insurance program for those older than 65 years, is paid by the federal government (our tax dollars). Medicare was running out of funds because of escalating health care costs until the BBA was passed. This Act saved finances for Medicare through cost-cutting measures and produced the first balanced budget for the U.S. government in over 30 years.[4] Medicare, managed by the **Health Care Financing Administration (HCFA)**, tends to be the trendsetter on how other insurance companies will pay. **Medicaid,** another governmental program, is an insurance plan designed for those of low economic status. It is administered by the state and supported by taxes.

To reduce the costs of health care, Medicare instituted the **Diagnostic Related Groups (DRGs)** for acute care hospitalization and recently implemented the **Prospective Payment System (PPS)** for inpatient rehabilitation facilities and skilled nursing facilities. Simply stated, both these payment systems (DRGs and PPSs) are based on the payment of one lump sum of money to cover the hospitalization or long-term inpatient costs for a patient per diagnosis, irrespective of the length of stay in the facility. In skilled nursing facilities, the **Minimum Data Set (MDS)** is a measurement tool that has been used to measure the cost of care of a patient in the facility. The MDS is then factored into the PPS that has been established for a diagnosis. Costs for physical therapy care are included within the DRG or PPS rate; however, rarely does the reimbursement rate meet the actual services provided to the patient. This shortfall has resulted in layoffs of PTs employed in skilled nursing facilities because the owner of the facility must cut costs as a result of reduced reimbursement via the PPS.

In an outpatient setting, a PT providing physical therapy care to a patient uses billing codes that are appropriate for the type of treatment provided to the patient. The bill is then sent to the insurance company (managed care network or indemnity plan) for reimbursement. The billing codes used for physical therapy services are not exclusive to PTs. These same billing codes are used by physicians and podiatrists. Monitoring overutilization of these billing codes is difficult because so many different health care providers use the codes. The regulations that are in place to monitor the cost, quality, and utilization of health care services by the patient and the health care professional are not adequate to control the system. Tighter restrictions must be developed to ensure that the consumer is receiving quality care at a reasonable cost.

Reimbursement is also affected by limiting the number of funded visits. The frequency of visits for outpatient physical therapy care is now regulated by the insurance agency, as opposed to the PT. A maximum number of visits is allocated by the insurance company on the basis of the patient's diagnosis, as well as a limit to the length of time that the patient can be treated. For example, it is common in our clinical practice to be limited by an insurance carrier to eight treatment visits or 2 months of treatment, whichever comes first. In some instances this amount of treatment can be sufficient, but not in the rehabilitation of a patient who has had a stroke or amputation. As a profession we have come to realize that treatment "doses" do not correlate with patient response and that in many cases more treatment does not necessarily produce greater functional gains.[9] However, to be denied requests for additional treatment visits based on our clinical judgment and the patient's response to treatment hurts the patient, especially when in some cases lack of rehabilitation can contribute to a fall or rehospitalization.

The limited number of physical therapy treatments for a particular diagnosis also has an impact on who provides the care. In the past, when a patient was treated two or three times per week, the PTA, under the therapist's supervision, could provide most of the interventions to the patient, with the therapist re-examining the patient once a week. Now, with limited treatments, the patient is seen only once a week over an 8-week period. Each visit with the therapist, now once a week, consists of re-examination to determine the change that has occurred over the past week and then progression of the treatment program by the therapist with emphasis on patient education. In this delivery model, the role of the PTA becomes diminished because the majority of the treatment session consists of re-examination and patient education.

Managed care networks are not the only health insurance agencies limiting outpatient care by restricting reimbursement. Medicare had a limit of $1500 for outpatient care, which included both physical therapy and speech therapy costs. Occupational therapy is allocated $1500 for services provided on an outpatient basis. In the case of a young patient with a knee injury referred for physical therapy, speech therapy would not be involved in the patient's rehabilitation, and therefore the $1500 would be fully accessible by physical therapy. However, a patient who had suffered a stroke and needed speech and physical therapy treatment would have used the $1500 quickly between the two rehabilitative services. The APTA successfully achieved a 2-year moratorium of the $1500 cap effective January 2000 that enables patients with Medicare coverage to receive the rehabilitative care needed without a monetary cap (Fig. 6–1). Data will continue to be collected over the next 2 years to maintain this moratorium and prevent reinstatement of a cap on Medicare benefits for physical therapy services.

Reform of the reimbursement system must *continue;* the question is how soon and to what extent. The issues described here are only a few of the many reimbursement problems that PTs face. PTs practicing in institutions such as hospitals and rehabilitation centers have previously been protected from these

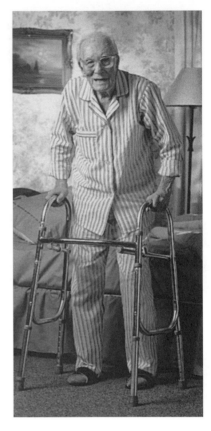

Figure 6–1. This advertisement by the APTA was run in popular magazines such as *Good Housekeeping* to educate the public about the monetary cap on rehabilitative services imposed by Medicare. This ad, as well as other lobbying efforts with the Health Care Financing Agency, resulted in a 2-year moratorium on the cap in January 2000. (Reprinted with permission of the American Physical Therapy Association.)

> **Thanks to the cap Congress put on rehabilitation services, Mr. Railey can make it to the sofa. He just can't make it out the door.**

reimbursement problems; private practice was the setting that was affected the most. Currently, hospital physical therapy operating budgets are being cut, and vacant PT positions are not being filled to decrease costs because of lack of reimbursement. PTs employed in skilled nursing facilities are being laid off because of diminished reimbursement with a PPS. The end result is that reimbursement problems affect both the consumer's ability to access physical therapy care and the provider's ability to provide quality care to meet the patient's needs.

Alliances

In addition to managed care, another major change that has occurred in health care reform is the formation of alliances. An **alliance** is a collaboration of several health care facilities and practices. For example, two hospitals could work together as an alliance without formally merging. By aligning, they can share resources, programs, and health care providers and negotiate contracts with the insurance companies as a larger entity. This arrangement makes the two hospitals stronger because of the multitude of services that they can provide under the alliance and yet maintain their independence as separate hospital corporations. An alliance could also be formed between a PT private practitioner and a hospital or between a private practitioner and other health care providers. The purpose of forming an alliance is to ensure the stability and quality of services that are provided and to market these services to insurance companies.

Resources have also been shared through formal mergers. Community hospitals have merged with large city hospitals, city hospitals have joined together, and home care agencies have been rolled in as well. The force behind these mergers has been the attempt of the chief executive officers (CEOs) of the hospitals to maintain the hospital's financial viability. Diminished reimbursement from Medicare and other third-party payers has forced CEOs to examine how to provide quality comprehensive health care with less financial resources. Mergers have resulted in a decrease in resources for capital expenses by eliminating the duplication of expensive diagnostic equipment for each hospital. They have also provided the opportunity for health care to be provided along a continuum, which has resulted in more efficient delivery of patient care. This **continuum of care** is important because it enables patients to stay within one system and receive tertiary, secondary, and primary care. Tertiary care is high-tech health care provided at a hospital that treats the most serious of patients, such as cardiac transplant recipients and neurosurgical patients. Secondary care is treatment by a specialist, but this care can be performed at a community hospital or even in an outpatient setting. Primary care is the treatment you receive from your family doctor, the primary care physician who is responsible for keeping you healthy.

6

Future of Physical Therapists in the Hospital Setting

The American Hospital Association conducted a study in 1992 of 6700 hospitals in the United States regarding vacancy rates of professional staff.[1] More than half the hospitals responded to the survey. The hospitals reported a decrease in vacancy rates for 20 of the 26 professions studied. One of the professions reported to have a decrease in vacancy was physical therapy. However, the decrease was insignificant at 0.3% from 1991 to 1992. According to the report, a 16.3% vacancy rate was reported in physical therapy, with a recruitment period for PTs usually exceeding 90 days.

Through alliances and mergers, many hospitals now provide a continuum of care. Although the number of PTs treating inpatients in acute care hospitals has not increased, the role of the PT in the health care system has expanded. The majority of health care is now provided in ambulatory care centers or through home care agencies. PTs play a role as primary care providers in some outpatient settings and also serve as case managers in some home care agencies. In both of these new roles the PT is the health care provider responsible for managing the patient's total care.

Guide to Physical Therapist Practice

During her two terms in office as president of the APTA, Marilyn Moffat, PhD, PT, FAPTA, was instrumental in the development and completion of the *Guide to Physical Therapist Practice.* This document was developed "to help physical therapists analyze their patient/client management and describe the scope of their practice."[10] The *Guide* is a companion document to *A Normative Model of Physical Therapist Education* and has been instrumental in educating legislators as well as insurance companies on the knowledge base and role of the PT in health care. The Guide has also served as the basis for PTs to define their role as primary care providers or case managers. In many education programs the Guide is required text for all students.

Direct Access

Background. Historically, the reconstruction aide worked closely with the physician and carried out orders for exercise, massage, or therapeutic modalities to be applied to the patient. Prescriptions were written by the physician that specified the type of exercise to be performed, the modality to be used, and the intensity and duration of the treatment. As education of the PT expanded, so too did the knowledge base and hands-on skills. However, as noted earlier in this chapter in the Historical Overview of Education, the education programs, under the auspices of the AMA, were not updated or revised until 1955.

As the educational preparation of the PT expanded after 1955, the provision of physical therapy to the consumer changed as well. In 1957, Nebraska became the first state to have direct access. Citizens of Nebraska could obtain treatment from a PT without seeing a physician first and being referred to the therapist. The second state to enact legislation for direct access was California in 1968. Legislation proliferated in the 1980s and early 1990s to enable PTs to practice with direct access in other states. In the states that allow direct access, PTs evaluate the patient, determine an appropriate treatment, and implement that treatment based on their findings.

Direct Access Today. At present, the consumer has direct access to a PT in 33 states. The concept behind direct access is to enable the consumer to have the *choice* of accessing a PT or a physician. If the PT determines that the patient's problem is outside the PT's scope of practice or that the patient needs further medical evaluation, the patient is referred to a primary care physician. Providing the consumer direct access to PTs contributes to the reduction of health care costs (by eliminating the physician office visit to obtain the referral) and expedites initiation of appropriate treatment. In states without direct access, patients may wait 4 to 6 weeks to see a physician, only to have the physician write a referral for physical therapy without conducting a comprehensive evaluation and then charging for a full office visit. On seeing the PT (4 to 6 weeks after injury), the acute problem may now have developed into a chronic problem with additional secondary problems (such as protective muscle spasms and contracture).

Direct access has worked effectively in the states in which it has been adopted. In states without such legislation, resistance to direct access has come primarily from the physician's professional organization. Concern has been raised that PTs do not have enough knowledge to diagnose problems that the patient has and, consequently, malpractice suits will result.

In reality, malpractice suits have not increased in states with direct access. Moreover, in states without direct access, a diagnosis is not typically noted on the physician's referral. The majority of patients referred to physical therapy from a physician have on the referral "Evaluate and Treat" or a symptom such as low back pain or knee pain. Neither of these reasons for referral are diagnoses that would aid the PT in determining a plan of care. The plan of care for the patient is developed after the PT completes the examination, evaluation, diagnosis, and prognosis.

The other unspoken concern of the physician's professional organization is that the number of patients in their care will be reduced if the PT has direct access. This concern has not been documented as a problem, or reality, in any of the states with direct access.

The Future of Direct Access with Health Care Reform. The key to direct access with health care reform was establishment of the **gatekeepers** or "gateways" into the health care system. Historically, the primary care physician has been the access (gatekeeper) into the health care system. It is the primary care physician who then refers patients to PTs, physician specialists, or other health care providers. Patients in managed care plans must enter the health care system through their primary care provider because it is less costly and often facilitates management of the patient's care to ensure the best outcome of treatment when multiple specialists are involved.

The limited number of physicians entering the field of primary health care opened the door for the nurse practitioner and the physician's assistant to serve as the entry point into health care, especially in rural settings. Some of the proposed federal legislation would enable any licensed health care provider practicing within the individual's scope of practice to be an entry point for the consumer into health care. If this type of legislation were passed, it would enable the consumer in any state to have direct access to physical therapy care. For example, in some HMOs the PT is the gatekeeper for musculoskeletal injuries. The PT also determines through examination, evaluation, and diagnosis whether other health care providers, such as a radiologist, are needed for further diagnostic procedures.

Physician-Owned Physical Therapy Service

As previously noted, the physician has in the past been the primary coordinator of the treatment that a patient receives. The physician ordered the necessary diagnostic work, requested consultations from other health care providers, and ordered the treatment regimen for the patient. With this responsibility and control, many physicians established clinics where they own all the diagnostic equipment, laboratory equipment, pharmacies, and physical therapy clinics. In this situation, physicians refer their patients to their own clinics. When such "self-referral" occurs, the patient has lost the choice of where to go for diagnostic work or treatment, and the potential for overuse of the services is created.

A **physician-owned physical therapy service (POPTS)** is an example of the overuse that can occur when a physician has a financial investment in a clinic. Two studies conducted in Florida and California have demonstrated that when the physician has ownership in physical therapy services, overuse of physical therapy care occurs and results in overspending of health care dollars.[12, 21] These two studies have shown that physicians who have ownership in a physical therapy clinic continue to refer patients for physical therapy care even when the patient has plateaued or reached established goals. Patients have also been *inappropriately* referred and treated in such clinical settings.

The AMA reported in the *American Medical News* that it is unethical for physicians to have a financial investment in a laboratory or clinic to which they refer.[11] Federal legislation (the Stark Law) has been enacted to prohibit patients receiving Medicare from being cared for in a laboratory or clinic in which the referring physician or a family member owns an interest. A related law effective January 1, 1995, expanded this limitation to Medicaid patients as well.

To avoid the unethical and potentially illegal situation of owning an interest in a physical therapy clinic, many physicians hire PTs to work as their employees. The same abuse of overutilization of physical therapy care can and does exist in this environment, but employment of a PT to work in the physician's office is currently not restricted in any way.

Encroachment and Human Resources

Encroachment. **Encroachment** is defined in *Webster's Dictionary* as "1. to trespass or intrude (on or upon the rights, property, etc., of another); 2. to advance beyond the proper, original, or customary limits."[24]

In the health care arena, encroachment occurs when one health care provider performs the skills and techniques of another health care provider.

Physical therapy is provided by PTs and PTAs. In the past, the shortage of qualified physical therapy professionals to meet the demands of the consumer led other health care providers to fill the void. This situation occurred most often with athletic trainers and occupational therapists. An example is the rehabilitation of a weekend athlete. If an individual injures a knee in a basketball game and edema (swelling), pain, and restricted mobility develop, that person should be treated by a PT. Because the injury occurred in a sporting event, the athletic trainer might say that the individual should be treated by an athletic trainer. Who is encroaching on the other's territory? Both providers should not be providing the same treatment to the patient and receiving reimbursement.

In another example, a PT and occupational therapist are treating an individual who had a stroke and are instructing the patient in bathtub transfers. In this duplication of services both units are receiving reimbursement. Who is encroaching on the other health care professional's territory?

These types of questions continue to be raised as each health care profession strives to maintain its own identity and professional integrity. The answers to some of these questions may differ depending on the different practice acts that regulate and govern health care professionals in each state. The bathtub transfer scenario could be performed by both the occupational therapist and the PT as long as they are both working on different outcomes for the patient. For example, the PT may be doing the transfer activity for the sole purpose of enabling the patient to be independent in the transfer. The occupational therapy goal would be more global and incorporate the activity of daily care so that the patient will be independent in bathing in the bathtub. To accomplish this goal, the patient must be able to perform the transfer as well as manage bathing activities in the tub.

The example of the weekend athlete with a knee injury may be addressed differently in each state. In New York, for example, the PT would be responsible for the acute rehabilitation of the weekend athlete's knee injury. However, either the athletic trainer or the PT could recondition the individual for return to recreational activities. The treatment provided by the PT would be reimbursed as physical therapy. According to the AMA (which establishes the Current Procedural Terminology [CPT] codes), the treatment provided by the athletic trainer cannot be reimbursed by accessing the examination and re-examination billing codes used by PTs. This situation becomes confusing and misleading to insurance agencies when they examine total expenditures for billing codes usually attributed to PTs. Physicians, podiatrists, and in the past, athletic trainers have used these billing codes, categorized as physical therapy costs, which has inflated the actual dollars spent for physical therapy care. In some states, chapters of APTA have attempted to change insurance regulations to require tracking of providers submitting bills attributed to physical therapy costs, but they have had limited success.

Human Resources. The biggest factor contributing to encroachment in different health care professions is the shortage of professionally trained personnel that may exist in a profession and the resulting inability of that profession to meet the service demands of the public. There had been a critical shortage of PTs up through 1997, even with the proliferation of schools graduating PTs. In 1992, physical therapy schools graduated 4850 new therapists, but 7000 vacancies still remained.[16] In June 1994, the APTA reported that there were 85,000 PTs in the United States, 2% of whom were retired or not working, which left approximately 83,300 physical therapists to fill 90,000 physical therapy jobs. In 1994, the U.S. Department of Labor predicted a growth of 88% in physical therapy by 2005. Projections indicated that most professions will grow by 22% from 1998 through 2005.[8]

More recent projections reflect a different trend. As stated previously in this chapter, the Vector Study commissioned by the APTA projected a mild surplus of PTs by 2000 (which has occurred) and a large surplus by 2005. This surplus is attributed by most in our profession to be due to the combined effects of managed care and the BBA, as well as the expansion of PT and PTA education programs. PTs are now encouraged to examine other areas in which we can be effective in health care, such as wellness and prevention. When therapists were in short supply, we were struggling just to meet the rehabilitative needs of those with injuries, illness, or disabilities. Time was too short for many practitioners to spend in the area of wellness and prevention. Now, therapists who are underemployed or unemployed are using their creative skills to develop and coordinate community health programs and health screening programs. Developing these skills may enhance the role that PTs play in the continuum of care and assist therapists in obtaining full-time employment.

Continuous Quality Improvement

Continuous quality improvement/total quality management (CQI/TQM) is "a method of examining and improving processes using data management tools."[25] Simply put, it means using data that are collected every day to improve the quality of a service that is provided. It has been a component of most hospitals for several years and has also been integrated into most physical therapy practice settings. TQM in a physical therapy clinic would consist of continual assessment of both how physical therapy care is being delivered and patient outcomes. In the early implementation of TQM, PTs would document the number of patient visits, cancellations, and no-shows. Now it has expanded to consider how efficiently the care is delivered, whether the patient achieves the desired outcome, and the patient's satisfaction with the care. **Customer satisfaction,** previously associated with the service received in hotels, restaurants, or stores, is now a major emphasis of health care systems.

As TQM developed in hospitals, it led to the advent of a new patient delivery model called **patient-focused care (PFC).** In this model, all departments in a hospital are decentralized, and professional staff members are assigned to work on multidisciplinary teams. Instead of the PT department's being located on one floor and all the patients' being transported to PT, the therapist is now stationed on a nursing unit with other health care providers to provide treatment to a core group of patients with similar problems. A good example is a PT working on a multidisciplinary team for orthopaedic surgical patients. All members of the team are on the floor with the patients, and all services that the patients need are brought to them. This system has decreased the wasted time that health care providers spend trying to find a patient because the individual left the nursing floor for tests or other reasons. The team coordinates the treatment to be provided to each patient at the beginning of every day, and responsibilities are shared among members of the team. Trained technicians are part of the team and carry out much of the basic care for the patient after instruction from the PT. Such care may include transfers of the patient and ambulation.

The PFC model has also brought with it the controversy of **cross-training** of health care professionals. This concept has sent a shock wave through most of the physical therapy professional community. Cross-training could include PTs' doing some physical therapy care, occupational therapy care, and nursing care for the patient. The concept of cross-training originally grew out of the inadequate supply of PTs available to work in hospitals; therefore, training occupational therapists and nurses to perform some of the physical therapy services was a necessity. In addition, cross-training affects not only physical therapy but also all health care professions. Skills from a variety of professions would be integrated to be provided by members of a multidisciplinary team.

The PFC model does introduce some cross-training of the members of the multidisciplinary team, but many PTs working in this model state that the important evaluative and treatment components of physical therapy have been retained by the PT. In many settings, therapists report that members of the multidisciplinary team have a better understanding and appreciation for the knowledge base of the PT.

A very positive development of the PFC model is the development of **critical pathways,** which are defined by Woods as "a guideline for patient care during hospital stay using 'milestones' to progress patients; a guide based on consensus, including only those aspects of care provided to affect patient outcomes."[25] The critical pathway is a planned sequence of treatment progression that is based on the patient's response and recovery. Initiating physical therapy treatment is an established part of the critical pathway, so a delay in receiving physician's orders does not occur. Likewise, the physical therapy progression of the patient is also a component of the pathway. Some therapists who use the system report that critical pathways are clearly defining the parameters of our practice and the role that the PT should play in rehabilitation of the patient.

6

RESEARCH

To address many of the issues that have been discussed in this chapter, evidence is needed to support the effectiveness of physical therapy care. Demonstrating improved patient outcomes as a result of physical therapy intervention will ensure the identity and integrity of our profession. Physical therapy is an art and a science, but clinical-based research is needed to substantiate the science component of the profession.

The major emphasis of physical therapy research must be in two areas: (1) establishment and utilization of measurement tools that are valid and reliable and measure patient outcomes and (2) the efficacy of physical therapy treatment.[14] The new terminology in all of health care is **evidence-based practice**, which ensures the consumer of health care that the treatment received is based on scientific research and evidence to substantiate outcomes.

The best environment for evidenced-based practice is in the physical therapy clinic. The research center established by the Foundation for Physical Therapy is an excellent example of advancing research in measurement and treatment efficacy. The University of Iowa was awarded a 3-year grant from the Foundation to establish a research center focusing on total hip and knee replacements and ultrasound treatment. The University of Pittsburgh received a 3-year grant from the Foundation in 1997 to examine low back injury. The research focuses on PT interventions for the prevention and treatment of low back pain. This type of focused research is needed to demonstrate the role that physical therapy plays in prevention and rehabilitation.

Clinicians who work with patients every day are another source of data collection for studying treatment outcomes. Unfortunately, the majority of practicing PTs have limited experience in research methodology. Stronger collaboration of physical therapy faculty with clinicians must be developed to facilitate clinical-based research. Another means to address this issue is to foster students in postprofessional physical therapy education programs to carry out clinically based research in conjunction with clinicians. To support postprofessional education, the Foundation for Physical Therapy has developed the program Doctoral Opportunities for Clinicians and Scholars (DOCS). The DOCS program has a new investigator scholarship award program and a three-level doctoral studies program. In 1999 the Foundation awarded more than $300,000 in the DOCS program to PTs in postprofessional education.

Summary _____ This chapter reviewed the current issues affecting physical therapy. Educational preparation of the PT remains an issue to be debated on the floor of the House of Delegates as the profession considers the DPT as the *required professional* degree. The role of the PTA has expanded from that of a technician to a paraprofessional. The practice settings continue to change with the advent of health care reform. PTs and PTAs will continue to work in hospitals, but the status of private practice as we know it today will continue to change with managed care. Legislation for direct access may become obsolete if health care reform enables the consumer to access any health care provider practicing within that individual's scope of practice. Any physician-owned physical therapy practice should become illegal with the enactment of federal legislation. Encroachment will continue until an adequate number of health care providers are available in each field to meet the consumers' demands.

All these issues, however, will not be resolved on their own. Resolution of most will require the active participation of PTs and PTAs in the local, state, and national levels of the APTA. Interaction with other members of the health care team will also be necessary to address common issues that face everyone affected by the rapid changes in health care.

References

1. American Hospital Association. One North Franklin, Chicago, personal communication.
2. American Physical Therapy Association Membership Database. Alexandria, VA, American Physical Therapy Association, 2000.
3. APTA Vision Sentence for Physical Therapy 2020 and APTA Vision Statement for Physical Therapy 2020, HOD 06-00-24-35. Alexandria, VA, American Physical Therapy Association, 2000.
4. Connolly J: APTA battles the BBA. PT—Magazine of Physical Therapy 1999;7(7):46–55.
5. Entry-Level Education, HOD 06-80-10-29. Alexandria, VA, American Physical Therapy Association, 1979.
6. Evaluative Criteria for Accreditation of Education Programs for the Preparation of Physical Therapists. Alexandria, VA, American Physical Therapy Association, 1996.
7. Fowler F: Beyond the Balanced Budget Act. Rehabil Econom 1998;7(3):90–91.
8. Growth of physical therapy to continue into next century. PT Bull 1994;9(18):2.
9. Guccione A: The effect of changes in the practice environment on employment patterns. PT—Magazine of Physical Therapy 1999;7(5):26–28.
10. Guide to Physical Therapist Practice. 2nd ed. Phys Ther 2001;81:9–744.
11. HCFA weighs option for wider referral ban. Am Med News 1994;37(23):1.
12. Joint ventures among health care providers in Florida, State of Florida, conducted by the

Florida Health Care Cost Containment Board in conjunction with the Department of Economics and Department of Finance, Florida State University, August 1991.

13. Managed care, managed fair. Am Med News 1994;37(19):13.
14. Model for Targeting Research Areas in Physical Therapy. Alexandria, VA, American Physical Therapy Association, 1994.
15. A Normative Model of Physical Therapist Professional Education: Version 97. Alexandria, VA, American Physical Therapy Association, 1999.
16. Physical Therapist Education Programs. Alexandria, VA, American Physical Therapy Association, 1992.
17. Pinkston D: Evolution of the practice of physical therapy in the United States. *In* Scully RM, Barnes MR (eds): Physical Therapy. Philadelphia, JB Lippincott, 1989.
18. Position on Physical Therapy Education Program Development and Expansion, HOD 06-99-28-30. Alexandria, VA, American Physical Therapy Association, 1999.
19. Rothstein J: Education at the crossroads: Which paths for the DPT? Phys Ther 1998;78:454–457.
20. Sahrmann S: Moving precisely? Or taking the path of least resistance? Phys Ther 1998;78:1208–1218.
21. Swedlow A, Johnson G, Smithline N, et al: Increased costs and rates of use in the California worker's compensation system as a result of self-referral by physicians. N Engl J Med 327:1502–1506, 1992.
22. Threlkeld J, Jensen G, Royeen C: The clinical doctorate: A framework for analysis in physical therapist education. Phys Ther 1999;79:567–581.
23. Vector Research Inc: Executive Summary, Workforce Study. Alexandria, VA, American Physical Therapy Association, 1997.
24. Webster's New World Dictionary, Second College Edition. New York, Simon & Schuster, 1986.
25. Woods EN: The restructuring of America's hospitals: What does it mean for physical therapy? PT—Magazine of Physical Therapy 1994;2(6):34–41.

6

Suggested Readings

Castro J: The American Way of Health. New York, Little, Brown, 1994.

An easy-to-read, informative book that details how health care has changed in our country and why we are faced with the issues that we have today. Many stories of different patients are presented to assist the reader in understanding the crisis that has existed.

Depoy E, Gitlin S: Introduction to Research: Multiple Strategies for Health and Human Services. St Louis, Mosby–Year Book, 1993.

This introductory text was written for members of all allied health professions and teaches the reader how to critically evaluate, implement, and respect a variety of research strategies.

House of Delegates Policies. Alexandria, VA, American Physical Therapy Association.

Updated annually, including new goals for the APTA.

PT Bulletin. Alexandria, VA, American Physical Therapy Association.

Contains short articles and letters to the editor that address current issues. Published weekly on-line (http://www.apta.org/Bulletin).

PT—Magazine of Physical Therapy. Alexandria, VA, American Physical Therapy Association.

The May issue of this monthly publication distributed to members of the APTA includes the annual report of the APTA.

Stewart D, Abeln S: Documenting Functional Outcomes in Physical Therapy. St Louis, Mosby–Year Book, 1993.

This text discusses a variety of documentation models that demonstrate the conceptual framework of clinical decision analysis. Examples of appropriate and inappropriate reporting are given along with the expectations of a variety of payers. Case studies are included.

REVIEW QUESTIONS

1. Explain the controversy over consideration of a DPT program. What issues does it raise?

2. Discuss both sides of the debate over PTA attendance at continuing education PT courses.

3. Why is it more difficult for PTs than physicians to establish a contractual relationship with an HMO?

4. Weigh the objections to direct access against its track record in states that legislate in its favor.

5. Explain the risks involved in a physician-owned physical therapy service.

6. What is "encroachment"? Discuss the issues that it raises and their impact on reimbursement for services.

7. Explain the advantages of developing physical therapy–specific billing codes from both the PT and consumer perspectives. Do you see any drawbacks?

8. Give balanced attention to analyzing the advantages and disadvantages seen in the patient-focused care model.

Part II

Practice

Greatness lies not in being strong, but in the right use of strength.
Harry Ward Beecher

Physical Therapy for Musculoskeletal Conditions

Barbara C. Belyea and Hilary B. Greenberger

KEY TERMS

accessory motion
active assisted range of motion
active free range of motion
active range of motion (AROM)

active resisted exercise

aerobics training

aquatic physical therapy

Bad Ragaz method

bursitis

closed-chain exercise/kinetic-chain exercise

cryotherapy

dysfunction

electrical stimulation

flexibility

flexibility exercise

fluidotherapy

fracture

functional exercise

goniometer

goniometry

Halliwick method

hot pack

hydrotherapy

hypermobile joint

hypomobile joint

infrared

joint mobilization

manual muscle testing (MMT)

massage

muscle endurance

muscular strength

myofascial release

nerve entrapment

objective examination

open-chain exercise/joint isolation exercise

paraffin treatment

passive range of motion (PROM)

proprioception

proprioceptor

range of motion (ROM)

range-of-motion exercise

resisted exercise

resisted test

short-wave diathermy

soft tissue mobilization

special tests

sprain

strain

strength

subjective examination

tendinitis

thermal agent

ultrasound

whirlpool

OBJECTIVES   After reading this chapter, the reader will be able to

- Identify the components of an initial examination
- Define and give examples of the various tests and measures used in physical therapy for musculoskeletal conditions
- List the general goals of a therapeutic exercise program
- Distinguish between active assisted range of motion, active free range of motion, and active resisted range of motion
- Define and give an example of an isometric, an isotonic, and an isokinetic exercise
- Explain the difference between open- and closed-chain exercise
- List four reasons why home exercise programs are important

Conditions that affect the musculoskeletal system are the primary domain of physical therapists who specialize in orthopaedic physical therapy. One of the largest clinical specialties within the physical therapy profession, orthopaedic physical therapy encompasses a wide array of therapeutic techniques and philosophies of treatment. Physical therapists practicing in the field of orthopaedics work in a variety of clinical settings and treat patients of diverse ages with a variety of physical and medical problems. This chapter will describe the types of patients seen by an orthopaedic physical therapist and present some of the examination techniques and interventions commonly used.

GENERAL DESCRIPTION

While the clinical interests or approaches to treatment may be diverse, the common thread throughout orthopaedic physical therapy is the focus on a patient's function. By examining the patient's functional ability, an orthopaedic therapist determines the cause and extent of any functional disability, referred to as a **dysfunction,** and works with the patient to return the individual to an optimal level of function. A person's function can be affected when a disruption occurs in the musculoskeletal system, either from traumatic injury or from repeated stress to tissue. Dysfunctions may be caused by a structural imbalance of either muscle or bone, by birth defects, by surgery, or by degenerative changes in the body.[14] Dysfunctions of the musculoskeletal system often result in symptoms of pain, stiffness, edema (swelling), muscle weakness or fatigue, or loss of **range of motion** (**ROM;** movement at a joint).

To conduct a comprehensive examination, generate an accurate diagnosis, and develop an appropriate plan of care, therapists must have an extensive understanding of anatomy, biomechanics, pathokinesiology, and exercise physiology. They must also be well vested in the application of various intervention techniques and be able to analyze clinical situations and problem-solve to determine which approach is the most appropriate for each patient situation. It is also critical for physical therapists and physical therapist assistants to have effective communication skills to establish good rapport with patients and provide the necessary information to gain the patient's compliance with the plan of care.

Development

Several factors continue to contribute to the growth of orthopaedic physical therapy. The development of sophisticated technology and new intervention techniques has opened opportunities for physical therapists who evaluate and treat this patient population. Changes in lifestyle have also contributed to the growth of orthopaedic physical therapy. Increasing interest and participation in physical fitness by the general population have resulted in an increase in musculoskeletal dysfunction secondary to overuse or traumatic injuries. The increased use of computers and other technical machinery requiring repeated motions has also had an impact on the incidence of overuse injuries in the upper extremity. Individuals who must sustain postures at a computer or machinery while performing repeated motions with their hands may be at risk for the development of muscle injury or nerve entrapment requiring intervention by a physical therapist. An increase in life span has also resulted in the

7

growth of this area of physical therapy as people are living longer and experiencing symptoms related to degenerative changes in their bodies.

A great deal of similarity exists between orthopaedic physical therapy and sports physical therapy. In both areas, the focus of physical therapy is to regain optimum function and return the patient to the previous level of function and activity. A sports physical therapist must therefore incorporate sport-specific activities into the treatment program to make sure that the patient can meet the physical demands of the sport with respect to strength, endurance, balance, and speed. An orthopaedic physical therapist may work with athletes but may also treat a variety of musculoskeletal conditions that are not related to sports activities.

COMMON CONDITIONS

Within the broad scope of orthopaedic physical therapy, a variety of patient problems may be treated. These conditions range from injuries sustained through athletic participation, work-related injuries, and dysfunction after orthopaedic surgical procedures to the degenerative changes that accompany the aging process. As previously stated, patients with musculoskeletal conditions referred for physical therapy may have pain, swelling, weakness, or loss of motion resulting from trauma to the musculoskeletal system. This trauma may include damage to bones or soft tissue such as muscles, tendons, joint capsules, ligaments, bursae, and fascia in the extremities or spine.

Overuse Injuries

Repeated stress to soft tissue can cause overuse injuries that may result in inflammation. The following examples describe some common conditions caused by overuse injuries.

Bursitis. **Bursitis is an inflammation of bursae**, which are fluid-filled sacs located throughout the body that serve to decrease friction between two structures. Bursae become irritated and painful when they are repeatedly pinched between two structures. A common example of this mechanism of injury occurs at the shoulder; the subacromial bursa may get pinched during repeated movements when the shoulder is in an overhead position, as with painting, reaching, or throwing motions.

Tendinitis. **Tendinitis is inflammation of a tendon**, which is a structure located at the ends of muscles that attaches muscles to bone. Repeated use of muscles can cause stress to the tendon and result in painful movement. Tendinitis is frequently seen in the patellar tendon at the knee in people who perform repeated jumping (e.g., dancers, basketball players) and at the elbow in people who do repeated or sustained gripping activities (e.g., carpenters, tennis players).

Nerve Entrapment. Pressure on a nerve, causing **nerve entrapment,** may result from a variety of sources and usually causes symptoms of tingling, pain, weakness, or any combination of these symptoms. A common condition of nerve compression at the wrist is referred to as carpal tunnel syndrome. Patients with carpal tunnel syndrome usually complain of numbness and pain in the hand and fingers, which commonly results from repeated activities with the wrist in a flexed position (e.g., musicians, computer keyboard operators).

Traumatic Injuries

Musculoskeletal injuries may also occur as a result of direct trauma. Bones, muscles, ligaments, and other soft tissue may be injured when they sustain a direct blow or when they are placed under excessive stretch. The following examples are just a few of the common conditions that can arise from direct trauma to the musculoskeletal system.

Ligament Sprain. Ligaments are supporting structures at joints that serve to stabilize the joint and prevent excess movement. When ligaments are overstretched, their fibers can tear and cause pain and instability at the joint. A common site of sprain is at the ankle when the lateral (outside) ligaments are overstretched. This injury occurs when a person lands on the foot in a turned-in position. Another common site of ligament sprain is the anterior cruciate ligament at the knee. Injuries to this ligament are usually the result of a twisting movement when the foot is planted, as seen with quick turns during running.

Fracture. Direct trauma to bone can result in a break, or **fracture,** of the bone. Fractures can occur in any bone in the body but are commonly seen at the wrist or the hip after falls. Elderly individuals are particularly prone to fractures because of changes in the structure of their bones resulting from inactivity, inadequate nutrition, and degenerative conditions. Fractures are best diagnosed through the use of radiographs.

Muscle Strain. A sudden contraction of a muscle or excessive stretch on a muscle can cause tearing of the muscle fibers, known as a **strain.** Muscle strains can occur in any area of the body and can range in severity. Low back strains can occur during improper lifting techniques, and cervical strains may be the result of a sudden movement of the neck, as with a whiplash injury. Complete rupture of the muscle may be seen in the ankle (Achilles rupture) or elbow (biceps rupture) and must be surgically repaired.

Surgical Conditions

Individuals who have had surgery are another group of patients commonly seen by the orthopaedic physical therapist. Injuries resulting from repeated stress, acute trauma, or disease processes may require surgical intervention for appropriate healing. The following are examples of orthopaedic surgery in which patients can benefit from physical therapy intervention to reduce pain and regain motion and strength to allow for optimal movement and function.

Total Joint Replacement. Degenerative changes at joint surfaces causing painful movement can be alleviated through surgical replacement of the joint surfaces. Joints most commonly replaced are weight-bearing joints, primarily the hips

7

and knees. A variety of plastic and stainless steel implants are used to effectively replace degenerated joint surfaces. Therapeutic intervention is necessary postoperatively to ensure maximum strength and function and to prevent complications such as dislocation.

Amputation. Surgical amputation is the removal of a portion of an extremity because of trauma, inadequate blood flow, or the presence of a malignant growth. Inadequate circulation can be a result of disease processes such as diabetes mellitus or peripheral vascular disease, whereas a growth may indicate the presence of cancer.

Medical Conditions

Other medical conditions may also affect the musculoskeletal system by causing weakness or loss of function. Systemic diseases such as rheumatoid arthritis, cancer, or acquired immunodeficiency syndrome may produce weakness or functional challenges that can be addressed by the orthopaedic physical therapist.

PRINCIPLES OF EXAMINATION

Treating a patient with a musculoskeletal injury requires the physical therapist to have an understanding of the injury to provide appropriate intervention. This understanding is accomplished by completing a thorough initial examination of the patient and, through the evaluative process, by developing an accurate diagnosis. Subsequent re-examinations are performed throughout the rehabilitative process to monitor patient progress toward established functional outcomes.

This section will discuss the following components of an initial examination: patient history, systems review, and tests and measures performed by the physical therapist. The history is part of the **subjective examination,** whereas the remaining parts constitute the **objective examination.**

Patient History

The history involves gathering information about the current and past health status of the patient. The information is obtained by interviewing the patient or the patient's family or by accessing the patient's medical record. It is a qualitative measurement based on the *patient's* perception of the problem and is therefore included in the "S" portion of the "SOAP" note (see Chapter 2).

The role of the therapist during the interview is to guide the patient through pertinent questions. This interaction allows the therapist to develop a rapport with the patient and to understand the patient's insight into and opinion of the problem. The interview also assists the therapist in appropriately directing the remainder of the examination. Often, the patient interview will give the therapist ample information to make a tentative physical therapy diagnosis. Questions asked during the interview include information on the cause of the condition, current symptoms, previous physical therapy treatments, past medi-

Box 7–1

Questions Typically Asked During The Subjective Component of an Initial Physical Therapy Evaluation

1. What brings you to physical therapy today?
2. What do you feel is your primary problem? Is it stiffness? Pain?
3. Was the onset of the problem slow or sudden? Was the problem caused by a specific incident or mechanism of injury?
4. Have you ever had this problem before? If so, were you treated for it? How long did it take to recover?
5. What provokes your symptoms? What relieves your symptoms?
6. Are your symptoms worsening or improving?
7. Are your symptoms constant or intermittent?
8. Can you describe your pain? Does your pain spread to other parts of your body?
9. What is your occupation?
10. Have you had any radiographs ("x-rays") taken?
11. Are you currently taking any medication for this problem?
12. Is there anything else you would like to tell me that I have not asked that would be pertinent to your problem?

7

cal history, and lifestyle as it pertains to work and recreation. Box 7–1 lists typical questions asked during the patient interview.

Frequently, the patient will be asked to draw the location of the pain on a body chart (Fig. 7–1). Pain scales are also often used to gauge the amount of pain that the patient is experiencing (Fig. 7–2). On completion of the history taking, the therapist should have gained information regarding the description and location of symptoms, nature of the disorder (acute vs. chronic condition), and behavior of the symptoms (what activities make the symptoms either better or worse).

Systems Review

Systems review provides additional information about the general health and fitness level of the patient separate from the specific reason that the patient has sought advice from a physical therapist. The information gathered during the systems review assists the therapist in developing an appropriate plan of care and identifying health problems that may require consultation or referral to another health care provider.

Tests and Measures

The objective portion of the examination refers to quantitative or qualitative measurements that are taken by the physical therapist. Specific numbers or grades may be assigned (quantitative measurement), as is the case with ROM

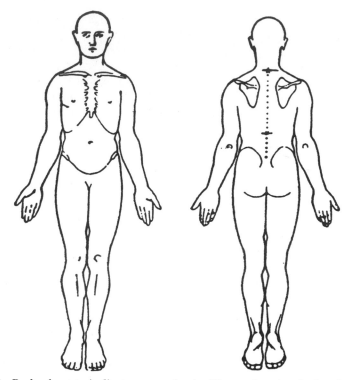

Figure 7–1. Body chart to indicate areas of pain. The patient is asked to indicate areas of pain with Xs, areas of numbness with slashes, and areas of tingling with plus signs.

or strength measurements. Other times, parts of the examination are performed by observing and describing patterns of movement, deformities, or both (qualitative measurement). The information derived from this portion of the examination is included in the "O" section of the SOAP note (see Chapter 2). The purpose of the objective examination is to establish baseline values and observations that can be used for comparison after a single treatment or a series of treatments. The physical therapist can then make appropriate changes in the plan of care based on the amount of progress or lack of progress found with repeated tests and measures.

This section will briefly describe the tests and measures performed in an orthopaedic physical therapy setting. The purpose is for introductory level students to become familiar with common terms used when working with a patient who has a musculoskeletal problem.

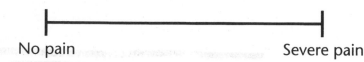

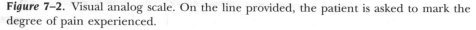

No pain   Severe pain

Figure 7–2. Visual analog scale. On the line provided, the patient is asked to mark the degree of pain experienced.

Observation. Observation is the "looking" phase of the examination. It may begin in the waiting room, where the therapist can observe the general attitude of the patient, general posture, and willingness to move. A perfunctory gait assessment may be made as the patient enters the examination area. Once the patient is appropriately undressed, a more detailed inspection can be made, including observation of obvious deformities such as an abnormal curvature of the spine, joint subluxations (a condition in which a joint partially dislocates), asymmetrical body contours, swelling, and color and texture of the skin. Many musculoskeletal injuries are a result of or are exacerbated by poor sitting and standing postures. Therefore, particular attention is paid to the standing and sitting posture of the patient.

Active Range of Motion **Active range of motion (AROM)** refers to the ability of the *patient* to *voluntarily* move a limb through an arc of movement. AROM provides the therapist with information regarding the quality of the movement (smooth vs. rigid movement), the willingness of the patient to move the limb, any pain produced during movement, and whether the patient has any limitations in the motion as compared with the unaffected side. An example of AROM of the shoulder in multiple planes is provided in Figure 7–3.

Passive Range of Motion. **Passive range of motion (PROM)** refers to the amount of movement at a joint that is obtained by the *therapist* moving the segment *without assistance from the patient*. In some instances, because of injury or prolonged immobilization, a joint may have less motion than is considered functional. This condition is referred to as a **hypomobile joint.** In other cases, such as a subluxing joint, the joint may have excessive motion, which is referred to as a **hypermobile joint.** PROM will also give the therapist an indication of the degree and pattern of pain, as well as the "feel" of the movement.

Many methods may be used to measure and document PROM. The most common measurement technique is called **goniometry** and is performed with a **goniometer.** Examples of different types of goniometers are illustrated in Figure 7–4. The amount of motion available at any joint is dependent on the structure of the joint. Additionally, norm values for joint ROM are dependent on several factors, including the age and gender of the patient.[3] Typically, a therapist will compare ROM values of the affected joint with those on the unaffected side. Figure 7–5 is an example of a physical therapist conducting a PROM measurement of a patient's knee flexion.

Strength. **Strength** can be defined as the amount of force produced during a voluntary muscular contraction. This contraction may be performed statically (no motion) or dynamically (through a complete ROM). When one is assessing the status of the muscles and tendons, a quick **resisted test** is used. This test allows the therapist to determine the general strength of a muscle group and assess whether any pain is produced with the muscle contraction. If it is determined from the resisted test that a muscle or muscle group is weak or painful, further testing is performed to isolate the specific muscle. To isolate and test specific muscles, **manual muscle testing (MMT)** is performed (Fig.

7

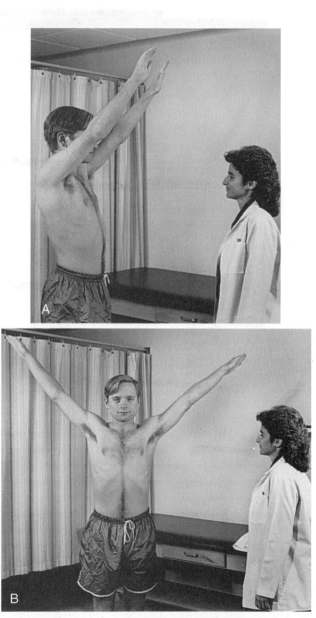

Figure 7–3. Examination of active range of motion at the shoulder. *A*, Shoulder flexion. *B*, Shoulder abduction.

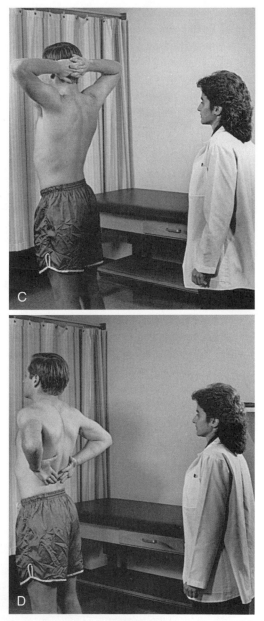

7

Figure 7–3 *Continued. C*, Shoulder external rotation. *D*, Shoulder internal rotation. (Courtesy of Dewey Neild.)

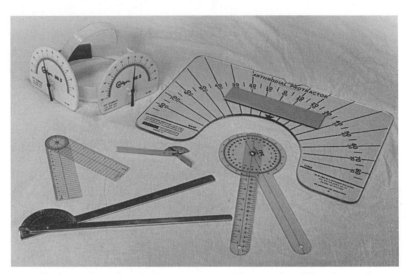

Figure 7–4. Variety of goniometers to measure joint angles. The size and type vary to measure long and short limb segments and the cervical region. (Courtesy of Dewey Neild.)

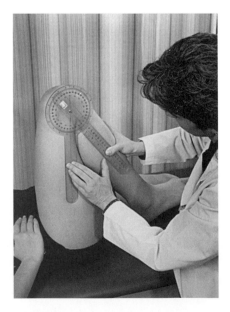

Figure 7–5. Physical therapist conducting a goniometric measurement of knee flexion. (Courtesy of Dewey Neild.)

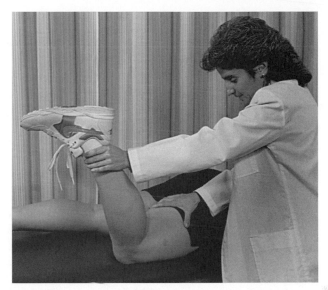

Figure 7–6. Physical therapists commonly perform manual muscle tests to determine muscle strength. Pictured is the manual muscle test for the hamstring musculature. (Courtesy of Dewey Neild.)

7

7–6). MMT allows the therapist to assign a specific grade to a muscle. This grade is based on whether the patient can hold the limb against gravity, how much manual resistance can be tolerated, and whether the joint has full ROM. Several systems of grading are widely used. One of the most common grading systems was initially described by Robert Lovett, MD, and later modified by Henry Kendall, PT, and Florence Kendall, PT.[9] This key to muscle grading is outlined in Table 7–1.

With the development of sophisticated technical equipment, many other methods are now available to measure strength, including hand-held devices and computerized instruments such as isokinetic devices. These machines allow the therapist to obtain strength curves of isolated muscles, as well as specific force values. These devices will be discussed in more detail in the treatment section of this chapter.

Flexibility. **Flexibility** refers to the ability to move a limb segment through a specific ROM. The amount of flexibility that an individual has at a given joint depends on a combination of two factors. First, the soft tissue surrounding the joint must be pliable to allow movement between the joint surfaces. This feature is referred to as **accessory motion** of the joint. Accessory motion refers to the ability of the joint surfaces to glide, roll, and spin on each other. Second, the muscle or muscles crossing the joint must be at an appropriate length to allow motion to occur. For example, the ability to stand up and touch your toes while keeping your knees straight would depend on the flexibility of the back and posterior hip muscles, as well as the ability of the spinal vertebrae to move.

Table 7–1
Key to Manual Muscle Testing Grades

	FUNCTION OF THE MUSCLE	GRADE	SYMBOLS	
No Movement	No contraction felt in the muscle	Zero	0	0
	Tendon becomes prominent or feeble contraction felt in the muscle, but no visible movement of the part	Trace	T	1
Test Movement	Movement in a horizontal plane			
	Moves through partial range of motion	Poor−	P−	2−
	Moves through complete range of motion	Poor	P	2
	Moves to completion of range against resistance or moves to completion of range against pressure	Poor+	P+	2+
	Antigravity position			
	Moves through partial range of motion			
Test Position	Gradual release from test position	Fair−	F−	3−
	Holds test position (no added pressure)	Fair	F	3
	Hold test position against slight pressure	Fair+	F+	3+
	Holds test position against slight to moderate pressure	Good−	G−	4−
	Holds test position against moderate pressure	Good	G	4
	Holds test position against moderate to strong pressure	Good+	G+	4+
	Holds test position against strong pressure	Normal	N	5

1993 Florence P. Kendall. Modified from Kendall FP, McCreary EK, Provance PG: Muscles Testing and Function, ed 4. Baltimore, Williams & Wilkins, 1993, p 189. Author grants permission to reproduce this chart.

Appropriate flexibility or balance of muscles is a key component of proper posture and body mechanics. Almost all musculoskeletal problems seen in the physical therapy clinic can be linked to muscle imbalances. For example, if the muscles surrounding the shoulder did not act synergistically (because of lack of flexibility), compensation may occur at joints distal and proximal to the shoulder, such as the elbow and cervical spine.

A physical therapist may perform a number of tests to determine flexibility. One common test for the lower extremity is called the 90/90 straight leg raise (Fig. 7–7). This test objectively measures hamstring flexibility, the muscle on the posterior aspect of the thigh.

Functional Tests. The ultimate goal in therapy is to return the patient to the previous level of activity, which may include anything from the ability to go grocery shopping independently to returning to athletic competition. In some types of injuries, returning to the previous level of activity is not feasible. In these cases, the ultimate goal would be to return the individual to the highest level of function achievable.

Traditionally, when we think of functional assessment, we refer to activities such as the patient's bed mobility, transferring between a variety of surfaces (e.g., moving from a sitting position in a wheelchair to a standing position), and the ability to perform activities of daily living (ADLs), such as hair combing, dressing, and bathing. Physical therapists may spend a large percentage of their time during the initial examination assessing the patient's ability to perform these ADLs. This activity becomes particularly important when working with

7

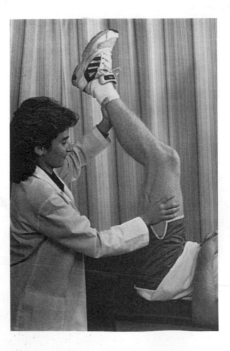

Figure 7–7. Example of a test for flexibility: the 90/90 straight leg raise. (Courtesy of Dewey Neild.)

Box 7–2

Examples of Activities of Daily Living

Eating

- Eat with spoon
- Eat with fork
- Cut with knife
- Open milk carton
- Pour liquid
- Drink from cup

Dressing and Undressing

- Reach clothes in closet
- Put on shoe
- Manage zippers
- Remove coat

Bathing/Grooming

- Turn on faucet
- Wash hands
- Dry with towel
- Manage cosmetics
- Brush teeth

Bed/Bathroom

- Get out of bed
- Transfer to toilet
- Reach objects on nightstand
- Sit up in bed

Transfer/Ambulatory Activities

- In and out of bus
- In and out of car
- Safe outdoor ambulation
- Endurance

Other Activities

- Propel wheelchair forward
- Propel wheelchair backward
- Manage elevator
- Hold book
- Dial a telephone
- Use scissors

postsurgical patients. An example would be a patient who is seen after a total joint replacement of the hip or knee. Box 7–2 lists examples of ADLs.

Recently, a surge of literature has appeared in the orthopaedic and sports physical therapy arena regarding the importance of functional testing for individuals returning to activities other than ADLs.[2, 3, 11, 16] These activities may include sports, gait, lifting tasks, and other multiplanar movements. Examples of functional tests for these activities include hop tests, jump tests, lunge tests, excursion tests, and balance tests. Gray has described these tests in detail.[7]

Special Tests. **Special tests** are used to examine specific joints to indicate the presence or absence of a particular problem. The purpose of these tests is to confirm or reinforce a physical therapy diagnosis. Because so many special tests are available for each joint, only those that appear to be indicated from the results of other tests and measures are performed. Examples of special tests include those that examine nerve compression (Phalen's test, Fig. 7–8A), tests for shoulder impingement (Hawkin's test, Fig. 7–8B), and tests for ligamentous knee injuries (Lachman's test, Fig. 7–8C).

Palpation. A comprehensive understanding of anatomy is essential for any physical therapist. In the clinical situation, the therapist uses the sense of touch, known as palpation, to assess what is occurring below the skin and what musculoskeletal structures are involved in an injury. When palpating an area of the body, the therapist is feeling for areas of pain and tenderness, areas of restriction, swelling, and whether structures are properly oriented.

Other Diagnostic Procedures. Depending on the patient's injury or complaint, other examination procedures may be performed to provide a more complete assessment of the patient. The patient may be referred to other personnel for these procedures. Such complementary procedures may include a variety of imaging techniques such as radiographs (x-rays), computed tomography (CT) scans, and magnetic resonance imaging (MRI). If the patient has had neurological damage, full sensory testing may be indicated. Additional tests for patients with cardiopulmonary conditions may include an assessment of lung capacity. Some of these tests are presented in more detail in Chapters 8 and 9.

PRINCIPLES OF EVALUATION, DIAGNOSIS, AND PROGNOSIS

Based on evaluation of the findings from the comprehensive examination, the physical therapist identifies the patient's limitations and determines the diagnosis and prognosis. As previously stated, most patients with musculoskeletal dysfunctions report symptoms of pain, loss of motion or strength, or edema. Once the problems have been identified, the therapist and patient develop goals to address each problem. Common goals are to decrease pain, decrease edema, increase strength, or increase motion. The ultimate goal for patients with musculoskeletal dysfunction is to achieve an optimal level of function, whether that means returning to work, returning to the athletic field, or resuming the ability to perform daily activities independently. Therapeutic goals should include the anticipated return of strength or function and the expected time frame for rehabilitation. Once goals have been established, the therapist then develops a plan of care designed to achieve these outcomes.

The plan of care is based on determining what intervention will most effectively improve a patient's function by decreasing pain, decreasing edema, increasing strength, or increasing motion. The intervention options and rehabilitation approaches available to the orthopaedic physical therapist are numerous. Some therapists may focus their treatment approaches on exercises, whereas others may incorporate physical agents or manual techniques. In most instances, a combination of techniques is most appropriate when designing a comprehensive plan to address the needs of a patient with musculoskeletal dysfunction. Whatever intervention is selected, the most important factor to consider when planning and implementing the treatment is to consider the goals of the patient and the desired outcome of therapy.

PRINCIPLES OF DIRECT INTERVENTION

The following discussion of intervention options is meant to introduce the reader to the typical indications and uses of various techniques. The techniques described include physical agents, manual techniques (including soft tissue and joint mobilization), and therapeutic exercise. The reader is referred to the

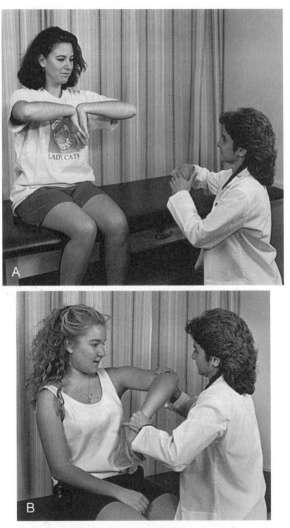

Figure 7–8. Examples of special tests. *A*, Phalen's test for nerve compression. *B*, Hawkin's test for shoulder impingement.

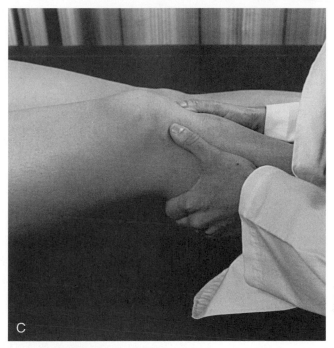

7

Figure 7–8 *Continued. C,* Lachman's test for anterior cruciate ligament instability. (Courtesy of Dewey Neild.)

reading list at the end of the chapter for sources that provide in-depth information regarding the application of these techniques.

Physical Agents

Many therapeutic agents are available for physical therapists to incorporate into rehabilitation programs when treating patients with musculoskeletal dysfunction. Based on the intended purpose and method of application, physical agents can be divided into two categories: thermal agents (thermotherapy) and electrical stimulation (electrotherapy). Thermal agents can be subdivided into agents that apply superficial heat, deep heat, and cold. The decision regarding which agent to use is based on a thorough examination of the patient's symptoms, the desired outcomes of therapy, and the therapist's knowledge of the physiological and clinical effects of each physical agent. Table 7–2 lists common physical agents used in physical therapy according to their *physical* effects and includes their *physiological* effects and clinical indications.

Thermal Agents. When a tissue in the body sustains an injury, an automatic response is initiated in an attempt to heal the tissue and return it to its preinjured state. These naturally occurring processes are referred to as inflammation and repair.[17] The inflammation and repair stages of tissue healing can be altered through the use of thermal agents or electrical stimulation.

Table 7–2
Summary of Common Physical Agents Used in Physical Therapy

PHYSICAL EFFECT	PHYSICAL AGENTS	PHYSIOLOGICAL EFFECTS	CLINICAL INDICATIONS
Superficial heat	Hot packs Infrared Paraffin Fluidotherapy Whirlpool	Increases blood flow Increases metabolism: promotes healing and removal of waste products Decreases pain Decreases stiffness	Muscle spasm Pain Joint stiffness Wound care
Deep heat	Ultrasound Short wave diathermy	Increases blood flow Increases metabolism: promotes healing and removal of waste products Decreases pain Decreases stiffness	Muscle spasm Pain Joint stiffness
Cold	Ice packs Ice massage Cold whirlpool Cold compression	Decreases blood flow Decreases metabolism Decreases edema Decreases pain	Acute injury Swelling Pain Muscle spasm Postexercise
Electrical stimulation	Transcutaneous electrical nerve stimulation (TENS) Iontophoresis Electrical stimulation for tissue repair (ESTR) Neuromuscular electrical stimulation (NMES)	Decreases pain Decreases edema Promotes wound healing Muscle re-education Decreases spasticity	Pain Edema Wounds Nerve regeneration Muscle weakness/imbalance

Thermal agents are used to modify the temperature of surrounding tissue and result in a change in the amount of blood flow to the injured area. Besides vascular changes, temperature changes also have an effect on the metabolism of the surrounding tissue, in addition to altering neuromuscular and connective tissue. Through the use of therapeutic changes in temperature, the healing process can be accelerated and the injured tissue restored to optimal strength and integrity.

The extent of the therapeutic changes caused by an alteration in tissue temperature depends on the intensity of the thermal agent applied, the length of time that the tissue is exposed to the agent, and characteristics of the tissue being treated. The therapist must continually monitor and re-examine the patient to ensure that the thermal agent selected is appropriate and that the treatment outcomes are being achieved.

Thermal agents can be classified as those that provide superficial heat, deep heat, or cold. Superficial heat modalities create an increase in blood flow to cutaneous tissue close to the surface, thereby reducing pain, reducing muscle spasm, allowing for increased motion, and promoting healing.[13] Examples of superficial heat agents include hot packs, infrared, paraffin, fluidotherapy, and whirlpools.

A **hot pack** is a pouch available in various shapes that is filled with silica gel and soaked in thermostatically controlled water (Fig. 7–9). Hot packs are applied to the affected body part with layers of towels to prevent overheating (see Fig. 2–12). Similar to a heat lamp, **infrared** uses infrared radiation to warm the superficial tissue and create a general feeling of relaxation and pain relief. **Paraffin treatment** involves dipping a patient's involved body part (usu-

7

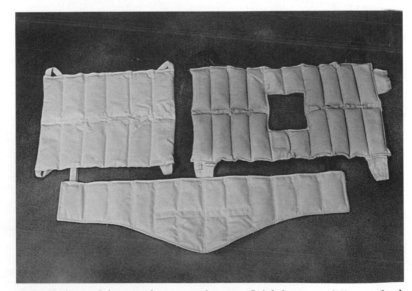

Figure 7–9. Variety of hot packs to apply superficial heat to different body areas. (Courtesy of Dewey Neild.)

ally hands or feet) into a mixture of melted paraffin wax and mineral oil that is maintained at a temperature of approximately 135°F (Fig. 7–10). The heat from the paraffin produces the relaxing and pain-reducing effects of other superficial heat treatments and also leaves the skin feeling warm and soft, which allows for greater comfort when performing ROM exercises. **Fluidotherapy** is the use of a self-contained unit filled with corncobs finely chopped into a sawdust-type substance. The particles are heated to the desired temperature and circulated by air pressure around the involved body part. In addition to receiving the effects of heating, the patient is also able to exercise while the treatment is in progress. A **whirlpool** makes use of the therapeutic effects of water by immersing the body part or entire body in a tank of water. Use of this physical agent is known as **hydrotherapy.** A variety of sizes of tanks are available, ranging from a small tank for the distal ends of extremities to a full-body tank known as a Hubbard tank. In addition to its heating effects, hydrotherapy has the added advantage of assisting with wound healing.

Deep heat modalities produce physiological effects similar to those of superficial heat agents, but at a greater tissue depth. Therefore, patients with deep muscle or joint dysfunction may receive more therapeutic benefit from the application of deep heat than from a superficial heating agent. Deep heat modalities include ultrasound and short wave diathermy. Ultrasound is the therapeutic application of high-frequency sound waves that penetrate through tissue and cause an increase in tissue temperature to promote healing and reduce pain (Fig. 7–11). Similar results are achieved with **short-wave diathermy,**

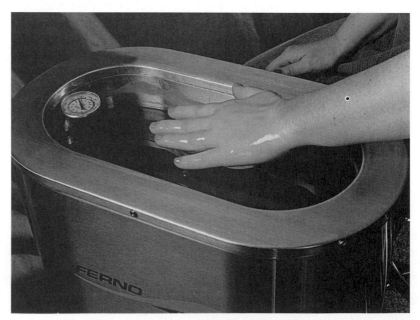

Figure 7–10. Paraffin tank to apply paraffin to a hand. (Courtesy of Dewey Neild.)

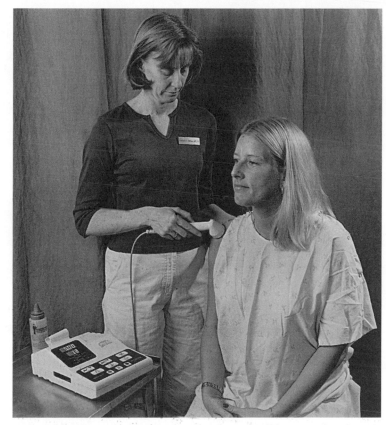

Figure 7–11. Application of ultrasound to produce deep heat in the shoulder region. (Courtesy of Dewey Neild.)

7

although diathermy uses electromagnetic energy to produce deep therapeutic heating effects.

In contrast to heating agents, therapeutic cold (**cryotherapy**) may be applied. Temperature differences produced by the application of cold agents cause a decrease in blood flow and decreased metabolism, which result in a decrease in swelling and diminished pain. Cold is the physical agent of choice in patients with acute injuries who have clinical symptoms of swelling, pain, or both (see Fig. 2–13). Cold may also be incorporated into a treatment protocol after exercise to help reduce postexercise soreness. Cryotherapy may take the form of commercial cold packs, ice massage, cold whirlpool, or cold used in conjunction with compression.

Electrical Stimulation. Physical therapists and physical therapist assistants may also use **electrical stimulation** as part of their plan of care to achieve therapeutic results. With the use of electrical stimulation units, electrodes are placed on the skin at specified locations to stimulate nerves, muscles, and other soft tissues in an attempt to reduce pain and swelling, increase strength and ROM,

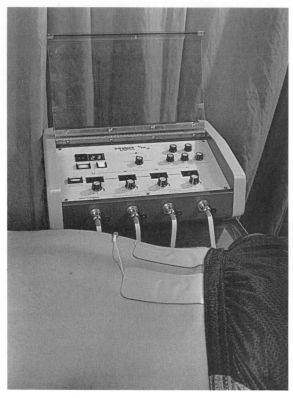

Figure 7–12. Use of transcutaneous electrical nerve stimulation (TENS) for the treatment of pain in the low back region. (Courtesy of Dewey Neild.)

and facilitate wound healing[18] (Fig. 7–12). The use of electricity to generate therapeutic benefits is not new, but the numerous electrotherapy devices on the market can make selection of the appropriate device confusing. The therapist must have a clear understanding of the desired effects from the electrical stimulation intervention and have knowledge of the appropriate parameters to use with regard to treatment intensity, voltage, and current type. Common physical agents used in electrotherapy are listed in Table 7–2.

Other Physical Agents. Additional physical agents that may be used in the treatment of patients with musculoskeletal dysfunction include mechanical traction, hyperbaric oxygen, biofeedback, laser therapy, and ultraviolet treatment. These modalities achieve therapeutic benefit through mechanisms different from those of thermal or electrical agents, but they may also be used to decrease a patient's pain or improve strength or motion in an attempt to maximize function.

Manual Techniques

Physical therapists working with patients with musculoskeletal dysfunction always have two tools at their ready disposal—their hands. Perhaps in no other patient population is touch so important as it is in the orthopaedic population.

Whether palpating a structure during an examination, providing manual force for a patient to resist against when exercising, or performing a mobilization to increase ROM, a therapist's hands are important therapeutic instruments. A variety of manual techniques are currently being used by orthopaedic physical therapists, and many of these techniques are the subject of clinical research to validate and clarify their purpose and clinical efficacy.

For the purpose of this text, manual techniques will be divided into two categories: soft tissue mobilization and joint mobilization. It is beyond the scope of this text to cover specific procedures and the schools of thought behind the various techniques. The reader is again referred to the reading list at the end of this chapter for further information regarding this topic.

Soft Tissue Mobilization. **Soft tissue mobilization** includes a variety of "hands-on" techniques designed to improve movement and function. The techniques are designed to decrease pain or swelling and relax muscle or fascia tension to create proper postural alignment and optimal muscle function.

Two common forms of soft tissue mobilization are massage and myofascial release. **Massage** involves the systematic use of various manual strokes designed to produce certain physiological, mechanical, and psychological effects. To achieve relaxation, Swedish massage strokes are used to help decrease pain or swelling, relieve tension, and improve the metabolism of surrounding tissue. More vigorous massage strokes may also be used before physical activity to stimulate and prepare the muscles for exertion. Another specific stroke known as transverse friction massage is useful in improving the flexibility and function of soft tissues such as muscles, ligaments, and tendons.[5]

7

Myofascial release involves manual stretching of the layers of the body's fascia, which is connective tissue that surrounds muscle and other soft tissue in the body[12] (see Fig. 2–10). Myofascial release techniques are thought to soften and loosen restrictions in muscles and fascia that are limiting normal movement. These techniques are unique in that the stretching force applied by the therapist depends on the response of the patient's tissues to the stretch. The therapist must be able to "feel" fascial tension diminish as stretch is applied and adjust the amount of stretch to the patient's comfort.

Joint Mobilization. In contrast to soft tissue mobilization, which focuses on stretching or relaxing soft tissue, **joint mobilization** techniques are used when a patient's dysfunction is the result of joint stiffness or hypomobility (limited motion). Based on knowledge of the anatomy of joint surfaces and the findings from joint examination, the therapist applies specific passive movements to a joint, either oscillatory (rapid, repeated movements) or sustained. Joint mobilization techniques are intended to reduce the pain and stiffness affecting movement and restore normal joint motion.

Therapeutic Exercise

Therapeutic exercise has been and continues to be the foundation of a rehabilitation program. This foundation is based on scientific principles and the knowledge that the human body has the ability to react and respond to physical stresses placed on it. In particular, the muscular and cardiovascular systems are adaptable, depending on the stresses and forces placed on them. When these systems are stressed with a program of progressive exercise, positive changes will occur such as improvement in strength and endurance. Likewise, the effects of abnormal stresses, such as prolonged bed rest, can lead to detrimental changes, including osteoporosis and muscle atrophy.[3]

The goals of therapeutic exercise are not only to facilitate and restore normal function in an individual but also to prevent an initial injury, educate the patient on how to prevent recurrence of an injury, and help maintain normal function. These goals are based on the results of the patient's examination and assessment of needs.

The level of sophistication of an exercise program should not be determined by the type of equipment that the clinic may have. Some of the most sophisticated exercises can be performed with very inexpensive equipment. With creativity, various pieces of equipment can be adapted to incorporate many of the goals of therapeutic exercise. This section will describe a variety of therapeutic exercise techniques that may be used with a patient who has a musculoskeletal dysfunction. These techniques include exercises to improve ROM, strength, flexibility, balance and coordination, cardiovascular endurance, and function.

Range-of-Motion Exercise. As mentioned earlier in the chapter, **range-of-motion exercise** can be categorized into two types: passive and active. PROM may be provided manually by the therapist or mechanically by a machine. This type of exercise might be used with (but is not limited to) patients who are restricted to bed rest, have paralysis of one or more limbs, or are in a coma. It may also be used when AROM is contraindicated. AROM can be subdivided into active assisted movement, active free movement, and active resisted movement. When performing **active assisted range of motion,** the patient may be assisted either manually or mechanically if the prime muscle mover is weak (Fig. 7–13A). Pendulum exercises in which the patient does not receive any support or resistance are an example of **active free range of motion** (Fig. 7–13B). In **active resisted exercises,** an external force resists the movement. The last category includes a variety of techniques, several of which are described in the next section.

Resisted Exercise. **Resisted exercise** is a form of active movement in which some form of resistance is provided.[10] The goals of a resisted exercise program are to increase muscular strength and endurance. **Muscular strength** refers to the maximal amount of tension that an individual can produce in one repetition. **Muscle endurance** refers to the ability to produce and sustain tension over a prolonged period.[6] If the goal is to increase strength, the program would concentrate on low repetitions with heavy resistance. If the goal is to increase endurance, the exercise program would concentrate on using low resistance for high repetitions. The type of exercise performed depends on the types of activities to which the patient is planning to return. When designing a program, the therapist must also consider the type or types of resisted exercise on which the patient should concentrate. Resisted exercise can be categorized into three

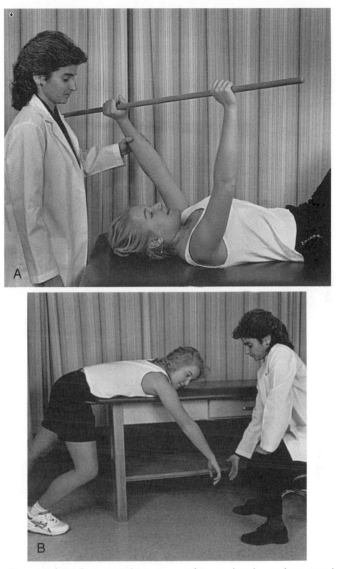

Figure 7–13. Range-of-motion exercises are used to maintain or improve joint motion. *A,* A cane can be used to conduct simple active assistive range-of-motion exercises for the shoulder. *B,* Pendulum exercises are effective active free exercises and require no special equipment. (Courtesy of Dewey Neild.)

types: isometric, isotonic, and isokinetic.[10] Definitions and examples of these types are outlined in Table 7–3. Typically, a combination of all three types of exercise is necessary to perform any type of functional activity.

In resisted exercise, resistance can be applied either manually by the therapist or mechanically by the use of equipment. Manual resistance can be applied to isolated muscle groups (as is the case with MMT positions), or it can be

Table 7–3
Classification of Resisted Exercises

TYPE OF EXERCISE	DEFINITION	EXAMPLE
Isometric	Muscle contraction without visible joint movement	Pushing against a wall
Isotonic		
Concentric	Muscle contraction that produces or controls joint motion resulting in muscle *shortening*	Flexing elbow with dumbbell in hand (biceps brachii muscle)
Eccentric	Muscle contraction that produces or controls joint motion resulting in muscle *lengthening*	Extending elbow with dumbbell in hand (biceps brachii muscle)
Isokinetic	A concentric or eccentric muscle contraction that occurs at a constant speed	Knee extensions using an isokinetic device

applied to patterns of movement that involve several muscle groups. An example of the latter is a technique called proprioceptive neuromuscular facilitation, which is described in Chapter 8. The use of manual resistance offers many advantages, the primary one being that it gives the therapist the ability to control the amount of resistance provided. This advantage is particularly useful when working with patients who are in the early stages of rehabilitation when ROM may need to be limited or the patient is able to tolerate only mild to moderate resistance. The disadvantage is that it is very difficult to quantify the amount of resistance provided, so it is also difficult for another therapist to replicate the same amount of resistance on that patient.

Many pieces of equipment can be used when applying mechanical resistance, from an inexpensive strip of elastic tubing (Fig. 7–14A) to very costly and highly technological isokinetic equipment (Fig. 7–14B). Other common and frequently used equipment in the clinic includes free weights (Fig. 7–14C), Nautilus machines, and pulley systems.

Flexibility Exercise. Patients recovering from a musculoskeletal injury frequently have decreased flexibility in the muscles crossing the involved joint. Conditions that may produce decreased flexibility include prolonged immobilization and tissue trauma. Many times, previous decreased flexibility may have contributed to or may have been the primary cause of the injury. Therefore, **flexibility exercise** is a very important component to address with the patient.

Soft tissue such as muscle has the ability to change length or adapt over time with stress. While a variety of techniques can be used to increase flexibility, research in this area indicates that no consensus has been reached on the most effective way to stretch. Furthermore, a stretching technique that works well for one patient may be ineffective for another.

Stretching techniques can be performed passively with an external force applied either manually or mechanically. Stretching can also be performed by actively inhibiting the shortened muscle. This technique, called contract-relax, requires the shortened muscle to actively contract before a stretching force is applied.[10]

Balance and Coordination Exercise. **Proprioception** is a term used to describe one's awareness of position and movement. The body is made aware of proprioception through various receptors found in the skin and joints. These **proprioceptors** respond to stimuli such as pressure, stretch, and position. After injury, particularly to the knee and ankle, there may be loss of proprioception and therefore loss of balance and/or coordination. Unfortunately, the paucity of well-documented tests to examine balance in patients with orthopaedic dysfunction makes it difficult to monitor changes in balance in a rehabilitation program. However, numerous exercises and equipment can be used to facilitate proper balance. One popular piece of equipment seen in the clinic is a balance board (Fig. 7–15). The patient progresses from a sitting to a standing position while shifting weight from side to side and front to back. This exercise can also be progressed from two-legged weight shift to one-legged weight shift (balancing on one leg). The exercise can be made more challenging by having patients close their eyes and incorporating upper extremity movement with and without weights.

Cardiovascular Endurance Training. Cardiovascular or **aerobics training** refers to exercise performed over a long period at low intensity.[10] Aerobic exercise typically involves large muscle groups used in a rhythmic type of activity. Many modes of exercise are available to improve cardiovascular endurance, including walking, running, stair climbing, cycling, cross-country skiing, and swimming. The physical therapist will choose the exercise modality that is most appropriate for the patient. For example, a patient who is recovering from a low back injury and has difficulty sitting may participate in a walking program rather than a cycling program. See Chapter 9 for a more detailed description of cardiovascular exercise.

Functional Exercises. As mentioned earlier in this chapter, the ultimate goal in physical therapy is to allow the patient to return to the previous level of function or highest level of function achievable. Therefore, it is imperative that exercises mimicking functional movements and activities be incorporated into the rehabilitation program. A **functional exercise** incorporates strength, flexibility, balance, and coordination. Incorporating all these factors allows patients to return to function with confidence because they know that they performed the same or very similar exercises in the clinic.

7

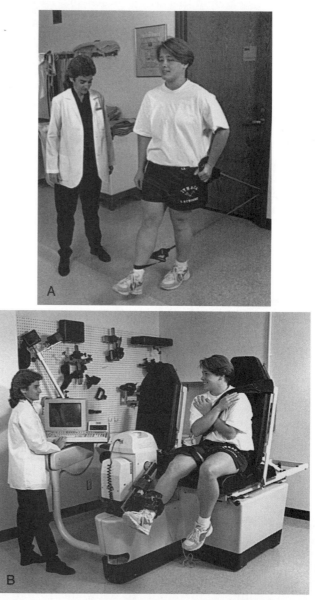

Figure 7–14. Different methods of using mechanical resistance for exercise. *A,* Elastic tubing is inexpensive and easy to use. *B,* Isokinetic equipment is generally very expensive and sophisticated.

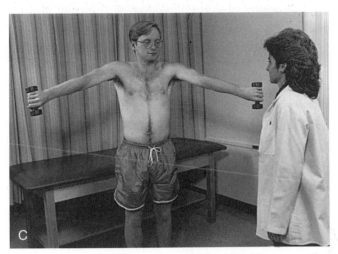

Figure 7–14 *Continued. C,* Free weights are readily available to produce mechanical resistance. (Courtesy of Dewey Neild.)

7

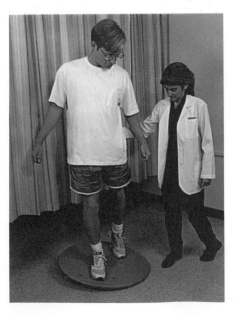

Figure 7–15. A balance board can be used for balance exercises. (Courtesy of Dewey Neild.)

The use of closed-chain or kinetic-chain exercises allows the patient to incorporate these functional movements. A **closed-chain exercise** or **kinetic-chain exercise** is an exercise in which movement at one joint affects movement at other joints (e.g., a two-legged squat). An **open-chain exercise** or **joint isolation exercise** is an exercise in which the end limb segment is free (e.g., biceps curl). Many of the exercises traditionally used to strengthen the lower extremity are those in which the foot is off the ground. An example would be the use of isokinetic equipment for thigh strengthening. However, the lower extremity typically functions with the foot on the ground. Closed-chain exercises are particularly important in the rehabilitation of the lower extremity. Therefore, exercises involving the movement of joints while the foot is on the ground facilitate proper proprioceptive feedback that mimics function (Fig. 7–16).

Aquatic Therapy. The use of water for therapeutic benefit dates back to the ancient Greeks and Romans, who used therapeutic baths for relaxation and pain reduction.[19] "Pool therapy" developed in the 1920s in the United States as part of the rehabilitation program for children with poliomyelitis (see Fig. 1–4). As polio declined with the introduction of vaccines, so did the therapeutic use of pools. Recently, however, **aquatic physical therapy** has been shown to be beneficial for a variety of orthopaedic dysfunctions. The popularity of aquatic therapy has grown significantly, and in 1992, the APTA established the Aquatic Physical Therapy Section.

The founding documents of this Section offer a comprehensive description of this form of therapy (Box 7–3).[1] The description indicates that this form of

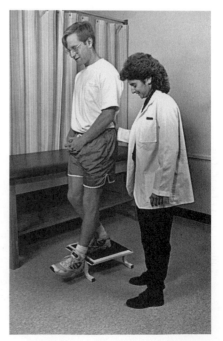

Figure 7–16. Functional exercises, such as descending a step, are designed to mimic daily activities. (Courtesy of Dewey Neild.)

Box 7–3 | **Description of Aquatic Therapy**

Aquatic Physical Therapy includes, but is not limited to, the rehabilitation, prevention, and overall wellness of a wide patient population. These patients, ranging from infants to the elderly, can benefit from safe and effective physical therapy intervention in the aquatic environment, addressing neurologic, orthopaedic, and other conditions. Aquatic physical therapy employs unique protocols but may also include swimming strokes in conjunction with specific treatment techniques. Aquatic physical therapy must be supervised and/or performed by a licensed physical therapist. Although various kinds of aquatic environments are utilized to perform these specific treatment techniques, aquatic physical therapy is not a modality, but a procedure requiring specific skill and training to implement the aquatic techniques correctly.

From APTA Aquatic Physical Therapy Section Statement of Purposes, Rationale, and Goals. Alexandria, VA, American Physical Therapy Association, 1992.

7

rehabilitation is effective for a variety of conditions, in addition to maintaining health and fitness in well individuals. As the description indicates, aquatic therapy is a specific intervention that requires the expertise and supervision of a trained specialist for the program to be safe and effective.

While general exercises and manual techniques may be performed in the water, highly specific techniques have also been developed.[15] In the **Bad Ragaz method,** the therapist uses proprioceptive neuromuscular facilitation techniques while the patient is suspended by rings in the water (see Chapter 8 for a description of proprioceptive neuromuscular facilitation). The **Halliwick method** uses a preswim stroke instruction and musculoskeletal rehabilitation. Therapists may also use other exercise techniques or treatment approaches such as Tai Chi or Shiatsu in the water to combine their therapeutic benefits with the effectiveness of the water environment.

The beneficial effects of aquatic therapy are largely dependent on the fundamental principles of physics,[8] such as the buoyancy, viscosity, and hydrostatic pressure of water. Both physiological and psychological benefits are derived from aquatic physical therapy. The physiological benefits include improved cardiovascular status, increased muscle strength and flexibility, decreased pain, and improved balance without the impact that occurs with exercises on land. Psychological benefits include general relaxation from the warmth of the water, the socialization process that may be associated with group sessions in a pool, and the increased patient confidence and level of satisfaction that accompany patient performance.

Certain contraindications and precautions must be considered when planning and implementing any aquatic therapy session (Box 7–4). These contraindications must be carefully considered to ensure the safety of the individual.

Box 7–4

Contraindications to Aquatic Therapy

- Fever
- Cardiac failure
- Urinary tract infections
- Open wounds

- Infectious diseases
- Contagious skin rashes
- Excessive fear of water

Adapted from Haralson KM: Therapeutic pool programs. Clin Manage Phys Ther 1985;5(2):10–13.

Home Exercise Programs

The use of therapeutic exercise in a rehabilitation program is an important and essential activity. Aside from the physical benefits derived from exercise, it also allows the patient to assume responsibility for care of the injury and encourages active participation in the rehabilitative process. For the same reasons, home exercise programs also become a very important aspect of patient care. Treatment in the clinic two or three times per week is not usually enough time to see the desired long-lasting effects of rehabilitation unless the patient is performing appropriate exercises, given by the physical therapist, at home. The inability of a patient to pay for physical therapy services (often because of lack of health care insurance coverage) may also limit the number of clinic visits, thus making home programs even more appropriate.

Patient Education

As mentioned earlier in the chapter, communication is a critical component of the orthopaedic physical therapy experience. The therapist's depth of knowledge and effectiveness in performing and interpreting the evaluation and the variety of treatment options available are of little value if the therapist does not share this information with patients and inform them of their role in the rehabilitation process. The patient and therapist must work together as a team and focus on the same goals and sharing of information to achieve optimal results.

It is the responsibility of the physical therapist and physical therapist assistant to educate the patient about exercises to perform at home, postures or positions to avoid during daily activities at work or home, and strategies to prevent the dysfunction from recurring (Fig. 7–17). To communicate effectively, the therapist must create a treatment atmosphere that ensures the patient's comfort and must also provide the necessary information in a clear manner that is easily understood.

It is important for the physical therapist and physical therapist assistant, when working with a patient, to treat the whole person rather than just an injured joint. Each patient comes to the therapist with a different set of values, different expectations, and a different background. All these factors must be considered to successfully and effectively treat a patient.

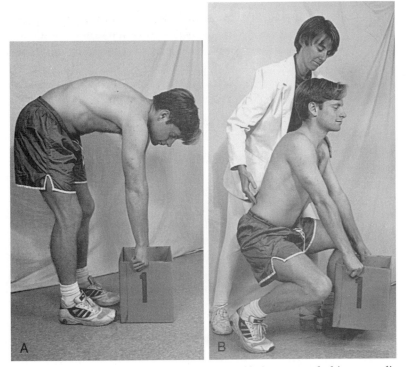

Figure 7–17. Patient education is essential to rectify improper habits regarding body movement and posture. *A,* Improper lifting can result in straining lower back muscles and ligaments. *B,* Instruction in proper lifting techniques can prevent injuries to the back. (Courtesy of Dewey Neild.)

Case Studies   *Jack—Low Back Pain*

Examination

History. Jack, a 36-year-old English-speaking male, is married and has a 2-year-old child. As an architect, he sits at a computer approximately 5 hours per day and drives 1 hour each way to work. His chief complaint is left-sided lower back pain that spreads into the buttock region and occasionally down the back of the thigh. Symptoms came on suddenly approximately 2 weeks ago after he bent down to pick up house keys; Jack had difficulty standing back up because of pain. He saw a physician, who recommended a course of muscle relaxants and rest. Jack states that the pain has gradually improved since its onset and rates the pain level a "4" on a scale of 1 to 10. The pain worsens when he lifts his daughter from the floor and with prolonged periods of sitting. Symptoms improve with walking. Jack has no complaints of numbness or tingling in the lower extremity but is currently unable to sit for more than 20 minutes without the onset of pain. Radiographs taken 1 week ago were "normal" according to Jack. Jack had a history of occasional low back discomfort after prolonged sitting, but no previous history of this type of pain. His medical/surgical history and family history were unremarkable. In social habits, Jack is sedentary but enjoys occasional weekend recreational activities.

Systems Review. Cardiopulmonary examination revealed a blood pressure of 136/88 mm Hg and resting heart rate of 86 beats per minute. The patient's integumentary system was unremarkable, and Jack had full ROM of the lower extremity. See below for detailed examination of the lumbar spine. Neuromuscular evaluation showed normal movement patterns of the lower extremities.

Tests and Measures. In tests of gait, locomotion, and balance, gait appears normal with equal weight bearing. In joint integrity and mobility testing, no swelling or temperature changes are noted over the lumbar erectors. Increased tone is seen bilaterally in the spinal muscles. Muscle performance testing finds the lower extremity to be within normal limits; however, the trunk muscles were not tested because of pain. A straight leg raise reproduces the thigh pain at 40 degrees. In standing posture, Jack has a posterior pelvic tilt with a slight lateral shift to the right, a forward head, and rounded shoulders. ROM testing demonstrates lumbar spine movements to be significantly limited in all directions; the chief complaint is exacerbated with flexion movements. Pain centralizes with lumbar extension in the prone position. Regarding sensory integrity, the lower extremity is intact to light touch bilaterally. Testing of reflex integrity reveals deep tendon reflexes (DTRs) of 2+ in the left extremity throughout (within a range of 0 to 4) and symmetrical.

Evaluation. The evaluation of Jack's dysfunction is low back pain peripheralizing to the left side with signs and symptoms indicative of low back derangement. Impairments include increased muscle tone of the lumbar erectors, pain with straight leg raise, poor posture, and decreased lumbar ROM. Functional limitations include a decreased ability to sit for prolonged periods. Regarding disabilities, Jack is unable to complete job tasks in a timely fashion because of a decreased ability to sit and is unable to participate in recreational activities.

Diagnosis. The patient presents with impairments in joint mobility, motor function, muscle performance, ROM, and reflex integrity secondary to intervertebral disk disorder.

Prognosis/Expected Range of Visits. Over the course of 4 to 8 weeks, Jack will return to his premorbid level of function with a minimal increase in symptoms. He is to be seen for 8 to 12 visits over the course of 3 months.

Short-Term Goals (2–4 Weeks). The following short-term goals are set: (1) pain reduced to 1 to 2 (out of 10), (2) abolishment of lateral shift, (3) 50% increase in all lumbar movements, (4) independence in a home exercise program, and (5) ability to demonstrate proper sitting posture throughout the treatment session.

Long-Term Goals/Outcomes (6–8 Weeks). For the long term, Jack's goals and outcomes are threefold: (1) functional limitations/disabilities—Jack should be able to sit for prolonged periods (up to 6 hours with breaks every hour) without symptoms, as well as return to leisure and recreational activities without symptoms; (2) patient satisfaction—services provided by the physical therapist are deemed acceptable by the patient; and (3) secondary prevention—the risk of impairment, functional limitation, and disability is reduced through adherence to an independent exercise program, and Jack understands and demonstrates strategies to prevent the recurrence of symptoms.

Plan of Care/Intervention. Jack's home exercise program will begin with lumbar extension exercises and progress to flexion exercises. He will be educated on proper sitting posture and body mechanics, including lifting techniques. Modalities (ultrasound, hot packs) and manual techniques (joint mobilization, soft tissue massage) are to be used as appropriate for pain relief. As pain resolves, exercises will increase to include functional movements and flexibility exercises. The importance of adhering to the home exercise program will be explained. Work site analysis will be performed, followed by recommendations to improve Jack's computer workstation.

Outcomes/Patient Status at Discharge. After 6 weeks of physical therapy, Jack was free of symptoms and all goals had been met. He was discharged with a comprehensive home exercise program. A recommendation was made to initiate a general fitness program at the local health club.

7

Alice—Fractured Radius

Examination
History. Alice, a 72-year-old widow and retired school teacher, lives alone. She is right hand dominant. Alice sustained a fractured right radius after slipping on ice 8 weeks ago. She was immobilized in a hand-to-midhumeral cast with her elbow positioned in 90 degrees of flexion and her arm supported in a sling for comfort. The cast was removed yesterday. Her chief complaints are stiffness and weakness throughout the upper extremity and an inability to perform daily activities such as getting dressed and preparing meals. Radiographs taken yesterday reveal "healing without complications." Alice has no past history of the current condition, and her medical and surgical history is unremarkable; she is in generally good health. Her family history is unremarkable. Regarding social habits, Alice walks 1 to 2 miles a day and enjoys cooking, gardening, and the outdoors.

Systems Review. Cardiopulmonary evaluation reveals a blood pressure of 140/90 mm Hg and a resting heart rate of 80 beats per minute. Integumentary examination reveals dry skin over the area covered by the cast. Musculoskeletal assessment discloses full ROM of left upper extremity movements and good range of strength in the left arm. See below for details of the right upper extremity. Neuromuscular evaluation of the left upper extremity reveals normal movement patterns.

Tests and Measures. Joint integrity and mobility testing demonstrate swelling over the dorsal aspect of the right wrist. In muscle performance testing, resisted tests reveal weakness in the following muscle groups: right shoulder abductors and external rotators, elbow flexors and extensors, and wrist flexors and extensors. Manual muscle tests revealed the following (see Table 9–1 for descriptions of grades; grades are based on a scale of 0 to 5):

Right biceps = 4−/5   Left biceps = 5/5
Right triceps = 3+/5   Left triceps = 5/5
Right hand grip = 15 lb   Left Hand Grip = 25 lb

Testing for pain reveals pain with movement of the right upper extremity. Alice's standing posture is with the head slightly forward and the shoulders rounded, and she holds her arm in a guarded position against her body. Muscle atrophy is noted throughout the upper extremity. ROM testing demonstrates limited and painful active movements of the right shoulder, elbow, and wrist. AROM of the right hand is within normal limits. PROM of the right upper extremity is as follows:

Shoulder: Flexion = 0–160 degrees
             Abduction = 0–60 degrees
             External rotation = 0–15 degrees
             Internal rotation = 0–70 degrees
Elbow: Unable to extend past 60 degrees of flexion
Wrist: Flexion = 0–45 degrees
             Extension = 0–45 degrees

Accessory motion is decreased at the right glenohumeral joint. Sensory integrity testing reveals the upper extremity to be intact to light touch bilaterally. In reflex integrity, Alice has upper extremity DTRs of 3+ throughout (within a range of 0 to 4) and symmetrical.

Evaluation. Alice has decreased ROM and strength secondary to immobilization after a wrist fracture. Impairments include swelling, decreased upper extremity strength, decreased upper extremity ROM, poor posture, and decreased accessory movement at the shoulder. Her functional limitation is a decreased ability to perform ADLs. Regarding disabilities, Alice is unable to participate in leisure activities, including cooking and gardening.

Diagnosis. The patient presents with impairments in joint mobility, muscle performance, and ROM secondary to immobilization following a Colles fracture.

Prognosis/Expected Range of Visits. Over the course of 8 to 12 weeks, Alice will return to her premorbid level of function with minimal limitation. She is to be seen for 6 to 18 visits over the course of 3 months.

Short-Term Goals (2–4 Weeks). Alice's short-term goals are as follows: (1) decrease swelling by 25%, (2) increase upper extremity strength to the next higher grade, (3) increase right grip strength to 18 lb, (4) increase ROM by 5 to 10 degrees in all limited movements, (5) increase accessory motion to nearly full range, (6) be able to demonstrate proper cervical and shoulder posture, and (7) demonstrate independence in her home exercise program.

Long-Term Goals/Outcomes (10–12 Weeks). Alice's long-term goals and outcomes are threefold: (1) Functional limitations/disabilities—Alice should be able to perform all ADLs independently and to return to all leisure activities; (2) patient satisfaction—services provided by the physical therapist are deemed acceptable by Alice; and (3) secondary prevention—the risk of impairment, functional limitation, and disability is reduced through adherence to an independent exercise program, and Alice should understand the importance of good posture as it relates to the shoulder.

Plan of Care/Intervention. Alice's home exercise program will progressively increase to enhance elbow and wrist ROM and strength. The program will include active assisted, active free, and active resisted exercises such as pendulum, pulley, and cane exercises (see Fig. 7–13). She will be educated on proper sitting posture and the relationship between proper posture and shoulder mechanics. Modalities (superficial heat) and manual techniques (joint mobilization) will be used as appropriate. Proprioceptive neuromuscular facilitation patterns will be incorporated to improve functional movements. As strength and ROM increase, simulated ADLs will be added to the treatment program.

Outcomes/Patient Status at Discharge. After 9 weeks of physical therapy, Alice had functional use of her right upper extremity and was able to return to all activities with minimal limitation. She was discharged with a comprehensive exercise program.

7

Summary ———

This chapter has presented the role that physical therapists and physical therapist assistants play in physical therapy for musculoskeletal conditions. Common conditions described were overuse and traumatic injuries and surgical and medical conditions. Components of the patient examination were presented. Treatment interventions focused on physical agents, manual techniques, therapeutic exercise, home programs, and patient education. The emphasis in physical therapy for musculoskeletal conditions is on evaluating a patient's function and developing a treatment program that will assist the patient in returning to optimal function in the environment, whether that be on the athletic field, at a work site, or at home.

References

1. APTA Aquatic Physical Therapy Section Statement of Purposes, Rationale, and Goals. Alexandria, VA, American Physical Therapy Association, 1992.
2. Bandy W: Functional rehabilitation of the athlete. Orthop Clin North Am 1992;1:269–281.
3. Barber SD, Noyes FR, Mangine RE, et al: Quantitative assessment of functional limitations in normal and anterior cruciate ligament–deficient knee. Clin Orthop 1990;255:204–214.
4. Bell BD, Hoshizak TB: Relationships of age and sex with range of motion of seventeen joint actions in humans. Can J Appl Sports Sci 1981;6:202.
5. Cyriax J: Textbook of Orthopaedic Medicine, vol 1, Diagnosis of Soft Tissue Lesions, ed 8. London, Bailliere Tindall, 1982.
6. Fox E, Mathews D: The Physiological Basis of Physical Education and Athletics. Philadelphia, WB Saunders, 1981.
7. Gray G: Developing the Lower Extremity Functional Profile. Adrian, MI, Wynn Marketing, 1994.
8. Haralson KM: Therapeutic pool programs. Clin Manage Phys Ther 1985;5(2):10–13.
9. Kendall FP, McCreary EK, Provance PG: Muscles Testing and Function, ed 4. Baltimore, Williams & Wilkins, 1993.
10. Kisner C, Colby LA: Therapeutic Exercise: Foundations and Techniques, ed 3. Philadelphia, FA Davis, 1996.

11. Lephart S, Perrin D, Fu F, et al: Relationship between selected physical characteristics and functional capacity in the anterior cruciate ligament–insufficient athlete. J Orthop Sports Phys Ther 1992;16(4):174–181.

12. Manheim CJ, Lavett DK: The Myofascial Release Manual. Thorofare, NJ, Slack, 1989.

13. Michlovitz SL: Biophysical principles of heating and superficial heat agents. *In* Michlovitz SL: Thermal Agents in Rehabilitation, ed 3. Philadelphia, FA Davis, 1996.

14. Moffroid M, Zimny N: Causes of movement dysfunction and physical disability. *In* Scully RM, Barnes MR (eds): Physical Therapy. Philadelphia, JB Lippincott, 1989.

15. Morris DM, Irion JM, Charness AL: Aquatic physical therapy as a procedure. Orthop Phys Ther Clin North Am 1994;3(2):231–249.

16. Noyes FR: Objective functional testing. *In* Noyes FR (ed): The Noyes Knee Rating System. Cincinnati, OH, Cincinnati Sports Medicine Research and Education Foundation, 1990.

17. Reed B, Zarro V: Inflammation and repair and the use of thermal agents. *In* Michlovitz SL (ed): Thermal Agents in Rehabilitation, ed 2. Philadelphia, FA Davis, 1990.

18. Robinson AJ, Snyder-Mackler L: Clinical Electrophysiology, Electrotherapy and Electrophysiologic Testing, ed 2. Baltimore, Williams & Wilkins, 1995.

19. Wynn KE: Lily ponds, warm springs and fortunate accidents. PT—Magazine of Physical Therapy 1994;2(12):44–45.

Suggested Readings

Bates A, Hanson N: Aquatic Exercise Therapy. Philadelphia, WB Saunders, 1996.

Provides easy-to-understand aquatic exercises referenced by joint and common musculoskeletal disorders.

Edmond S: Manipulation and Mobilization: Extremity and Spinal Techniques. St Louis, Mosby–Year Book, 1993.

This is a clinically applicable text that describes manual therapy techniques of the extremities and spine.

Evans R: Illustrated Essentials in Orthopedic Physical Assessment. St Louis, Mosby–Year Book, 1994.

Hundreds of tests can be used for making conservative care diagnoses of disorders of the nervous and orthopaedic systems. This manual describes them in a clearly illustrated, sequential fashion. Organization of the text is by region and specifically by initial signs, symptoms, and indications.

Hall M, Thein-Brody L: Therapeutic Exercises: Moving Toward Function. Philadelphia, Lippincott, Williams & Wilkins, 1998.

Offers a comprehensive approach to therapeutic exercise based on the disablement model, with an emphasis on the role that exercise plays in improving functional limitations.

Hecox B, Mehreteab TA, Weisberg J: Physical Agents: A Comprehensive Text for Physical Therapists. E Norwalk, CT, Appleton & Lange, 1994.

Discusses the physiological effects and application procedures for commonly used physical agents, including heat, cold, light, water, ultrasound, and electrotherapy.

Kennedy R: Mosby's Sports Therapy Taping Guide. St Louis, Mosby–Year Book, 1995.

This practical manual offers step-by-step procedures for taping and wrapping. With over 170 illustrations and clear, descriptive instructions, this is a comprehensive manual about sports taping for the prevention of injuries and care of athletes.

Magee D: Orthopedic Physical Assessment, ed 3. Philadelphia, WB Saunders, 1997.

An excellent text detailing the evaluation of joints, with good descriptions of special tests.

Manheim CJ, Lavett DK: The Myofascial Release Manual. Thorofare, NJ, Slack, 1989.
Photographs and illustrations demonstrate a variety of myofascial techniques used in treatment, in addition to a discussion of evaluation and an extensive reference list.

Michlovitz SL: Biophysical principles of heating and superficial heat agents. *In* Michlovitz SL (ed): Thermal Agents in Rehabilitation, ed 3. Philadelphia, FA Davis, 1996.
Presents the foundation and methods of application for thermal agents, with an emphasis on clinical decision making. This edition also includes extensive references.

Prentice WE: Rehabilitation Techniques in Sports Medicine. St Louis, CV Mosby, 1990.
A comprehensive text discussing the implementation and profession of rehabilitation programs for sports-related injuries.

Richardson J, Iglarsh ZA: Clinical Orthopaedic Physical Therapy. Philadelphia, WB Saunders, 1994.
A regional approach to evaluation and treatment of joints. Differential diagnoses and common pathologies at each joint are also discussed.

7

Robinson AJ, Snyder-Mackler L: Clinical Electrophysiology, Electrotherapy and Electrophysiologic Testing, ed 2. Baltimore, Williams & Wilkins, 1995.
Provides basic theoretical background and clinical applications for electrotherapy based on desired therapeutic outcomes.

Tappan FM: Healing Massage Techniques: Holistic, Classic, and Emerging Methods, ed 2. E Norwalk, CT, Appleton & Lange, 1988.
Describes a variety of techniques and methods of massage, including the history of massage, general principles, and clinical rationale.

REVIEW QUESTIONS

1. What is the difference between active ROM and passive ROM?

2. Without looking at the text, how many questions can you come up with that may be helpful in a patient interview?

3. How would quantitative and qualitative measurements fit into the "SOAP" note?

4. Research some physical therapy books in your school's library to find examples of resisted tests and manual muscle testing. What, in your observation, is the main difference?

5. Try the following study technique: Photocopy Table 7–2 and block out the second column ("Physical Agents") with a folded strip of paper.

Can you fill in the applicable agents? Repeat this exercise by filling out column 3 instead ("Physiological Effects") or column 4 ("Clinical Indications"). Performing this exercise will reinforce the uses and effects of physical agents.

6. Describe the difference in purpose between exercising for muscular strength and exercising for muscular endurance.

7. Explain why closed-chain exercises are usually preferable in lower limb rehabilitation, as opposed to open-chain exercises.

A sense of history and an appreciation of why things happened can provide a perspective in understanding the present and in projecting the future.
Lucy Blair, PT

Physical Therapy for Neuromuscular Conditions

Shree Pandya

KEY TERMS

akinesia

amyotrophic lateral sclerosis (ALS)

angiography

bradykinesia

Brunnstrom's approach

computed (axial) tomography (CAT or CT)

electroencephalography (EEG)

electromyography (EMG)

expressive aphasia

hypertonia

hypotonia

lumbar puncture

magnetic resonance imaging (MRI)

motor control

motor development

motor learning

multiple sclerosis (MS)

nerve conduction velocity (NCV) study

neurodevelopmental treatment (NDT)

paraplegia

Parkinson's disease

perception

proprioceptive neuromuscular facilitation (PNF)

quadriplegia

receptive aphasia

rigidity

Rood's approach

sensation

spinal cord injury (SCI)

stroke or cerebrovascular accident (CVA)

tone

traumatic brain injury (TBI)

tremor

OBJECTIVES   After reading this chapter, the reader will be able to

- Discuss the role of the physical therapist in the management of patients with neuromuscular disorders
- Describe some of the common neuromuscular conditions in which physical therapists play an essential role
- Compare the different roles that a therapist may play depending on the patient's condition and problems

GENERAL DESCRIPTION   At the beginning of the last century one could learn about the human nervous system from autopsy tissue samples only. Today, with new technologies, the brain can be seen in action in living human beings. The 1990s were declared the decade of the brain by the U.S. Congress. During this period, tremendous progress was made in the areas of neuroscience, clinical neurology, and genetics. As the function of the brain and nervous system is better understood, physical therapists are able to devise and provide effective techniques and explain the efficacy underlying previously developed techniques.

Patients with problems related to disorders of the neuromuscular system make up a large proportion of individuals treated by physical therapists today. Disorders of the neuromuscular system can be inherited or acquired. Acquired disorders may result from trauma or disease, be secondary to disorders affecting other body systems, or occur as part of the normal aging process. In addition, many disorders whose causes are still unknown or not well understood affect the neuromuscular system.

Neuromuscular disorders can affect people at any age. For example, inherited disorders such as Friedreich's ataxia or spinal muscular atrophy are present from birth. Traumatic disorders such as spinal cord injuries (SCIs) or brain injuries are most often caused by motor vehicle accidents, and the age groups most commonly involved range from the teens to the thirties. Disorders such as multiple sclerosis (MS), Parkinson's disease, and Lou Gehrig's disease (amyotrophic lateral sclerosis [ALS]) are manifested most often between the thirties and sixties. The two most common neuromuscular disorders encountered with age are stroke (paralysis secondary to disruption of blood flow within the brain) and Alzheimer's disease. Thus, when working with patients with neuromuscular problems, therapists are likely to encounter persons of any age, both sexes, and all races.

Depending on the cause of the disorder, the condition may be lifelong or temporary. It may be reversible, static, or progressive. The patient may go through periods of "plateaus" (i.e., relative stability) interspersed with progression. Because of the lengthy course of most neuromuscular disorders, physical therapists have extended contact with their patients and play a critical role in their care. Depending on the condition, the stage of illness, and the reason for referral, the frequency of treatment will vary. For example, patients may be treated as often as two times per day for an hour each session in the rehabilitation or hospital setting, or two or three times per week if the patient is past the acute stage and is being seen in the home or an extended care facility. If the therapist sees the patient on a consultation basis or for education regarding personal care and management, these visits may be as infrequent as monthly, quarterly, or yearly.

From the description just presented it is apparent that physical therapists who work with this population encounter diversity in their clients, work settings, and the types of services that they provide. This situation is a major change from the early days of physical therapy practice and even from 20 years ago, when physical therapists practiced under physician's orders only and followed prescriptions for massage, electrotherapy, thermal agents, hydrotherapy, and exercise. Today, the physical therapist is an autonomous member of the health care team and in many states practices under direct access. As described in the patient/client management model, therapists are involved in examination, evaluation, diagnosis, prognosis, intervention, prevention, education, consultation, coordination, and any number of other related activities (see Chapter 2). The next section provides a brief overview of some of the most common neuromuscular disorders and the role of physical therapy in the care and management of patients with these disorders.

8

COMMON CONDITIONS

Stroke

Stroke or **cerebrovascular accident (CVA)** refers to neurological problems arising from disruption of blood flow in the brain. This disruption may be caused by hemorrhage (bleeding) or blockage from a clot that results in ischemia (decreased oxygen). The type and severity of symptoms will depend on the area of brain tissue involved. The most common symptom is a complete paralysis or partial weakness on the side opposite the site involved. Depending on the site of the lesion, the paralysis may be accompanied by symptoms such as difficulty speaking or understanding the spoken word, visual problems, and neglect of the affected side. Approximately 30% of patients die during the first month. Of the survivors, approximately 30% to 40% will have severe disability.[9] A major psychological problem after stroke is depression, which can have a great impact on management. Recovery from stroke occurs most rapidly during the first 6 months, but functional gains can be seen for 2 years or longer. Currently under investigation are several medications that have thrombolytic properties, such as tissue plasminogen activator (tPA), medications that have neuroprotective properties such as glutamate antagonists, or calcium channel blockers, which have the ability to halt or reverse the cascade of events after ischemia. Some (such as tPA) are effective only if given within the first 3 to 6 hours after the stroke. Hence, a key issue is to educate the public regarding the symptoms of a stroke and have them seek immediate attention for this "brain attack," just as they would for a "heart attack."

The purpose of physical therapy is to facilitate and enhance the functional recovery occurring in response to the resolution of neurological changes. Once functional recovery plateaus, the therapist and assistant will teach the patient and family to adapt and compensate for the residual deficits in order to function at the optimal level possible within the constraints of the condition.

Figures 8–1 and 8–2 illustrate the preventive and functional training aspects of management of a patient with left-sided paralysis secondary to stroke.

Traumatic Brain Injury

Traumatic brain injury (TBI) is most often caused by motor vehicle accidents or is due to falls and violence.[7] Because of the nature of the injury, the brain trauma may be associated with fractures, dislocations, lacerations, and the like. The groups most commonly affected are children (from bicycle accidents) and young adults (from car accidents), with traumatic brain injury being the most common cause of death and disability in this age group. Early management is focused on preservation of life and prevention of further damage. The diffuse nature of the brain injury usually results in problems with multiple brain functions and mechanisms. A complex picture is common, with varying deficits in motor and sensory capabilities, intellectual and cognitive functions, and emotional and psychological functions. Because of the complexity and variability of problems that may be encountered with each patient, management and treatment require an individualized plan and a multidisciplinary team approach in which each team member plays a specific and significant role. Currently, not enough data are available on long-term outcomes or valid and reliable measures that may help predict outcomes. Hence, this area provides several opportunities for research to answer questions important to patients and their families. TBI

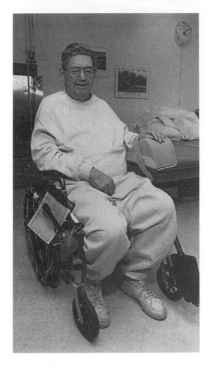

Figure **8–1.** Positioning for a patient with a stroke to prevent secondary problems in the shoulder and hand on the paralyzed (left) side.

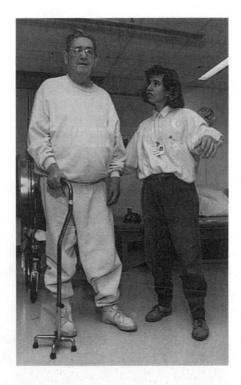

Figure **8–2.** Gait training for a patient with left-sided paralysis caused by a stroke.

8

is also an area where prevention through education is *key*. Wearing helmets when riding a bike and using seat belts when riding in a car can make a difference between life and death.

Spinal Cord Injury

Spinal cord injury, like TBI, most often results from motor vehicle accidents, falls, violence (especially gunshot wounds), and sports (diving and football). The age group most often affected is between 15 and 25 years of age, and men are affected four times as much as women.[12] Spinal cord damage can also be precipitated by other diseases and conditions, and in these instances, older patients are affected more commonly. Depending on the level of injury, all limbs may be affected **(quadriplegia),** or the lower part of the trunk and legs may be affected **(paraplegia).** If the lesion is complete, no residual sensory or motor function can be found below the level of the lesion (-plegia). When the cord is not completely severed, some distal motor and sensory functions may be preserved (-paresis).

As with TBI, SCI may be accompanied by multiple injuries, and the early goal of management is preservation of life and prevention of further damage to neural tissue. Further damage is prevented through internal immobilization of the area by fusing the vertebrae with bone grafts, rods, and wires—or externally with devices such as body jackets or casts. Medications are used to prevent further damage to neural tissue and enhance repair and recovery.

While this healing process occurs, it is important to maintain mobility in the joints of the extremities, strength in the unaffected muscles, cardiorespiratory capacity, and endurance. Figure 8–3 illustrates one of the types of body jackets used to provide stability. The patient is working on strengthening the upper extremity and trunk muscles. Once medical and orthopaedic clearance is obtained, more vigorous functional training is begun.

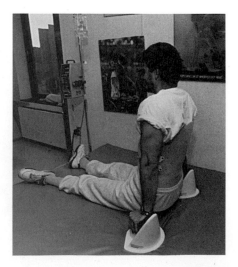

Figure 8–3. Patient with spinal cord injury in a body jacket working on upper body strengthening.

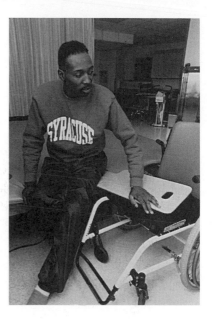

Figure 8–4. Patient with paraplegia working on mat table-to-wheelchair transfers.

As illustrated in Figures 8–4 and 8–5, the patients are learning mat table-to-wheelchair transfers and wheelchair manipulation skills. Simultaneously, equipment needs and environmental adaptations need to be identified. For example, most patients use a wheelchair as a primary means of mobility, and they need to be custom-ordered for each patient with specific size and adaptation requirements. Figure 8–6 shows a patient with quadriplegia using an electric wheelchair for mobility and a special device that allows him to write. The home will need to be made wheelchair accessible with ramps and other modifications. Thus, a therapist plays a major role not only in the treatment but also in the rehabilitation of patients with SCI by providing family education and consultation on many related issues.

Multiple Sclerosis

Multiple sclerosis (MS) is a disease in which patches of demyelination in the nervous system lead to disturbances in the conduction of messages along the nerves. The condition is most often manifested between the ages of 15 and 45 years and affects women more often than men. The specific cause is still unknown. MS can cause a variety of symptoms, depending on the location of the patches of nerve demyelination. Common symptoms include visual problems, sensory problems such as tingling and numbness, weakness, fatigue, problems with balance, and speech disturbances. The course in the early stages is unpredictable. Eventually, the course may take one of four forms[8]: (1) benign, in which the disease seems to go into remission and the patient is relatively symptom-free, with no functional disabilities; (2) exacerbating-remitting, in which the patient undergoes periods of worsening followed by periods

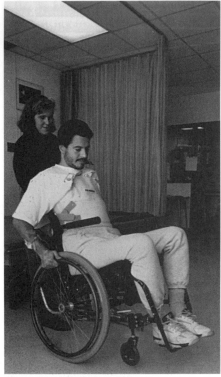

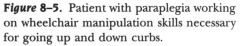

Figure 8–5. Patient with paraplegia working on wheelchair manipulation skills necessary for going up and down curbs.

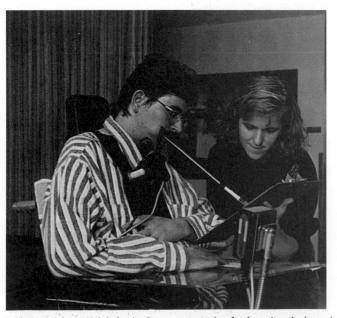

Figure 8–6. Patient with quadriplegia in a customized electric chair using a special device that enables him to write.

of improvement; (3) remitting-progressive, which is similar to the exacerbating-remitting form except that improvement after the episode of worsening is not as complete and each occurrence leaves a residual problem or increase in problems that causes general progression of the disease; and (4) progressive, in which the disease progresses unremittingly and causes severe disability.

The role of the therapist with this group of patients is more consultative and educational. Patients may benefit from active treatment during an acute exacerbation, but otherwise they require periodic evaluation and recommendations because of their changing functional needs.

Parkinson's Disease

Parkinson's disease is a progressive condition first described by James Parkinson in 1817. It is also referred to as paralysis agitans and idiopathic (cause unknown) parkinsonism and is commonly seen with advancing age. Parkinson's disease is characterized by a classic triad of symptoms. **Tremor** (alternating contractions of opposing muscle groups), usually affecting the hands and feet, tends to occur at rest (e.g., when the part is not being used or moved). **Rigidity,** a disturbance in muscle tone, is manifested as resistance when the limbs are passively moved. **Bradykinesia,** or slowness of movements, and/or **akinesia,** a poverty of movements, completes the triad.[2]

This condition results from a deficiency in dopamine, a neurotransmitter (chemical messenger) produced in a region of the brain called the substantia nigra. The specific cause of this depletion is unknown. Even though a cure does not yet exist, medications that restore neurochemical balance are available and help alleviate the symptoms. Unfortunately, the effectiveness of the medications diminishes over the years, and the symptoms continue to worsen. Currently, neural cell transplantation is under investigation as an option for a more permanent treatment or cure.

The tremor, rigidity, and bradykinesia have a great impact on the patient's ability to maintain balance and perform activities such as walking, stair climbing, and reaching. Patients tend to have a stooped posture, walk with short, shuffling steps, and lose reciprocal arm movements. The role of the therapist is to educate the patient and family about the secondary problems that result from the basic deficits and teach the patient compensatory strategies to maintain function and prevent or minimize further problems.

Amyotrophic Lateral Sclerosis

Amyotrophic lateral sclerosis (ALS), also known as Lou Gehrig's disease (after the famous baseball player), is a rapidly progressive neurological disorder associated with the degeneration of motor nerve cells. Its cause is unknown. The median age at onset is in the fifties.[4] ALS is characterized by weakness, atrophy (loss of muscle bulk), and fasciculations (muscle twitches). The weakness can be present in limb muscles and cause difficulty in functional activities or can be present in the muscles involved in speech, swallowing, and breathing and cause difficulty in communication, feeding, and respiration. Regardless of

8

where it begins, eventually all muscles are involved. Currently, no cure is available for this disease, and the survival time is about 4 years from diagnosis to death. Recently, some medications have been shown to slow progression of the disease and prolong life by several months.

The role of the therapist is to provide preventive and supportive care for the secondary problems of weakness, recommend appropriate devices and equipment to keep the patient as independent as possible, and educate the family and caregivers regarding handling of the patient. (See also Chapters 11 and 12 for additional neuromuscular conditions common to specific age groups.)

PRINCIPLES OF EXAMINATION

The goal of physical therapy is to improve or maintain functional movements and prevent decline. Functional movements include not only the activities of daily living (dressing, eating, bathing, etc.), but also those necessary for educational, vocational, and recreational purposes. Thus, likely candidates for physical therapy are individuals with disorders of movement or function resulting from involvement of the neuromuscular system.

To assess the cause of movement dysfunction, the contributing factors need to be examined individually and collectively. Most patients with neurological problems are referred to physical therapy after extensive evaluation by a neurologist, physiatrist, or both. The first step in patient evaluation is to review all the pertinent medical records and data. The therapist will need to make note of not only the current conditions and problems but also any previous problems or current comorbid conditions that will affect the prognosis. The therapist will also need to note psychological, emotional, and social factors that may have an impact.

A therapist needs to be familiar with and understand the results and implications of special tests used by physicians to arrive at the medical (etiological or pathological) diagnosis. Some of the tests commonly used include radiography (use of x-rays on photographic film), **computed (axial) tomography** (**CAT** or **CT**—computer synthesis of x-rays transmitted through a specific plane of the body), **magnetic resonance imaging** (**MRI**—creation of computer images by placing the body part in a magnetic field), angiography, lumbar puncture, and electrodiagnostic tests.[1] CT scans and MRIs have become available only during the past two decades as a result of improved (CT) and new (MRI) technologies. They have revolutionized diagnostic capabilities by providing three-dimensional and cross-sectional images of internal structures, including the brain and spinal cord. These tests provide better visualization and differentiation of tissues such as bone, nerve cells, and blood as they relate to the brain and spinal cord. **Angiography** involves injecting radiopaque material into blood vessels to better visualize and identify problems such as occlusion (blockage) of blood vessels, aneurysms, and vascular malformations.

Lumbar puncture is a procedure used for three main purposes: (1) to measure intracranial pressure, (2) to inject a radiopaque substance for a myelogram, or (3) to obtain a sample of cerebrospinal fluid for examination. The procedure is performed under local anesthesia. A needle is inserted in the space between the L3 and L4 vertebrae until it reaches the subarachnoid space, and then, depending on the purpose of the lumbar puncture, the appropriate procedure is performed. Cerebrospinal fluid is examined for its chemical and cellular content—that is, the specific type and number of cells present. It is also used to identify or obtain bacteriological or viral cultures.

Electrodiagnostic tests are also very helpful in identifying the specific neurological disorder. **Electroencephalography (EEG)** involves recording the electrical potential/activity in the brain by placing electrodes on the scalp. This test is essential in the diagnosis and management of patients with seizure disorders. **Electromyography (EMG)** involves recording the electrical activity in muscle during a state of rest and during voluntary contraction. It helps differentiate disorders primarily related to muscle pathology and those secondary to nerve or neuromuscular junction disorders. A **nerve conduction velocity (NCV) study** involves recording the rate at which electrical signals are transmitted along peripheral nerves. These studies help clarify and differentiate disorders that affect the axons as opposed to those that affect the myelin sheath covering the axons. In many cases, the physical therapist performs the diagnostic tests, such as an EMG or NCV, and provides information directly to the individual.

Knowledge of these tests and the results not only gives the therapist a better understanding of the disorder and its implications and progression but also enables the therapist to respond appropriately to questions that the patient may have about these procedures.

The next step in the evaluation is an interview with the patient or a family member or caregiver. The interview gives the therapist an opportunity to hear firsthand the sequence of events that brought the patient to therapy. It allows the therapist to ask specific questions that will provide information about the patient's premorbid (prediscase) lifestyle and functional level, as well as assess the patient's cognitive and communicative capabilities. The interview also provides the patient and family members with an opportunity to voice concerns and hopes about what the individual wants to achieve through therapy. This interchange between patient and therapist is extremely important in setting realistic short- and long-term goals and expectations. It is a process that will occur periodically as conditions change and goals are met. (See also Subjective Examination in Chapter 7.)

8

Cognition

Functions such as orientation, attentiveness, long- and short-term memory, reasoning, and judgment can be impaired in disorders of the central nervous system and can have a major impact on the patient's ability to function in daily activities and return to school or work. If these impairments are present, they may be more thoroughly evaluated by a neuropsychologist, who can then also act as a resource for other team members regarding strategies to manage the problems. For example, patients with TBI often exhibit behavioral problems. To address these problems successfully, it is important that everyone in contact with the person respond similarly to such behavior and give consistent responses. The specific strategies chosen would be determined by discussion among the team of care providers and the neuropsychologist and would be based on an evaluation and understanding of the underlying phenomena.

Communication

Communication is another area that will have a major impact on how the therapist works with the patient. If the patient exhibits a diminished ability to receive and interpret verbal or written communication (**receptive aphasia**) or has an impaired ability to communicate by speech (**expressive aphasia**), the therapist again will have to use specific strategies to work with the patient successfully. For example, when working with patients with receptive aphasia, the therapist may need to physically mime or demonstrate to the patient what is expected or required and to use gestures to augment the words.

The specific components of the physical therapy examination will be determined by various factors such as the current state of the patient, concurrent conditions, mental and emotional status, age, and other factors. The examination will include some or all aspects of the components described in the next sections.

Functional Activities

The examination may begin with the therapist's asking the patient to first demonstrate or describe activities and movements that the patient can perform and then describe activities that are difficult or that the patient is unable to perform. The most common activities of daily living involve the ability to move and change positions in bed; to get in and out of bed, a chair, and the like; to stand, walk, and climb stairs; and to get up from the floor in case of a fall. In short, these activities involve the ability to assume and maintain a posture and to function in different positions and environmental conditions. Several components are responsible for the smooth and efficient performance of even the simplest and most routine activities. A problem with even a single component can impair function.

Motor Control

The first component to examine in the evaluation of **motor control** is whether the patient is capable of performing voluntary, isolated activity of a specific muscle or whether the patient is capable of performing only movements that are linked together involuntarily. For example, very often in the early stages of recovery after a stroke, a patient is unable to isolate and restrict the activity of bringing the hand to the mouth without the automatic and involuntary activity of raising the shoulder. A second step is to determine whether the patient is able to isolate and *control* specific muscle activity and movements (able to start, stop, reverse, change speed, change direction, regulate force, etc.) and, if so, how well this movement is controlled. A third step is to determine whether the patient exhibits any involuntary movements. Do they occur at rest or with activity? Do the nature and intensity of the involuntary movements change with activity and are the movements detrimental to the patient's overall functioning? Finally, is the patient exhibiting any reflex reactions caused by damage to specific parts of the nervous system? For example, when damage occurs to the cortex, the patient may exhibit certain reflex reactions that are indicative of control exerted by the brain stem. These automatic reactions will prevent the patient from exerting independent and isolated control and thus affect function (see also Chapter 11).

Tone

Tone is tension exerted or maintained by muscles at rest and during movement. In certain conditions, tone is disturbed and a patient may exhibit **hypotonia** (low tone) or **hypertonia** (high tone). This disturbance in tone may be evident at rest, during activities, or in both conditions. The following questions will need to be answered before making a decision regarding any interventions: Is the tone disturbance at a level that affects posture and function? What factors seem to increase or decrease it? Does it have a beneficial or detrimental effect on the patient's ability to function?

Sensation and Perception

Both sensation and perception are essential for normal movement. **Sensation** is the ability to receive sensory input from within and outside the body and transmit it through the peripheral nerves and tracts in the spinal cord to the brain, where it is received and interpreted. Sensory information most essential for movement is visual, vestibular, tactile, and proprioceptive in nature. **Perception** is the ability to both integrate various simultaneous sensory inputs and respond appropriately. It is the ability to respond appropriately that is most often affected in patients with brain lesions, and it has a tremendous impact on movement and function.

Flexibility

Flexibility of the soft tissues, such as muscles and tendons, and alignment and mobility of the joints are important to evaluate. Therapists perform manual tests and use goniometers to help quantify the degree of restriction of movement (see Chapter 7).

Systems Review

The therapist will also perform a quick check of the other body systems such as the cardiopulmonary system. The purpose of this review is to evaluate the role, if any, that problems in these other systems may be playing in the overall functional limitations of the patient.

PRINCIPLES OF EVALUATION, DIAGNOSIS, AND PROGNOSIS

From the preceding brief descriptions, it is apparent that movements and activities that seem so simple are the result of very complex and interconnected mechanisms. Sometimes it takes therapists several sessions to diagnose the movement disorders and functional limitations and identify the components that are responsible. Based on the findings of this detailed evaluation, a plan of care can be drawn up to meet the goal of enhancing movement and function.

PRINCIPLES OF DIRECT INTERVENTION

The human nervous system is an incredible system that because of its plasticity and redundancy is capable of adaptation and modification after injury or disease. The peripheral nervous system also has the additional capacity of regeneration. Creative treatment approaches are necessary to accommodate these characteristics of the nervous system. This is the challenge and reward of working with patients with neuromuscular disorders.

Early approaches to neurological physical therapy focused on poliomyelitis. This disease causes paralysis of muscles from damage to motor nerve cells. It was one of the conditions responsible for the growth and development of physical therapy in the 1920s and 1930s.[10] As the poliomyelitis epidemics subsided, therapists started working with patients with other neurological conditions, such as stroke and cerebral palsy. As therapists worked with these patients, they found that treatments such as hot packs, massage, stretching, and strengthening exercises—which had worked so well with the polio patients—were not appropriate or sufficient for patients with other neurological problems. Therefore, between the 1940s and 1970s several therapists developed a variety of treatment and handling approaches based on their observations of motor behavior in their patients. They also found that they could influence motor behavior with a variety of sensory inputs (e.g., visual, auditory, thermal, tactile, proprioceptive). To understand and explain the phenomena they were observing, they turned to the literature available at the time. The work of neurophysiologists such as Jackson, Sherrington, and Magnus provided some explanations and influenced treatment philosophies. These early approaches are briefly described.

Proprioceptive Neuromuscular Facilitation

Proprioceptive neuromuscular facilitation (PNF) is one of the earliest techniques developed by Dr. Kabat, a neurologist associated with the physical therapists Margaret Knott and Dorothy Voss. Working with patients with MS and cerebral palsy, Dr. Kabat observed that the "one muscle–one joint" approach used in the treatment of patients with polio was not applicable to this group. From his observations of normal human movement, he emphasized that most human activities require multidimensional movements; that is, various muscles at various joints complement and enhance one another's activities. He also observed that motor performance could be facilitated and enhanced by providing the patient with sensory stimuli at specific locations and times within a movement.[17] Such techniques, as their name implies, emphasize proprioceptive (joint and position sense) stimuli, but they also use tactile, visual, and auditory stimuli. These techniques are currently used to enhance movement and motor control not only in patients with neuromuscular problems but also in patients with musculoskeletal problems.

Rood's Approach

Margaret Rood recognized and emphasized the importance of sensory stimuli in arousing, calming, and modulating motor responses. She used a variety of stimuli to influence motor behavior. In addition, she recognized and emphasized the importance of the autonomic nervous system in modulating motor responses.[14]

Brunnstrom's Approach

Signe Brunnstrom worked with patients who had suffered damage to the nervous system from a CVA. She made detailed observations regarding the movement patterns that these patients exhibited as they recovered and was thus able to precisely describe the natural history of recovery of movement and function after a stroke. Based on her observations, as well as her extensive research and interpretation of the literature available, she made specific recommendations (**Brunnstrom's approach**) regarding the sequence of movements and activities that would facilitate recovery and function.[11] Her observations have been replicated, and her recommendations regarding treatment continue to be used.

8

Neurodevelopmental Treatment

Neurodevelopmental treatment (NDT) was developed by Berta Bobath and Karel Bobath, her husband. Berta Bobath worked extensively with children with cerebral palsy and adult patients with stroke. Her theories and treatment approach are based on observations in these patient populations and her interpretation of the works of Jackson, Sherrington, and others. Her hypothesis, especially in regard to adult patients with stroke, asserts that because of the damage caused by the stroke, the patient is unable to direct the nerve impulses appropriately.[3] This defect results in abnormal patterns of coordination in posture and movement and abnormal qualities of tone.[11] The aim of treatment is to inhibit the abnormal patterns of movement and facilitate integrated, automatic reactions and voluntary functional activity.

Techniques based on all these approaches continue to be used to improve motor control. Their efficacy is still being established and researched. No specific technique has proved to be more effective than others, and therapists continue to mix and match them depending on patient needs.

Current Approaches

Over the past 20 years, our understanding of life span **motor development**[16] (age-related processes of change in motor behavior), motor control (neural control of posture and movement), and **motor learning** (process of acquisition or modification of movement) has increased tremendously. This increased understanding has led to a review and re-evaluation of the earlier techniques—those that emphasized inhibitory and facilitatory input and modifying motor behavior through handling.[15] Because they are based on principles of motor learning and skill acquisition, current approaches put less emphasis on passive handling of the patient.[6] They recommend more active involvement by the patient, especially in terms of problem solving and finding appropriate solutions.[5] These approaches emphasize the need for the therapist to create the appropriate environment for learning and the appropriate use of feedback to facilitate learning. Shumway-Cook and Woollacott recommend that assessment and treatment of clinical problems be based on a systems model of motor control in which a more "task-oriented approach is used."[13] They suggest that movement results from a dynamic interplay between perceptual, cognitive, and action systems. They also believe that it is critical to recognize that movement emerges from an interaction between the individual and the task and the environment in which the task is being carried out.

Besides these specific techniques, therapists may choose options that are specifically targeted to the impairments and dysfunction. These techniques include stretching or strengthening exercises to improve flexibility and strength. Other options may be more compensatory or adaptive. For instance, the therapist may teach a patient with impaired sensation in the soles of the feet to rely more on the eyes and visual system for maintenance of balance; another may initiate the use of braces to improve walking in the case of irreversible paralysis of leg muscles. The therapist may also recommend environmental modifications to help the patient function better. Thus, a therapist is constantly challenged to be as creative as possible in treating and managing movement-related problems of function caused by disorders of the nervous system.

Case Study

Jim—Rehabilitation Following Spinal Cord Injury _____

Jim is an 18-year-old who sustained a gunshot wound to his thoracic spine. The shot ruptured his spine and caused damage to the spinal cord that resulted in paralysis below the waist. He also sustained abdominal injuries that required surgery. Jim is now medically stable and has been referred to therapy to begin the long process of rehabilitation.

The first task of the team members (which include a physiatrist, nurse, psychologist, social worker, and physical and occupational therapists) is to complete detailed evaluations. This process may take several days because each team member is working within the constraints imposed by the patient's physical and emotional condition. When all the information is gathered, a team meeting is scheduled to discuss the information with the patient and his family and to start setting some short- and long-term goals.

Even as they were carrying out their evaluations, the team members had already started treatment and management to maintain mobility, increase strength in the uninvolved muscles, and educate the patient about problems arising from loss of sensation. The nurses had initiated a program to manage bowel and bladder function. The psychologist had begun helping Jim cope with the trauma of this unexpected event and the loss of body image and body functions. The social worker was starting to determine Jim's needs on discharge and whether these needs could be met by his family and in the current home environment.

During the next several weeks, the physicians will continue to check Jim thoroughly for any change in or return of sensory or motor activity because that will determine the final prognosis. Other team members will continue to work with Jim to teach the new skills necessary to function within the new reality. The physical therapist will play a major role in teaching and training him in these new skills. The therapist will also be involved in ordering equipment, such as the appropriate wheelchair and cushion, to meet the needs of his lifestyle. The therapist will make recommendations to the family for a ramp to gain access to the house. The family may need to widen doorways and remove carpeting to make wheelchair mobility and access easier. They may need to adapt or build a bathroom and bedroom on the main floor level to meet Jim's needs. They may be able to get some financial help or may end up bearing the complete financial burden themselves.

Not only is Jim dealing with many physical and psychological challenges, but the family also is dealing with many emotional issues. As the therapist trains the family to assist Jim, family members will frequently be very open during these sessions and voice their fears and concerns. The therapist's role is then to provide not only technical support for the physical needs but also psychological and emotional support for both the patient and the family.

Summary ———

The goal of neuromuscular physical therapy is to treat problems of movement and function that result from damage to the nervous system. If the problems are untreatable and progressive, the goal is to teach the patient and caregivers to accommodate and compensate for the problems and prevent secondary complications. To achieve these goals, therapists need to evaluate the components necessary for movement and assess their role in the dysfunction. Based on the findings, the therapist—in conjunction with the patient, family, and other caregivers—will draw up a plan of care with appropriate short- and long-term goals and specific strategies to meet these goals. This process of evaluation, assessment, and treatment will occur periodically as goals are met. If goals become unachievable because of physical, psychological, or social factors, re-evaluation of goals and strategies becomes necessary.

The ultimate objective is to help rehabilitate the patient to function at the highest level attainable within the constraints of the condition.

References

1. Adams RD, Victor M: Special techniques for neurologic diagnosis. *In* Adams RD, Victor M (eds): Principles of Neurology. New York, McGraw-Hill, 1989.

2. Bannister R: Parkinsonism and movement disorders. *In* Bannister R (ed): Brain and Bannister's Clinical Neurology. Oxford, Oxford Medical Publications, 1992.

3. Bobath B: Adult Hemiplegia: Evaluation and Treatment. Oxford, Butterworth-Heinemann, 1990.

4. Brooke M: Diseases of the motor neurons. *In* Brooke M (ed): A Clinician's View of Neuromuscular Diseases. Baltimore, Williams & Wilkins, 1986.

5. Carr JH, Shepherd RB: A Motor Relearning Program for Stroke. Rockville, MD, Aspen, 1987.

6. Carr JH, Shepherd RB: Movement Science, Foundation for Physical Therapy in Rehabilitation. Rockville, MD, Aspen, 1987.

7. Leahy P: Traumatic head injury. *In* O'Sullivan SB, Schmitz TJ (eds): Physical Rehabilitation Assessment and Treatment. Philadelphia, FA Davis, 1994.

8. O'Sullivan SB: Multiple sclerosis. *In* O'Sullivan SB, Schmitz TJ (eds): Physical Rehabilitation Assessment and Treatment. Philadelphia, FA Davis, 1994.

9. O'Sullivan SB: Stroke. *In* O'Sullivan SB, Schmitz TJ (eds): Physical Rehabilitation Assessment and Treatment. Philadelphia, FA Davis, 1994.

10. Pinkston D: Evolution of the practice of physical therapy in the United States. *In* Scully RM, Barnes MR (eds): Physical Therapy. Philadelphia, JB Lippincott, 1989.

11. Sawner K, Lavigne J: Brunnstrom's Movement Therapy in Hemiplegia. Philadelphia, JB Lippincott, 1992.

12. Schmitz TJ: Traumatic spinal cord injury. *In* O'Sullivan SB, Schmitz TJ (eds): Physical Rehabilitation Assessment and Treatment. Philadelphia, FA Davis, 1994.

13. Shumway-Cook A, Woollacott MH: Motor Control: Theory and Practical Applications. Baltimore, Williams & Wilkins, 1995.

14. Stockmeyer SA: An interpretation of the approach of Rood to the treatment of neuromuscular dysfunction. Am J Phys Med 1967;46:900–961.

15. Umphred DN: Merging neurophysiologic approaches with contemporary theories. *In* Lister MJ (ed): Contemporary Management of Motor Control Problems. Alexandria, VA, Foundation for Physical Therapy, 1991.

16. VanSant AF: Life span motor development. *In* Lister MJ (ed): Contemporary Management of Motor Control Problems. Alexandria, VA, Foundation for Physical Therapy, 1991.

17. Voss DE, Ionta MK, Myers BJ, et al: Proprioceptive Neuromuscular Facilitation, ed 3. Philadelphia, Harper & Row, 1985.

Suggested Readings

The following is a list of books published for patients and their families to gain a better understanding of the causes, clinical features, diagnostic procedures, treatment and management principles, and roles of the various team members in caring for patients with the noted disorders.

Caroscio JT (ed): Amyotrophic Lateral Sclerosis: A Guide for Patient Care. New York, Thieme, 1986.

Duvoisin RC (ed): Parkinson's Disease: A Guide for Patients and Their Families, ed 3. New York, Raven, 1991.

Faye-Pierson J, Toole JF (eds): Stroke: A Guide for Patients and Their Families. New York, Raven, 1987.

Philips L, et al (eds): Spinal Cord Injury: A Guide for Patients and Their Families. New York, Raven, 1987.

Ringel SP (ed): Neuromuscular Disorders: A Guide for Patient Care. New York, Raven, 1987.

Schienberg LC (ed): Multiple Sclerosis: A Guide for Patients and Their Families. New York, Raven, 1983.

REVIEW QUESTIONS

1. Why might the physical therapy plan of care change several times for a patient recovering from a stroke?

2. List the kinds of information you might hope to gain from interviewing the patient and family. What other insights does the interview provide?

3. Contrast the differing roles that the physical therapist and physical therapist assistant may assume, depending on the nature of the patient's neurological condition (e.g., contrast the physical therapist's roles in the care of patients with the following: spinal cord injury, stroke, Parkinson's disease, and amyotrophic lateral sclerosis).

4. Describe the purposes of at least three diagnostic tests in neuromuscular disorders. How do they differ in procedure as well?

5. What purpose do body jackets, braces, assistive devices, and environmental modifications serve in neuromuscular rehabilitation?

8

Those aspects of physical therapy commonly referred to as cardiopulmonary physical therapy are fully recognized as fundamental components of the knowledge and practice base for all entry-level physical therapists.
E.A. Hillegass, PT, and H.S. Sadowsky, PT

Physical Therapy in Cardiopulmonary Conditions

Ray A. Boone

GENERAL DESCRIPTION
   Prevalence
   The Cardiovascular System
   The Pulmonary System
   Cardiovascular and Pulmonary System
      Integration

COMMON CONDITIONS
   Cardiovascular Diseases
   Lung Diseases

PRINCIPLES OF EXAMINATION
   Cardiovascular Diagnostic Tests and
      Procedures
   Pulmonary Diagnostic Tests and Procedures

PRINCIPLES OF EVALUATION, DIAGNOSIS,
AND PROGNOSIS

PRINCIPLES OF DIRECT INTERVENTION
   Medical Management
   Surgical Management

KEY TERMS

angina

angioplasty

arteriosclerosis

blood gas analysis

cardiac catheterization

cardiac muscle dysfunction

cardiac pacemaker

chronic obstructive pulmonary disease
(COPD)

conducting airways

congestive heart failure (CHF)

coronary artery bypass grafting (CABG)

coronary heart disease (CHD)

dyspnea

echocardiography

electrocardiogram (ECG)

embolus

exercise stress testing

expiration

heart failure

inspiration

ischemia

myocardial infarction

obstructive lung disease

postural drainage

pulmonary function test

respiration

restrictive lung disease

spirometer

target heart rate (THR)

training zone

ventilation

OBJECTIVES   After reading this chapter, the reader will be able to

- Describe the normal anatomy and physiology of the cardiopulmonary system
- Define and describe the effects of common diseases that alter normal function of the cardiopulmonary system
- Outline how the functions of the cardiopulmonary system are evaluated both normally and when disease is present
- Discuss how physical therapists examine, evaluate, and provide interventions to individuals who have cardiopulmonary disease

**GENERAL
DESCRIPTION**

Prevalence

Less than 30 years ago, people with cardiopulmonary conditions had little hope of leading normal lives. In fact, in certain instances exercise was considered deleterious to such people. Today, the physical therapist and physical therapist assistant play major roles as team members for these patients to enhance their function and improve the quality of their daily lives.

Common cardiopulmonary conditions are described later in this chapter; however, it is important to recognize the prevalence of these conditions in the United States. Some form of cardiovascular disease (CVD) develops in 1 in 3 men and 1 in 10 women before the age of 60, and it has recently been estimated that nearly 60 million Americans have one or more types of this disease.[3] CVD is the leading cause of death in American males and females and has been annually since 1900 except for 1918 (Fig. 9–1). About every 33 seconds an American will die of CVD. As a subgroup of CVD, coronary heart disease (CHD) accounts for nearly half of the deaths from CVD (Fig. 9–2). Current estimates indicate that over 12 million Americans have CHD. Another 4.6 million have congestive heart failure (CHF).[3]

Further estimates reflect the prevalence of myocardial infarction (MI), or heart attack. In 1999 it was estimated that 1,100,000 people would have a new or recurrent MI, with 650,000 being a first MI and 450,000 being recurrent MIs. At least 250,000 people die within 1 hour of having an MI. These sudden deaths are usually caused by an abnormal rhythm developing in the heart after the infarction. About two thirds of all those who have a heart attack do not

9

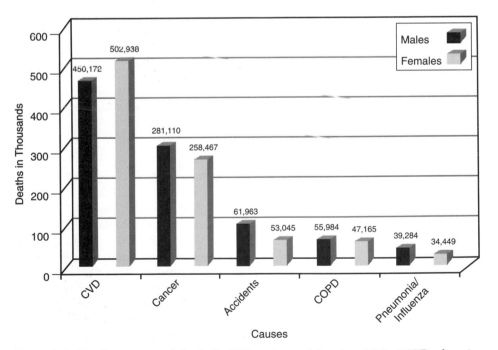

Figure 9–1. Leading causes of death for U.S. males and females, 1997. COPD, chronic obstructive pulmonary disease; CVD, cerebrovascular disease. (Data from Cardiovascular Diseases. Retrieved from *http://www.americanheart.org/statistics/03.html*, American Heart Association, 1999.)

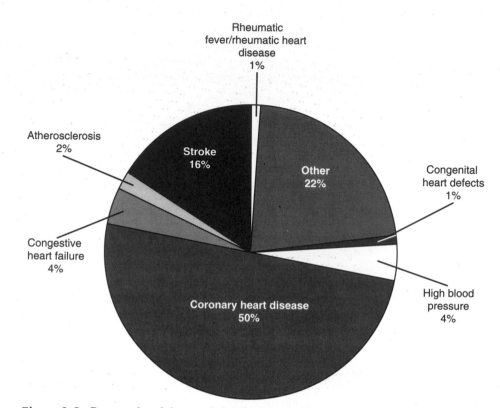

Figure **9–2.** Percent breakdown of deaths in the United States from cardiovascular diseases, 1997. COPD, chronic obstructive pulmonary disease; CVD, cerebrovascular disease. (Data from Cardiovascular Diseases. Retrieved from *http://www.americanheart.org/ statistics/03.html*, American Heart Association, 1999.)

completely recover to their previous functional levels; however, 80% of those younger than 65 return to work.[17]

Data available from the National Center for Health Statistics indicate that in 1995, an estimated 16.4 million Americans suffered from chronic obstructive pulmonary disease (COPD).[17] This disease is more common in men than women; however, the incidence in women has more than doubled since 1979 while remaining relatively stable in men. COPD is composed of many diagnostic groups, the most common being emphysema and chronic bronchitis. Chronic bronchitis affects people of all ages, whereas emphysema is more concentrated in the elderly. Of the nearly 2 million people with emphysema in 1995, 93% were 45 years of age or older, whereas of the 14.5 million people with chronic bronchitis, only 37% were 45 years of age or older.[26]

The annual cost to our economy to care for individuals with heart or lung disease is tremendous. Medicare provided $26.1 billion in payments to its beneficiaries in 1996 for hospital expenses from CVD.[3] For individuals with COPD, $13.6 billion was expended on direct health care costs in 1998.[26]

Both heart and lung diseases are chronic diseases. Various types of medically trained personnel become involved in caring for people with these problems. Physical therapists and physical therapist assistants who work with patients with cardiopulmonary disease must have a thorough understanding of the normal anatomy and physiology of these systems. With this knowledge, appropriate treatment programs can be developed.

The Cardiovascular System

Heart. In an adult, the heart is found in the center of the chest (mediastinum), with the base located superiorly and the apex inferiorly and left of center. The major portion of the heart is made up of muscle tissue referred to as the myocardium. This tissue is layered with muscle fibers running in multiple directions.[29]

The heart has two pairs of matched chambers. The two atria are thin-walled chambers, whereas the two ventricles have much thicker muscular walls (Fig. 9–3).[22] These chambers are separated by valves that direct the blood through the chambers in a specific pattern.

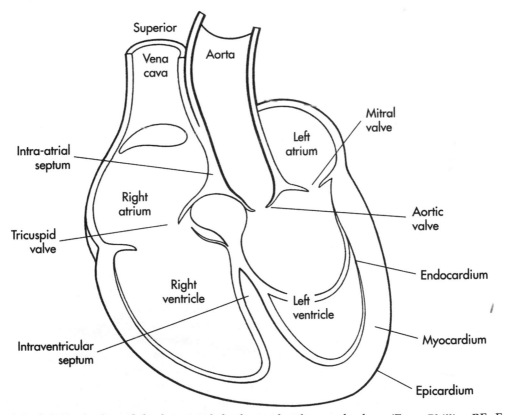

Figure 9–3. Schematic view of the heart and the heart chambers and valves. (From Phillips RE, Feeney MK: The Cardiac Rhythms, ed 2. Philadelphia, WB Saunders, 1980.)

9

The right atrium receives venous blood from the body through the superior and inferior venae cavae. With atrial contraction (atrial systole), the blood then passes through the tricuspid valve into the right ventricle (Fig. 9–4A).[22] The left atrium receives oxygenated blood through the pulmonary veins coming from the lungs. During atrial systole, this oxygenated blood passes through the bicuspid (mitral) valve into the left ventricle (Fig. 9–4B).

Once the right and left ventricles have received blood from their respective atria, ventricular contraction (ventricular systole) occurs. This contraction results in an increase in pressure in the ventricular chambers, which causes the tricuspid and bicuspid valves to close tightly and prevents blood from passing back into the atria. As ventricular contraction continues, venous blood leaves the right ventricle through the pulmonic or semilunar valve and flows into the lungs to be reoxygenated. Oxygenated blood leaves the left ventricle through the aortic valve into the aorta to be transported to the body through the systemic circulation.

It is significant that the ventricles have thicker muscular walls than the atria.

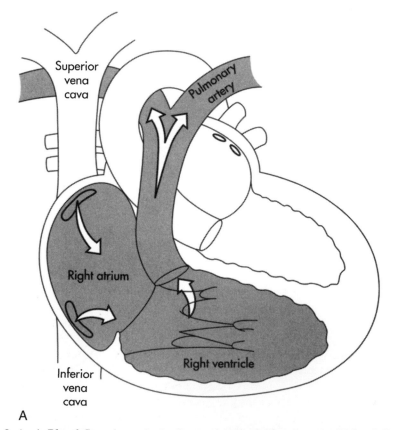

Figure 9–4. *A,* Blood flow through the heart chambers: deoxygenated blood flow from the right atrium to the right ventricle to the lungs through the pulmonary artery.

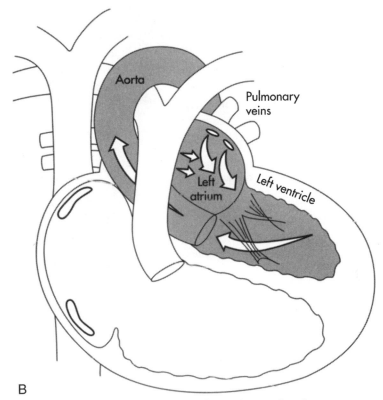

B

Figure 9–4 *Continued. B,* Blood flow through the heart chambers: oxygenated blood returning to the left atrium from the lungs via the pulmonary veins, moving into the left ventricle, and exiting through the aorta. (From Phillips RE, Feeney MK: The Cardiac Rhythms, ed 2. Philadelphia, WB Saunders, 1980.)

This greater muscle mass, especially in the left ventricle, must provide enough force to overcome the resistance to flow that blood encounters as it moves through the peripheral arteries.[21]

Conduction. The myocardium contains special types of tissue responsible for conducting the electrical impulse causing the myocardium to contract in a synchronized pattern. This synchronized depolarization and repolarization of cardiac muscle results in efficient movement of blood through the chambers of the heart and through the coronary and peripheral vessels.

These specialized tissues are called nodal and Purkinje fibers (Fig. 9–5).[25] The sinoatrial node (SA node) initiates the impulse (sinus rhythm) and is sometimes called the pacemaker of the heart. Once a signal is initiated by the SA node, it travels quickly through the walls of the atria on special tracts to the atrioventricular node (AV node). The impulse also travels to the muscle fibers of the atria and causes them to contract. The AV node transports the signal to the bundle of His, which is where the Purkinje fibers start to spread out into the muscle fibers of the ventricles. For every heartbeat or contraction, the

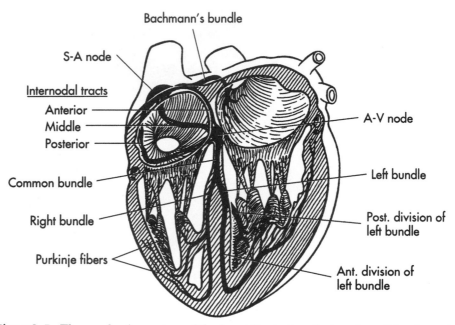

Figure 9–5. The conduction system of the heart illustrating the location of the sinoatrial (S-A) and atrioventricular (A-V) nodes. (From Sanderson RG, Kurth CL: The Cardiac Patient: A Comprehensive Approach, ed 2. Philadelphia, WB Saunders, 1983.)

depolarization signal that causes the myocardium to contract must travel through this conduction system.

Both the SA and AV nodes receive autonomic nerve fibers via the sympathetic and parasympathetic systems. These nerve fibers release special neurotransmitters that influence the rate of contraction and myocardial contractility. The ability to influence the heart's rate and contractility is extremely important because this mechanism allows the central nervous system to tell the heart how to respond to increases in demand, such as those made during exercise.[21]

Coronary Arteries. The myocardium receives its blood supply from two major vessels, the right and left coronary arteries (Fig. 9–6).[19] These arteries arise from the ascending aorta, which is the major artery leaving the left ventricle and carrying blood to the body (see Fig. 9–3). In general, the right and left coronary vessels supply the right and left sides of the heart, respectively; however, this arrangement can vary a great deal among individuals. If something occurs that causes blockage of a coronary vessel, it is important to determine exactly how that blockage alters blood flow to the individual's myocardium. When blockage occurs, the person has had a heart attack (MI).

Peripheral Circulation. The blood vessels that make up the peripheral circulation are arteries, capillaries, and veins, and disorders in these vessels can result in cardiopulmonary dysfunction. Physical therapists and physical therapist assis-

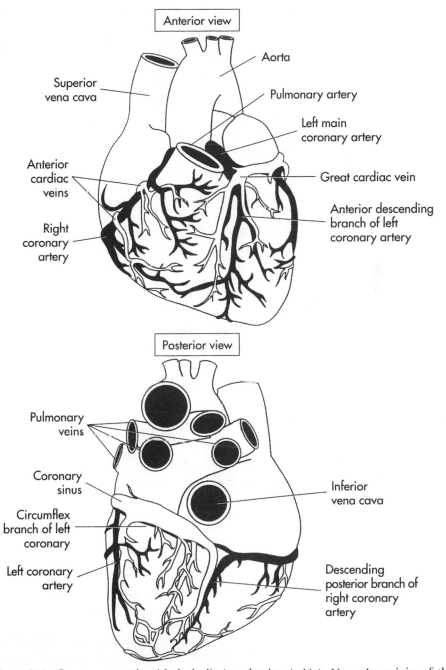

Figure 9–6. Coronary arteries (*dark shading*) and veins (*white*). Note the origin of the arteries from the aorta. (From McArdle WD, Katch FI, Katch VL: Exercise Physiology—Energy, Nutrition, and Human Performance, ed 3. Philadelphia, Lea & Febiger, 1991.)

9

tants work with a variety of patients who have disabilities caused by pathological changes in the peripheral circulation.

The arteries, the largest in diameter being the aorta, and the arterioles have elastic fibers and smooth muscle in their walls. If the smooth muscle contracts, the diameter of the vessel is decreased, which causes an increase in the resistance to blood flow through the vessels. Arterioles are often referred to as "resistance vessels." Changes in resistance to blood flow in the peripheral circulation directly affect how hard the heart has to work to pump blood through the body. A disease called arteriosclerosis, which is often referred to as "hardening of the arteries," causes plaque to build up on the inner wall and decreases the elasticity of the vessel, with subsequently higher resistance to blood flow.

Capillaries are the smallest vessels in the peripheral circulation. They connect arteries to veins and can be so small that they will allow only one red blood cell to pass through at a time. Their walls are only one cell thick, which allows for efficient exchange of oxygen and carbon dioxide. Nutrients and waste products also pass through the wall. Capillaries are often referred to as "exchange vessels."

The veins, which return blood to the heart from the body, have much less elastic fiber and smooth muscle in their walls. The larger veins can act as a blood reservoir and are often called "capacitance vessels."

The Pulmonary System

Respiration. **Respiration** is the process of exchanging oxygen and carbon dioxide between the air we breathe and blood cells that pass through the lungs. **Ventilation** is the process of exchanging air between the atmosphere and the lungs through inspiration and expiration.[7] The mechanics of inspiration and expiration depend on many factors, including the structure of the lungs, chest, and muscles. **Inspiration** occurs when the muscles of ventilation, the most important being the diaphragm, contract to cause an increase in the space within the thoracic cavity. This expansion causes air pressure to drop inside the lungs, which causes air to move into the lungs. **Expiration** is the reverse of this process.

If increased amounts of oxygen need to be delivered to the body, such as during exercise, the amount of air that must flow into and out of the lungs must markedly increase. When this situation occurs, the muscles of ventilation must work extensively. When disease affects the lungs, the results can be the same. In this case, however, the body is not requiring more oxygen. The ability of air to normally move into and out of the lungs is compromised because of blockage of the tubes that conduct the air. This obstruction results in high resistance to airflow and increased work for the muscles of ventilation.[27]

Conducting Airways and Lungs. **Conducting airways** are the passageways and tubes that transport air into and out of the lungs. The upper conducting airway includes the nose, pharynx, and larynx. This component of the air transport system cleans and humidifies the air and terminates at the beginning of the

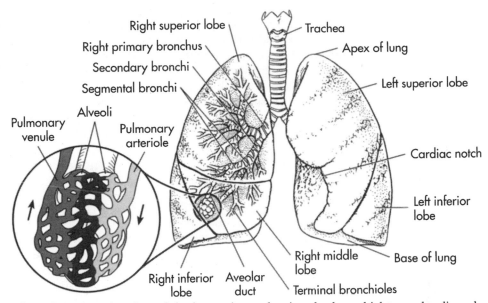

Figure 9–7. Anterior view of the lower airway showing the bronchial tree, alveoli, and the pulmonary circulation. (From Van De Graaff KM, Fox SI: Concepts of Human Anatomy and Physiology, ed 2. Dubuque, IA, WC Brown, 1989.)

trachea. The lower conducting airway is made up of the trachea and bronchiole system (Fig. 9–7).[27] The bronchiole system consists of tubes branching from the main bronchus out to the terminal bronchioles. It is here that the conduction system ends and air enters into the alveolus, where gas exchange takes place. The alveolus is surrounded by capillaries that contain deoxygenated blood coming from the right ventricle of the heart. It is at this junction that oxygen and carbon dioxide are exchanged, with the reoxygenated blood returning to the left atrium. The lungs are compartmentalized into a system of lobes, which are present because of the structure of the bronchial airway system (see Fig. 9–7). A special membrane, the pleura, covers the outer surface of the lungs and the inner surface of the chest wall. The pleura is extremely important to the process of ventilation and maintenance of the continuity of the lungs.[29]

Cardiovascular and Pulmonary System Integration

When considering the importance of how the cardiovascular and pulmonary systems interact with each other, all one has to do is realize that when disease affects one system, eventually the other system will also be affected. For example, if arteriosclerosis develops in the coronary vessels, the amount of oxygen going to the heart muscle will be decreased. With time, the heart muscle begins to fail and will not pump blood to the lungs and body efficiently. Eventually, this insufficiency results in an increase in blood volume and pressure in the lungs, which in turn causes a decrease in lung efficiency and, finally, permanent damage.

9

The degree of success that physical therapists or physical therapist assistants have in establishing appropriate examination or intervention procedures for individuals with cardiovascular or pulmonary disease depends in part on how well they understand how each system functions and interacts. The following section briefly describes common cardiovascular and lung diseases that are treated by physical therapy.

COMMON CONDITIONS

Cardiovascular Diseases

Two major categories of disease processes influence the myocardium: ischemic conditions and cardiac muscle dysfunction.[14]

Ischemic Conditions. **Ischemia** occurs in the presence of insufficient blood flow and results in inadequate oxygenation of tissues because of a blocked blood vessel. In CVD, **arteriosclerosis** (hardening of the arteries) affects the coronary vessels and is commonly called **coronary heart disease. Angina** is the condition in which chest pain occurs from ischemia of the heart muscle.

The etiology of arteriosclerosis, which can affect all vessels of the body, is not completely understood. It has been made clear, however, that the severity of the arteriosclerotic process can be influenced by many risk factors (Table 9–1).[13] Some of these factors cannot be changed, such as having a family history of CHD. However, most of these risk factors can be altered or eliminated completely by changing behavior. Physical therapists and physical therapist assistants help patients with cardiac dysfunction try to alter their behavior as they progress through the rehabilitation process.

Cardiac Muscle Dysfunction. **Cardiac muscle dysfunction** refers to various pathologies associated with heart failure.[14] **Heart failure** occurs when a disease process or congenital defect either directly or indirectly causes a decrease in

---

Table 9–1
Risk Factors that Promote the Development of Coronary Heart Disease

MAJOR RISK FACTORS	MINOR RISK FACTORS
Cigarette smoking	Family history
Hypertension (high blood pressure)	Diabetes
Elevated cholesterol	Age
	Gender
	Stress
	Obesity
	Sedentary lifestyle

Data from Heart and Stroke Statistical Update. Dallas, American Heart Association, 1998.

the pumping capability of the heart muscle. These disease processes can occur either acutely or over time. An example of an acute change in the heart's pumping capability is the occurrence of a **myocardial infarction** (heart attack). In this case, one of the coronary arteries suddenly becomes blocked by an **embolus** (clot). When embolism occurs, blood flow to heart muscle beyond the embolus stops, and that part of the heart muscle no longer receiving blood dies. If this embolus causes an interruption in blood flow to a large amount of heart muscle, death can result.

If an individual survives a heart attack, other symptoms may develop that further complicate the condition. One of the major complications after infarction is an abnormal rhythm in the sequence of heart muscle contraction (abnormal conduction). This problem makes the heart contraction very inefficient. If the left ventricle is seriously damaged from the infarct, it may not contract strongly enough to move the blood through the body appropriately. This deficiency can cause the blood to back up into the lungs, or it may seriously limit function, such as the heart's ability to respond to an increase in physical activity.

When the heart muscle is compromised to the point that it cannot move blood volume effectively, **congestive heart failure** will develop. This disorder can occur acutely or chronically. When CHF is present, the ventricles are not adequately pumping the appropriate volume from their chambers. When the right ventricle is not contracting efficiently, blood volume backs into the venous system and fluid collects in the liver, abdominal cavity, and legs. If the left ventricle does not contract appropriately, an abnormal amount of blood volume remains in the lungs and results in fluid collection. The right ventricle then has to work harder because it must try to push blood into the lungs against increased resistance. This increased workload will eventually lead to compromised function of the right ventricle (see Fig. 9–4A).

A person with CHF has many clinical problems. If fluid collects in the lungs, breathing becomes more difficult and the blood is not oxygenated appropriately. If fluid has collected in the legs, walking becomes more difficult. Because of increasing difficulty in performing activities, the patient would have to expend more energy to accomplish simple tasks. With increased energy expenditure, the heart would have to work harder to support simple functional activities. A physical therapist responsible for exercising a patient with these types of problems must have a thorough understanding of how these disease processes compromise function in order to develop an appropriate treatment program.

Lung Diseases

Diseases of the lung are generally classified as being obstructive or restrictive. If pathological changes in the lung cause an abnormality in airflow through the bronchial tubes, the process is defined as **obstructive lung disease**, whereas if pathological changes cause the volume of air in the lungs to be reduced, the process is defined as **restrictive lung disease**.[14] How lung diseases are classified

9

is still the subject of a great deal of controversy. What is most important is that the common diseases that change lung function eventually demonstrate both obstructive and restrictive characteristics.[2]

Chronic Obstructive Pulmonary Disease. **Chronic obstructive pulmonary disease** is a group of disorders that produce certain specific physical symptoms. These symptoms include chronic productive cough, excessive mucus production, changes in the sound produced when air passes through the bronchial tubes, and shortness of breath **(dyspnea).** The specific disorders that can produce these changes include chronic bronchitis (inflammation of the bronchi), emphysema (trapping air in the alveoli), and peripheral airway disease (collapsing of terminal bronchioles). Other disorders sometimes included in this disease group include bronchial asthma (spasm-like contraction of bronchi resulting in air trapping) and cystic fibrosis (dysfunction of mucous glands, causing blockage of bronchi).[2] Differences between these obstructive diseases include their etiology (cause), pathology (what tissues are affected and how they are changed), and management. However, all of them cause similar symptoms in varying degrees.

The signs and symptoms that develop as COPD progresses include bronchial wall abnormalities causing a decrease in lumen size and alveolar destruction. This process results in air's being trapped in the lungs, which causes the lungs to become hyperinflated, and in a decrease in gas exchange in the alveoli, which results in hypoxemia (below-normal oxygenation of blood). Hypoxemia occurs when the lungs cannot adequately supply oxygen to or retrieve carbon dioxide from the red blood cells as the cells pass by the alveoli.

As resistance to airflow increases because of the decreasing lumen size of the bronchioles, the thorax enlarges as a result of air trapping. This enlargement of the thorax causes the respiratory muscles to work harder. With time, the effectiveness of the respiratory muscles decreases. With chronic hypoxemia, changes begin to occur in the function of the heart, in blood pressure, and in the thickness of the blood. All these changes can lead to respiratory failure.[2, 14]

Restrictive Lung Diseases. Restrictive lung diseases cause a decrease in the ability of the lungs to expand, which results in a decrease in the volume of air that can move into and out of the lungs. The most common cause of this disease process that affects lung tissue directly is idiopathic, or unknown. Other causes include chronic inhalation of air pollutants such as coal dust, silicon, or asbestos. Infections such as pneumonia, cancer of the lung, and changes in heart function (causing chronic fluid collection in the lungs) can also result in restrictive changes. Diseases or trauma to the nerve supply to the muscles of ventilation or disease of the muscles themselves can also result in decreased movement of the chest wall. Thus, many disease groups and structural changes in the chest wall can cause restrictive changes.

The signs and symptoms that develop as restrictive disease progresses include some of the same changes seen in COPD, including shortness of breath and chronic cough. However, in the case of restrictive lung disease, the cough is nonproductive (does not bring mucus out of the lungs). Other changes include tachypnea, or an increase in the rate of breathing, which results in a marked increase in the amount of energy expended on breathing. This increased energy cost can be so severe that it results in weight loss and an emaciated appearance. Patients with restrictive lung disease are also subject to the problems associated with hypoxemia.[2, 14]

PRINCIPLES OF EXAMINATION

The examination performed by physical therapists and physical therapist assistants is an inclusive process that involves not only the patient but also the family and other caregivers who are participating in the overall care of the patient. It includes a review of the patient's past medical and social history, review of the body systems, and tests and measures to gather data about the patient's condition. Areas reviewed include not only physical parameters but also functional, psychological, social, and employment conditions. The tests and measures that are selected to examine a patient/client depend on various parameters, including the age of the patient/client; severity of the problem; stage of recovery (acute, subacute, chronic); phase of rehabilitation (early, intermediate, late, return to activity); and home, community, and work status.[12] Table 9–2 describes tests and measures commonly performed when examining patients with cardiopulmonary conditions.[12]

Other diagnostic tests of the cardiovascular and pulmonary systems beyond the scope of the physical therapist often require invasive techniques and generally place the patient at a certain amount of risk. It is essential that physical therapists understand the results of these tests to understand the severity of the pathology and establish an appropriate plan of care.

Cardiovascular Diagnostic Tests and Procedures

9

Invasive Procedures. Various pieces of equipment can be used to assess how the heart is functioning or how adequately blood is flowing through an artery. Invasive procedures used to evaluate heart function require some type of instrument to be placed in the body or injection of dye into the blood. One of the most common invasive procedures used to assess heart function is **cardiac catheterization.** The procedure requires passing a catheter (a flexible tube) into an artery in the leg until it reaches the heart. The catheter can then be placed in the chambers of the left heart or in the coronary arteries or pulmonary veins. The catheter can have a special sensory device on the tip to measure pressure; thus, its use allows assessment of how much pressure is being generated in chambers of the heart. This measure in turn evaluates the strength of myocardial contraction. Dye can be released directly into the coronary arteries from the catheter, and a special type of imaging technique can then record how well blood flows through the vessels and demonstrate where blockage has occurred. The catheter could also have a small camera in the tip to allow viewing of the heart chamber valves and the inside of the coronary vessels. Other types of invasive procedures may also be performed, all of

Table 9–2
Description of Common Tests and Measures for Patients with Cardiopulmonary Conditions

FUNCTION/CHARACTERISTIC	DESCRIPTION
Home, work, and community (job/play/school)	Analysis of the home and/or work environments to determine the level of functional capacity needed to perform safely within these environments. Examination of the patient's capacity to function at an appropriate level of social interaction with various populations, e.g., family, peers, strangers
Ergonomics and body mechanics	Determination of the dynamic capabilities required of the patient to safely perform within various environments, e.g., home, work, school, leisure
Aerobic capacity and endurance	Assessment of cardiopulmonary performance during controlled exercise and functional activities. Can include measuring oxygen consumption, heart and respiratory rates, blood pressure, dyspnea, and blood gases; electrocardiogram; and heart and lung auscultation
Ventilation and respiration	Assessment of pulmonary function, arterial blood gases, airway clearance efficiency, and perceived exertion and dyspnea during and after exercise; measurements of strength and endurance of muscles of ventilation and of chest wall mobility and expansion
Anthropometric characteristics	Determination of body fat composition
Muscle strength and endurance	Assessment of functional muscle strength and endurance as they relate to exercise protocols
Posture	Assessment of posture abnormalities and their effect on energy cost during movement
Range of motion	Assessment of limitations in joint range of motion and impact on energy cost during movement

Data from Guide to Physical Therapist Practice. 2nd ed. Phys Ther 2001; 81:9–744.

which require highly trained personnel and sophisticated equipment. These procedures are expensive and generally involve some risk to the patient.[25]

Noninvasive Procedures. Noninvasive procedures are also used to assess heart function. Some of the more common procedures include echocardiography, electrocardiography, and exercise testing. **Echocardiography** is the use of high-frequency ultrasound to assess the size of the heart chambers, the thickness of the chamber walls, and the motion of the chamber walls and heart valves. Generally, the transducer (device that produces the ultrasound and records the returning echo) is placed on the chest wall. However, in some cases the transducer is placed in the esophagus to improve the accuracy of its recording and allow assessment of the posterior aspect of the heart.[25]

One of the most common and inexpensive methods of noninvasive evaluation of heart function is the **electrocardiogram (ECG).** Physical therapists who work with individuals being monitored by ECG must be able to interpret normal and abnormal ECG readings. This ability requires a basic understanding of the anatomy and conduction system of the heart (see Fig. 9–5).

As previously discussed, the conduction system is responsible for initiating depolarization or contraction of the heart muscle. When the conduction and muscle tissues depolarize, a change in electrical potential occurs across the individual cell membranes. This minute electrical change is detected by special electrodes placed on the skin of the anterior chest wall, and the "signal" can be recorded by an ECG machine (Fig. 9–8).[14]

The ECG assesses the heart's rate and rhythm (Fig. 9–9).[14] When the heart is functioning normally, it produces a consistent ECG pattern. As seen in Figure 9–9, different components of the waveform are assigned names and represent specific events in the heart cycle. For example, the P wave represents atrial depolarization, and the QRS complex represents ventricular depolarization (contraction). If the heart does not depolarize in a normal way or if part of the heart muscle is not functioning correctly, characteristic changes would be seen in the ECG. Other heart problems that can be assessed by ECG include heart muscle hypertrophy and the presence of MI.[8]

Exercise stress testing is a noninvasive method of determining how the cardiovascular and pulmonary systems respond to controlled increases in activity. This technique of assessment is most frequently used to diagnose suspected or established CVD. However, it is also valuable in other applications, such as assessing a patient's performance after coronary artery bypass surgery or heart valve replacement. Often, the exercise stress test is used to assess someone's functional status or help prescribe limitations for occupational activities.[1]

A physical therapist can be involved in administering an exercise stress test. Generally, the therapist is required to have special training in the techniques of testing, especially if the testing protocol requires the patient to exercise at maximum capability. At a minimum, the physical therapist must be able to interpret the data recorded during a stress test to establish a patient's appropriate level of exercise prescription, which should include a specific description of exercise intensity, duration, frequency, and mode.

9

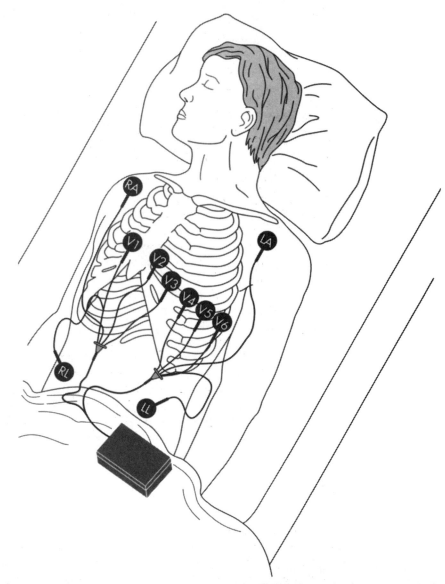

Figure 9–8. Electrode placement for electrocardiogram monitoring. (From Hillegass EA, Sadowsky HS: Essentials of Cardiopulmonary Physical Therapy. Philadelphia, WB Saunders, 1994.)

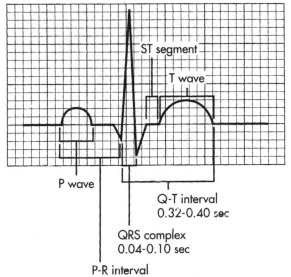

Figure 9–9. Normal electrocardiogram tracing during a single heart cycle. (From Hillegass EA, Sadowsky HS: Essentials of Cardiopulmonary Physical Therapy. Philadelphia, WB Saunders, 1994.)

Several methods can be used to administer an exercise stress test, the most common including walking on a treadmill and riding a bicycle ergometer. Generally, the actual testing procedure includes the following:

- Continuous ECG monitoring
- Heart rate monitoring (from the ECG)
- Blood pressure monitoring
- Heart and lung sounds
- Feedback from the patient by reporting symptoms

In many stress test laboratories, analysis of expired gas (air) from the lungs is accomplished by having the subject breathe into a collection device. This technique permits a determination of the amount of oxygen that the patient used during the test.[1, 14]

When an exercise test is performed on a treadmill or bicycle ergometer, the exercise intensity or "protocol" used is very specific and has been tested in many laboratories (Table 9–3).[9] The advantage of following a protocol is that the results of the test can be compared with the results of thousands of other patients on whom the same test has been performed. This comparison helps determine the status of the patient.

Pulmonary Diagnostic Tests and Procedures

As with cardiovascular diagnostic testing, both invasive and noninvasive procedures have been developed to assess lung function and the severity of pulmo-

Table 9–3
Bruce Treadmill Protocol

STAGE OF EXERCISE	TIME OF EACH STAGE (min)	SPEED OF TREADMILL (mph)	GRADE OF TREADMILL (%)
I	3	1.7	10
II	3	2.5	12
III	3	3.4	14
IV	3	4.2	16

Adapted from Ellestad MH, Myrvin H: Stress Testing Principles and Practice. Philadelphia, FA Davis, 1986.

nary disease. Physical therapists are not generally involved in performing these assessments; however, the information that is provided must be used by physical therapists so that appropriate evaluation and treatment procedures are established.

Chest Imaging. Chest imaging is the most common noninvasive method of assessing abnormalities of the lungs. Within the last decade, new technology has enhanced the use of what are commonly called x-rays (radiographs). For example, computed tomography (CT scan) is a technique that uses x-rays to take pictures of small slices of the chest and lungs and then a computer to put these individual images into a single picture.

Magnetic Resonance Imaging. Magnetic resonance imaging (MRI) uses the same principle as the CT scan except that the energy source used to take the picture is not x-rays but magnetic waves.[20]

Even though highly technical equipment can provide a great deal of information concerning the condition of the lungs, the standard chest radiograph is often the first diagnostic test used. A physical therapist must be competent in interpreting a standard chest radiograph. Therefore, the therapist must have a thorough understanding of normal anatomy and disease processes that affect the lungs to assess this common diagnostic procedure.

Pulmonary Function Tests. A **pulmonary function test** is an assessment of the effectiveness of the respiratory musculature and the integrity of the airways and lung tissue. The testing procedure can help classify the lung disease pattern into obstructive or restrictive by assessing

- Lung volumes
- Lung capacities
- Gas distribution
- Gas diffusion
- Gas flow rate

Generally, in a pulmonary function test the patient blows as hard as possible with the biggest breath into a machine called a **spirometer.** This device measures the various volumes and airflow rates, which are then compared with a normal scale. The degree of change from normal helps assess the seriousness of the obstructive or restrictive disease.[6]

Blood Gas Analysis. **Blood gas analysis** involves assessing arterial blood to determine the concentration of oxygen and carbon dioxide. This measure helps determine how well the lungs are being ventilated or whether the patient has any deficits in respiration. Another parameter that is assessed is the acid balance of the blood. If the lungs are having difficulty maintaining appropriate levels of oxygen and carbon dioxide, the blood generally becomes more acidic. In humans, blood must be maintained at a very specific acid level. Small changes in this acid level can result in severe reactions, possibly even death.[5]

PRINCIPLES OF EVALUATION, DIAGNOSIS, AND PROGNOSIS

The evaluation process results in establishing a diagnosis and prognosis. A diagnosis is a description of a specific disease by assessing the clinical signs, symptoms, or syndromes resulting from various pathological conditions. Prognosis estimates the maximum level of improvement that the patient will experience while progressing through the treatment process.[7] During the process of establishing a diagnosis and prognosis the physical therapist also develops a "plan of care." This plan establishes the specific outcomes that the patient should be able to demonstrate at the end of the treatment process. It also includes an estimate of how long and how frequently the treatment process will need to be administered to reach the established goals and outcomes, as well as the criteria for discharge.

PRINCIPLES OF DIRECT INTERVENTION

As a team member, the physical therapist will be treating a patient in conjunction with several other personnel (e.g., doctors, nurses, nutritionists, psychologists, occupational therapists, social workers, and exercise physiologists). Each of these specialists will be applying specific management procedures. Therefore, the physical therapist must be aware of all the treatments that the patient is receiving and develop the treatment plan accordingly.

Medical Management

One of the major forms of treating heart and lung disease is medical or pharmacological management. Each year new pharmacological agents become available to treat very specific components of the complex symptoms that develop in individuals with cardiopulmonary disease. Generally, drugs used to treat cardiopulmonary disease relieve or improve symptoms but do not eradicate the disease.

Understanding the effects of drugs used to treat specific heart diseases is extremely important. Many of these drugs can alter the ability of the heart to respond to exercise. For example, drugs that alter how the sympathetic nervous system influences the heart can result in a decreased heart rate and prevent the rate from increasing in response to exercise. Other drugs used to treat the

9

heart can help control the rhythm of contraction, increase or decrease the rate, and increase or decrease the strength of myocardial contraction. They can also improve coronary blood flow or help decrease the resistance to blood flow, thereby decreasing the work that the heart must perform.[4]

Medical management of symptoms caused by pulmonary disease focuses primarily on promoting bronchodilation and decreasing inflammation. Drugs producing bronchodilation improve airflow through the bronchial tubes, which helps oxygen reach the alveolus and thereby decreases the work of breathing. Anti-inflammatory agents help control the results of infection or inflammation. As in the case of cardiac drugs, pulmonary drugs can have adverse effects, including alteration of heart function, gastrointestinal distress, nervousness, muscle tremor, headache, anxiety, sweating, and insomnia.[4]

Surgical Management

As in drug management, surgical management of cardiopulmonary disease does not generally alter the disease process, but it improves the quality of life by relieving symptoms. In the case of CHD, the arteriosclerotic process is not stopped, but coronary artery blood flow can be improved through surgery, which in turn enhances heart performance.

Two methods are commonly used to improve coronary blood flow to the heart, angioplasty and bypass surgery. **Angioplasty,** which is the process of mechanically dilating the coronary artery, does not require surgically opening the chest. A catheter is placed through an artery in the leg and then positioned in the coronary vessel blocked by arteriosclerotic plaque. A balloon is then inflated or laser light is used to destroy the plaque.[28]

Coronary artery bypass grafting (CABG) requires surgically opening the chest wall and grafting a small artery or a leg vein from the aorta to a point beyond the blockage or plaque. This technique bypasses the blockage and thereby re-establishes blood flow to the heart through the previously blocked vessel. Several vessels may be bypassed during the same surgery.[28]

Another major surgical intervention is heart transplantation, which is performed only when the heart has failed and all other therapies have been tried. A patient selected for heart transplantation is screened very carefully. The patient is generally younger than 60 years, free of other diseases or infection, and emotionally stable with strong family support. The two major problems that a heart transplant patient faces is infection and rejection. If the patient overcomes these problems, the survival rate at the end of 1 year is greater than 80% and after 5 years it is greater than 50%.[15, 30]

Surgical intervention is also required for inserting a pacemaker. A **cardiac pacemaker** is an electronic device that produces a pulse that controls heart depolarization. In other words, it replaces the function of the SA node. This intervention is generally done to control severe cardiac arrhythmias. The electrodes can be inserted through a vein in the arm up to the heart and placed on the inner surface of the heart. The generator is then placed below the skin on the anterior chest wall and sutured in place. When a pacemaker is present in a patient, the physical therapist and physical therapist assistant must monitor the patient closely during exercise. Most pacemakers used today can produce variable rates in response to exercise; however, if maximum-intensity exercise is performed, careful monitoring is mandatory.[23]

Surgical management is not as frequently used for common lung diseases as it is in the management of cardiac diseases. Resection of lung disease generally applies to removal of malignant and benign tumors, fungal infections, cysts, tuberculosis, fistulas, or bronchiectasis. Pathological changes that occur from obstructive or restrictive diseases generally do not require surgery. However, when surgery on the heart or lungs is performed, the physical therapist and physical therapist assistant play a major role in preoperative and postoperative care.

When the chest wall is opened, the patient must generally be placed on a machine that breathes for the individual and, in the case of heart surgery, a machine that pumps the blood because the heart is stopped. This very serious interruption of the normal function of the heart and lungs results in certain changes that will have to be managed no matter what surgical procedure is performed.[10] Box 9–1 identifies some of the problems a patient will have preoperatively and postoperatively that must be managed by a physical therapist.[16]

Physical Therapy Cardiac Rehabilitation Procedures

The physical therapist is responsible for establishing an appropriate level of intensity, duration, frequency, and mode of exercise for an individual with cardiac disease, which means monitoring the patient's cardiovascular response to the exercise to ensure the patient's safety. In addition, the therapist must review all the medical data obtained from invasive and noninvasive testing procedures to select an appropriate level of activity for the patient's program.

To help the physical therapist accomplish this activity, individuals with cardiac disease are generally classified according to the severity of the condition. Table 9–4 presents two classification systems that use functional and therapeutic terms to determine the patient's basic condition and the type of activity in which the individual might engage.[11]

Other guidelines used by the physical therapist to help establish appropriate cardiac rehabilitation activities include phases of recovery. Cardiac rehabilitation is typically divided into inpatient and outpatient stages. The inpatient stage is often referred to as phase I (acute), whereas the outpatient stage is generally broken down into phase II (subacute), phase III (intensive rehabilitation), and phase IV (ongoing rehabilitation).[14, 18, 28] This classification system varies a great deal and often remains specific to a program. For instance, phase IV is frequently combined with phase III.

The person would participate in phase I of the cardiac rehabilitation program as an inpatient. Table 9–5 lists the kinds of exercises and activities of daily living that a physical therapist or physical therapist assistant would supervise or monitor.[28] The therapist or assistant must monitor the ECG, heart rate, blood

9

Box 9–1

Factors Influencing Recovery Following Chest Surgery

Preoperative Factors

> Risk factor profile
> Underlying pulmonary or heart disease
> Other medical problems

Factors During Operation

> Pulmonary collapse and hypoxemia
> Direct trauma to heart or lungs
> Heart arrhythmias
> Danger of emboli (clots) in lungs
> Damage to the mucous membrane of the lungs
> > Poor humidity to lungs
> > Reaction of lungs to anesthesia
> Drying of pleura

Postoperative Factors

> Atelectasis (collapse of alveoli)
> > Narcotics to suppress pain
> > Incisional pain preventing deep breathing
> > Inactivity promoting shallow breathing
> Inability to clear lung secretions due to decreased coughing
> > Pain
> > Weakness

Adapted from Howell S, Hill J: Acute respiratory care in open heart surgery. Phys Ther 1972;52:253–260.

pressure, and other physiological parameters to ensure that the patient stays within the predetermined safety range. It is important to note that the patient is involved in educational activities, including risk factor modification, understanding the medications being taken, and discharge planning. This education program could also include flexibility exercises and learning how to take one's own pulse.

After discharge, the individual participates in the outpatient phases of the cardiac rehabilitation program. These phases focus on exercises that will gradually and safely increase the individual's functional capacity. The early stages of outpatient rehabilitation (phase II) are performed under supervision and monitored closely. Generally, patients attend outpatient cardiac rehabilitation programs that have representatives of the entire rehabilitation team (e.g., occupational therapy, physical therapy, nutrition). During phase II, close physi-

Table 9–4

Functional and Therapeutic Classifications of Patients with Diseases of the Heart

FUNCTIONAL CLASSIFICATION		THERAPEUTIC CLASSIFICATION	
Level	Description	Level	Description
I	Patients with cardiac disease, but without resulting limitations of physical activity. Ordinary physical capacity does not cause undue fatigue, palpitation, dyspnea, or anginal pain	A	Patients with cardiac disease whose physical activity need not be restricted in any way
II	Patients with cardiac disease resulting in slight limitation of physical activity. Patients are comfortable at rest. Ordinary physical activity results in fatigue, palpitation, dyspnea, or anginal pain	B	Patients with cardiac disease whose ordinary physical activity need not be restricted but who should be advised against severe or competitive effort
III	Patients with cardiac disease resulting in marked limitation of physical activity. Patients are comfortable at rest. Less than ordinary physical activity causes fatigue, palpitation, dyspnea, or anginal pain	C	Patients with cardiac disease whose ordinary physical activity should be moderately restricted and whose more strenuous efforts should be discontinued
IV	Patients with cardiac disease resulting in an inability to carry out any physical activity without discomfort. Symptoms of cardiac insufficiency or anginal syndrome may be present even at rest. If any physical activity is undertaken, discomfort is increased	D	Patients with cardiac disease whose ordinary physical activity should be markedly restricted
		E	Patients with cardiac disease who should be at complete rest or confined to bed or chair

Data from Functional and Therapeutic Classifications of Patients with Diseases of the Heart. Dallas, American Heart Association, 1999.

9

Table 9–5
Seven-Step Inpatient Rehabilitation Program for Myocardial Infarction

STEP	SUPERVISED EXERCISES	ACTIVITIES OF DAILY LIVING	EDUCATIONAL ACTIVITIES
1	Active and passive ROM of all extremities, in bed; teach patients ankle plantar flexion and dorsiflexion, repeat hourly when awake	Partial self-care, feed self, dangle legs on side of bed, use bedside commode	Orientation to CCU, personal emergencies, social service aid as needed
2	Active ROM of all extremities, sitting on side of bed	Sit in chair 15–30 min 2–3 times/day; complete self-care in bed	Orientation to rehabilitation team, program; smoking cessation, if needed; educational literature, if requested; planning transfer from CCU
3	Warm up exercises, stretching, calisthenics; walk 50 ft and back at slow pace	Sit in chair, go to ward class in wheelchair, walk in room	Normal cardiac anatomy and function, what happens with myocardial infarction
4	ROM and calisthenics; walk length of hall (75 ft) and back, average pace; teach pulse counting	Out of bed as tolerated, walk to bathroom, walk to ward class with supervision	Coronary risk factors and their control
5	ROM and calisthenics, check pulse counting, practice walking few stair steps, walk 300 ft twice daily	Walk to waiting room or telephone, walk in ward corridor	Diet, energy conservation, work simplification techniques (as needed)
6	Continue above activities; walk down flight of stairs (return by elevator), walk 500 ft; instruct on home exercises	Tepid shower or tub bath with supervision, go to occupational therapy, cardiac clinic teaching room, with supervision	Heart attack management; medications; exercise; family, community adjustments on return home
7	Continue above activities; walk up flight of steps, walk 500 ft; continue home exercise instruction, present information regarding outpatient exercise program	Continue all previous ward activities	Discharge planning: medications, diet; return to work; community resources; educational literature; medication cards

CCU, cardiac care unit; ROM, range of motion.
Data from Functional and Therapeutic Classifications of Patients with Diseases of the Heart. Dallas, American Heart Association, 1999.

cian management is always available. Depending on the severity of the problem, the patient will attend supervised training sessions three to four times per week for 10 to 12 weeks. If recovery has continued well, a stress test will be performed to help determine whether the patient has improved or responded to the exercise program.

Progression to phases III and IV involves more independent and aggressive activities. To proceed to these levels, the individual must (1) be able to self-monitor the exercise program, (2) have no contraindications to exercise, and (3) be emotionally stable.[5] These phases include a gradual increase in exercise intensity. Periodic checkups by the professional team occur most frequently in phase III. Once phase IV has been attained, the patient should be functioning at the maximum safe capacity.

During the outpatient phases of the cardiac rehabilitation program, the exercises emphasize aerobic training that includes rhythmic activity of large muscle masses. Appropriate aerobic training involves a warm-up period, a peak period, and a cool-down period. The length of time for these periods may vary with the status of the patient, but generally the warm-up and cool-down phases should be at least 8 to 10 minutes each. The peak period should last 20 to 60 minutes. It is during the peak period that the patient must reach and maintain a target heart rate (THR).[2, 14]

A **target heart rate** is calculated as a percentage of the individual's maximum heart rate. The maximum heart rate can be accurately determined only by a maximum stress test. However, it is commonly *estimated* by subtracting one's age from 220. The THR is then determined to establish a person's **"training zone,"** or minimum and maximum heart rates that must be achieved to produce an aerobic training effect. The percentage of the maximum heart rate that is selected will depend on the individual's level of fitness, symptoms, and ECG findings. If the person is a patient with cardiac disease and is very deconditioned, the training zone levels would be small, perhaps only a maximum of 120 beats per minute or 20 to 30 beats per minute above resting levels.[14] By contrast, a training zone for a young athlete may fall between THRs of 60% to 85% of that person's maximum heart rate capacity. To produce a "training effect" or a change in aerobic capacity, this individual would have to reach a heart rate in the established "training zone." The important thing to remember is that as aerobic capacity improves, the amount of work that the heart has to perform at a specific exercise intensity decreases. This improvement in aerobic capacity in turn improves the patient's functional capacity without causing the heart to be overworked.[17]

Other factors to consider when establishing an aerobic training program besides the intensity of exercise (how hard a patient works during a single exercise period) and the duration of exercise (how long each exercise period should last) include the mode of exercise (what the patient does, such as walking, jogging, bicycle riding) and the frequency of exercise (how many times a day or week the patient exercises).[1] The mode of exercise must allow for aerobic performance, which includes rhythmic contraction of large muscle groups over several minutes (20 to 60 minutes). Running, swimming, walking,

9

and bicycle riding all promote this type of activity. An individual with cardiac disease, however, may not be able to sustain 20 minutes of exercise at one time; therefore, several periods of exercise throughout the day would be more appropriate. The frequency of exercise may also be determined by the patient's condition. Normally, in the latter phases of their program, individuals with cardiac disease must generally perform a minimum of 20 minutes of exercise three to five times per week to promote or maintain aerobic training.[19]

The physical therapist and physical therapist assistant must continuously monitor the patient during all phases of the exercise program. Appropriate monitoring includes assessing heart rate, blood pressure, and respiratory rate responses to the specific exercise intensity. This monitoring is quite important, especially in the early phases of rehabilitation, to ensure that the patient does not exercise at an unsafe level. As the patient progresses, the therapist must teach self-monitoring for safe participation in activities, thus moving the patient one step closer to independent activity. When the patient can function independently at maximum functional capability, the therapist's responsibilities have been met.

Physical Therapy Pulmonary Rehabilitation Procedures

As with patients who have cardiac dysfunction, the physical therapist is responsible for establishing an appropriate level of exercise programming for individuals with pulmonary disease. The intensity and duration of the program must be at an appropriate level to promote a training effort that will enhance the patient's ability to perform daily functions aerobically. Aerobic performance occurs when the active muscles receive all the oxygen they need to perform their task. To select the appropriate intensity and duration of exercise, the physical therapist must review the results of all examination procedures performed on the patient. From these data and the physical therapy evaluation, the appropriate exercise program can be established. It is important to remember that during aerobic exercise the physical therapist and physical therapist assistant must monitor the patient's cardiovascular response to the exercise, such as the heart rate, blood pressure, and breathing rate and depth, as well as elicit feedback on how the patient feels. In this way, excessive exercise that could put the patient at risk is prevented.

Other components of physical therapy treatment for patients with pulmonary disease include secretion removal techniques, respiratory muscle training and breathing techniques, and energy-saving techniques.

Secretion removal techniques are performed in patients who produce excessive mucus in the bronchi of the lungs as seen in obstructive pulmonary disease. The technique applied to promote mucus removal is called **postural drainage.** The patient is placed in a certain position ("posture") to passively drain fluid from a specific portion of the lung. Percussion (or clapping), vibration, and shaking are applied by the therapist to specific areas of the chest wall overlying specific lobes of the lung (Fig. 9–10).[24] Percussion promotes movement of mucus through the bronchial tubes. Having the patient assume

Trendelenburg's (inverted) position and cough immediately after the percussion or vibration procedure also helps move mucus out of the different sections of the lungs.

Producing a good cough is essential for maintaining normal lung function in everyone. If the respiratory muscles are weakened or do not work properly, the efficiency of the cough mechanism is reduced. This reduced cough efficiency can occur in both the obstructive and restrictive disease patterns. It also occurs in patients who have experienced trauma, such as an individual with quadriplegia after spinal cord injury or patients who have had thoracic surgery.

The physical therapist can help the patient enhance coughing in three ways: by strengthening both the primary and secondary muscles of respiration, by changing the breathing pattern, and by teaching the patient how to use different devices to support the chest wall so that the expiration force generated during coughing is enhanced.[10]

Patients are taught energy-saving techniques so that they can perform their daily activities more efficiently, thereby decreasing the demand on the pulmonary system. The physical therapist determines the activity needs for the patient in the home or work environment and then helps select assistive devices that can be used to perform certain tasks. Examples of such devices include a bathtub seat for showering in a seated position or a long shoehorn to help make putting on shoes easier. The therapist also teaches these patients how to divide an activity into components so that each part of an activity is performed in stages. This technique is sometimes referred to as pacing.[2, 10, 14]

The physical therapist and physical therapist assistant engage in direct intervention during pulmonary rehabilitation. They also participate in helping modify the patient's risk factor profile, such as promoting weight management, good nutrition, smoking cessation, and a positive psychological state. They must be prepared to monitor the activities of other health care professionals and ensure that their treatment program is integrated into a comprehensive care plan. The primary goal for pulmonary rehabilitation is to help the patient achieve the highest functional level allowed by the pulmonary impairment.

9

The "Well" Individual

A discussion of cardiopulmonary physical therapy would not be complete without reviewing the concept of the "well" individual (individual without a diagnosis of any cardiopulmonary disease). These individuals may be candidates for fitness programs aimed at improving their functional work capacity. A physical therapist or physical therapist assistant needs to be prepared to offer guidance to this type of person. Generally, these exercise programs focus on a specific purpose for starting exercise. Such purposes may include stress reduction, weight management, improvement in physique and body image, alteration of cardiac risk factors, or enhancement of functional capacity.[14]

The aging population represents a large group of "well" individuals who can benefit from exercise but have a tendency to be sedentary. Specific cardiopulmonary changes occur with aging, one of the most specific being a decrease

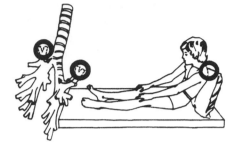

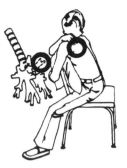

UPPER LOBES Apical Segments

Bed or drainage table flat.

Patient leans back on pillow at 30° angle against therapist.

Therapist claps with markedly cupped hand over area between clavicle and top of scapula on each side.

UPPER LOBES Posterior Segments

Bed or drainage table flat.

Patient leans over folder pillow at 30° angle.

Therapist stands behind and claps over upper back on both sides.

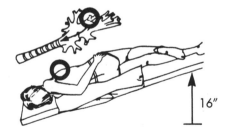

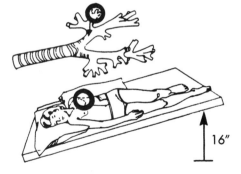

RIGHT MIDDLE LOBE

Foot of table or bed elevated 16 inches.

Patient lies head down on left side and rotates 1/4 turn backward. Pillow may be placed behind from shoulder to hip. Knees should be flexed.

Therapist claps over right nipple area. In females with breast development or tenderness, use cupped hand with heel of hand under armpit and fingers extending forward beneath the breast.

LEFT UPPER LOBE Lingular Segments

Foot of table or bed elevated 16 inches.

Patient lies head down on right side and rotates 1/4 turn backward. Pillow may be placed behind from shoulder to hip. Knees should be flexed.

Therapist claps with moderately cupped hand over left nipple area. In females with breast development or tenderness, use cupped hand with heel of hand under armpit and fingers extending forward beneath the breast.

A

Figure 9–10. Positions and guidelines for performing postural drainage to remove fluid from the lungs. See also Figure 2–11*A* and *B*. (From Rothstein JM, Roy SH, Wolf SL: The Rehabilitation Specialist's Handbook. Philadelphia, FA Davis, 1991.)

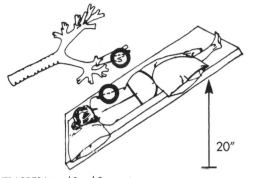

LOWER LOBES Lateral Basal Segments

Foot of table or bed elevated 20 inches.

Patient lies on abdomen, head down, then rotates 1/4 turn upward. Upper leg is flexed over a pillow for support.

Therapist claps over uppermost portion of lower ribs. (Position shown is for drainage of right lateral basal segment. To drain the left lateral basal segment, patient should lie on his right side in the same posture.)

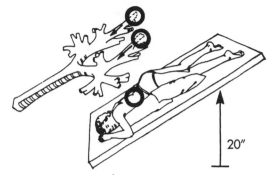

LOWER LOBES Posterior Basal Segments

Foot of table or bed elevated 20 inches.

Patient lies on abdomen, head down, with pillow under hips. Therapist claps over lower ribs close to spine on each side.

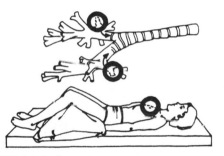

UPPER LOBES Anterior Segments

Bed or drainage table flat.

Patient lies on back with pillow under knees.

Therapist claps between clavicle and nipple on each side.

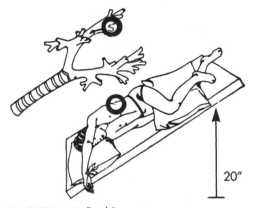

LOWER LOBES Anterior Basal Segments

Foot of table or bed elevated 20 inches.

Patient lies on side, head down, pillow under knees.

Therapist claps with slightly cupped hand over lower ribs. (Position shown is for drainage of left anterior basal segment. To drain the right anterior basal segment, patient should lie on his left side in same posture.)

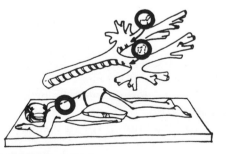

LOWER LOBES Superior Segments

Bed or table flat.

Patient lies on abdomen with two pillows under hips.

Therapist claps over middle of back at tip of scapula on either side of spine.

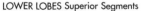

B

Figure 9–10 *Continued*

in the safe maximum heart rate. It is well established that the heart rate is inversely related to age. As one grows older, the maximum heart rate declines. At the same time, the pulmonary system demonstrates a decline in both static and dynamic measurements. However, while endurance training in the elderly cannot reduce cardiac changes, it can reduce pulmonary changes.[19]

Just as an individual with cardiac or pulmonary disease needs an examination, so does the "well" individual. This examination should include reviewing the risk factor profile, including smoking and family history. The physical therapist should examine the functional status of the musculoskeletal system. The performance results of an exercise stress test, body composition (percentage of body fat), strength, and flexibility should also be reviewed. Any preexisting conditions, such as orthopaedic abnormalities, must also be considered. An important aspect of the examination is to determine the individual's specific interests. Does the individual like to swim, run, or ride a bicycle? Understanding the person's interests could help the therapist design a program more likely to induce compliance with the exercise routine.

Box 9–2 presents a summary of benefits gained from aerobic and strength-training programs.[14] This type of information can be used to encourage a sedentary person to engage in a regular exercise program. However, appropriate assessment and monitoring must accompany any regular exercise.

Case Studies   *Joe—Myocardial Infarction* _____

Clinical History. Joe is a 60-year-old man who retired after 30 years as a high school math teacher. He had not experienced any previous symptoms of heart disease, such as chest pain or shortness of breath, but had been taking medicine over the past 3 years for mild high blood pressure, which was well controlled. His risk factor profile included the following:

• Family history—mother and older brother died of heart disease
• Smoking—between the ages of 16 and 40, one pack per day
• Sedentary—has not engaged in any regular exercise program since the age of 50
• Obesity—has "been carrying" an extra 30 lb since his mid forties

One week ago he was admitted to the emergency room after 1 hour of severe chest pain. The ECG demonstrated severe abnormalities indicating a change in the function of the anterolateral part of his heart. He was rushed to the operating room, where cardiac catheterization revealed major blockage in different sections of his left coronary artery. Angioplasty was performed on two areas of artery blockage, and it improved blood flow through the left coronary artery by 90%.

Cardiac Rehabilitation. After surgery, Joe was admitted to the cardiac care unit. He was prescribed medications that helped control his heart rate, improve the strength of the heart's contractions, and prevent arrhythmias. The physical

Box 9–2

Benefits of Aerobic Exercise and Strength-Training Programs

Benefits of an Aerobic Exercise Program

Improvement in aerobic capacity
  Increased efficiency to extract oxygen in trained muscles
  Increase in stroke volume
  Decrease in resting heart rate
  Decrease in submaximal heart rates
Change in body composition (loss of fat)
Decreased clotting factors in blood
Decrease in resting blood pressure in hypertensive individuals
Altered method of cholesterol transport
  Increase in high-density lipoproteins (HDLs)
  Slight decrease in low-density lipoproteins (LDLs)
Decrease in various fats produced by the body
Increase in using carbohydrates as an energy source
Improvement in psychological well-being
  Improved response to stress
  Decrease in physiologic responsiveness to stimuli
  Improved self-image
Decrease in risk for developing heart disease owing to elimination of a number of the risk factors

Benefits of a Strength-Training Program

Increase in strength of trained muscles
Increase in utilization of anaerobic metabolism
  Improved ease in performing many activities of daily living especially with upper body strength training
Increase in bone mass
Increase in size, endurance, or both, of trained muscles
Improvement of body image and self-esteem

9

Adapted from Hillegass EA, Sadowski HS: Essentials of Cardiopulmonary Physical Therapy. Philadelphia, WB Saunders, 1994.

therapist assessed the patient's status and, after conferring with the cardiologist and ward nurse, initiated the activities outlined in Table 9–5. The physical therapist reported the following results at the end of the exercise period:

1. Resting heart rate (beats per minute): 86 while lying in bed, 98 while sitting, 105 while standing, 135 while performing activities of daily living such as brushing teeth at the bedside.

2. Blood pressure: 130/90 while lying in bed, 110/80 while sitting, 110/65 while standing, 100/60 while performing daily activities.
3. ECG: no indication of any change in pattern except when performing daily activities. This change demonstrated possible mild ischemia.

After 2 days in the cardiac care unit, Joe was transferred to the ward. After appropriate examination, the physical therapist initiated the exercise and education programs for ward activities listed in Table 9–5. After the first 2 days of this exercise routine, the patient demonstrated appropriate physiological responses to the exercises. The physical therapist assistant assumed the responsibility for the ambulation and range-of-motion exercises. The patient was discharged after 1 week of hospitalization. He had an understanding that the medicine he took was to help prevent arrhythmias. He had learned how to take his own pulse and was instructed to not engage in any activities that caused his heart rate to exceed 135 beats per minute. At the time of discharge, he was instructed to move his bed to the first floor of his home to avoid a flight of stairs.

Outpatient Program. Joe returned to the outpatient cardiac rehabilitation program conducted in the physical therapy department 3 days after discharge. He reported that he had not had any difficulty at home; however, further inquiry revealed that he did not engage in any activity other than activities of daily living and walking around the house.

The physical therapist initiated phase II of cardiac rehabilitation by determining how long Joe could walk on a treadmill at his preferred rate before reaching the THR of 135 beats per minute. This rate was established by the cardiologist at the time of discharge as the maximum exercise heart rate that Joe could reach. Over the next three outpatient visits (1 week), the physical therapist established the following exercise routine to be performed at home twice daily.

1. 15 minutes of warm-up and stretching
2. 20 minutes of stationary bicycle riding
3. 15 minutes of cool-down exercises

Joe remained on this exercise program for 3 more weeks. During that time he came to the cardiac rehabilitation program to meet with a nutritionist and a psychologist. He then underwent an exercise stress test on a treadmill, which revealed that he could safely reach a maximum heart rate of 146 beats per minute before incurring serious changes in heart function. Phase III cardiac rehabilitation was then initiated and included bicycle riding and fast walking with increasing intensity, duration, and frequency. At the end of 6 weeks of monitored phase III activities, another stress test revealed that Joe could reach a safe maximum heart rate of 160 beats per minute. His resting heart rate and blood pressure were now within normal limits, he lost 20 lb, and his diet was cholesterol-free. He was no longer taking any cardiac medication. The cardiologist approved Joe's transfer into phase IV cardiac rehabilitation with 3-month checkups by the physical therapist and another stress test in 1 year.

Martha—Chronic Obstructive Pulmonary Disease

Clinical History. Martha is a 58-year-old homemaker with a history of shortness of breath on exertion. She admits to a 25-year history of smoking, but stopped 5 years ago. She states that she has a productive cough in the morning. Recently, she was admitted to the hospital with a temperature of 102°F and a productive cough. Severe upper respiratory tract infection was the diagnosis. This was Martha's third such admission in the past year. After discharge, the physician requested a full pulmonary examination and initiation of rehabilitation to reduce the frequency of hospitalization.

The results of pulmonary testing revealed that her ability to forcefully expire a normal volume of air in 1 second was markedly decreased even though the total volume of air in her lungs remained near normal. The carbon dioxide concentration in her blood was elevated and the amount of oxygen was below normal. A chest radiograph demonstrated mild inflammation of the bronchial tubes.

Physical therapy examination of her chest revealed that her breathing pattern depended mostly on the diaphragm with very little chest wall motion. The angle between her ribs and sternum has increased, which indicates that her lower chest wall has permanently expanded beyond normal. There is evidence that her accessory muscles of ventilation around the neck and shoulders contract during quiet inspiration. When Martha was placed on a treadmill and asked to walk at 3 mph with no grade, she demonstrated a further drop in the oxygen saturation of her blood, shortness of breath, and mild wheezing.

Pulmonary Rehabilitation. The results of the examination led to a diagnosis of moderate obstructive lung disease accompanied by physical deconditioning. The primary goals for Martha's rehabilitation program would be to achieve a daily walk or jog of 30 continuous minutes without shortness of breath, improve her functional capacity, and perform pulmonary hygiene to assist with clearing of her lungs each morning.

The physical therapist instructed Martha in the appropriate postural drainage positions that she will use for 10 minutes on each side of the chest before getting out of bed in the morning. She was taught breathing exercises that will help mobilize her lower chest wall, increase the strength of her diaphragm and intercostal muscles, and improve her ability to perform a forceful cough. Martha must also learn specific diet modifications and how to monitor for symptoms that might occur if her blood oxygen concentration drops too severely.

Martha's exercise program includes progressive walking. The heart rate achieved when shortness of breath requires her to stop will be used as the maximum heart rate. Warm-up and cool-down periods will occur before and after the continuous walking period. The duration, intensity, and frequency of the exercise program will be increased until she can achieve 30 continuous minutes of walking without shortness of breath. In conjunction with the exercise program, the physical therapist must educate the patient on how she will monitor herself safely and perform the exercise routine independently.

9

Summary ———— Cardiopulmonary physical therapy has, over the past two decades, become an inherent part of the knowledge and practice base of the physical therapist. A thorough understanding of the anatomy, physiology, and function of the cardiopulmonary system is essential to develop the skills necessary to make appropriate clinical decisions for proper examination, management, and progression of patients with cardiopulmonary diseases. It is also essential for all physical therapists and physical therapist assistants to remember that no matter what the diagnosis, when exercise is applied as an intervention, the cardiopulmonary response to that exercise must always be monitored.

Physical therapists who work with individuals with cardiopulmonary disease must also be acutely aware of their role as team members. Whether guiding a physical therapist assistant in applying appropriate exercise intensity or whether discussing maximum exercise intensity levels with a cardiologist, the physical therapist must always take into account the total management program that the patient with cardiopulmonary disease is experiencing.

References

1. American College of Sports Medicine: Guidelines for Exercise Testing and Prescription, ed 4. Philadelphia, Lea & Febiger, 1991.
2. Brannon FJ, Foley MW, Starr JA, et al: Cardiopulmonary Rehabilitation: Basic Theory and Application, ed 2. Philadelphia, FA Davis, 1993.
3. Cardiovascular diseases. Retrieved from *http://www.americanheart.org/statistics/03cardio.html*, American Heart Association, 1999.
4. Ciccone CD: Pharmacology in Rehabilitation. Philadelphia, FA Davis, 1996.
5. Cohen S (ed): Blood Gas and Acid Base Concepts in Respiratory Care. New York, American Journal of Nursing Company, 1976.
6. Cohen S (ed): Pulmonary Function Tests in Patient Care. New York, American Journal of Nursing Company, 1980.
7. Dorland's Medical Dictionary, ed 27. Philadelphia, WB Saunders, 1988.
8. Dubin D: Rapid Interpretation of EKG, ed 3. Tampa, FL, Cover Publishing, 1974.
9. Ellestad MH, Myrvin H: Stress Testing Principles and Practice. Philadelphia, FA Davis, 1986.
10. Frownfelter DL: Chest Physical Therapy and Pulmonary Rehabilitation, an Interdisciplinary Approach, ed 2. Chicago, Year Book, 1987.
11. Functional and Therapeutic Classifications of Patients with Diseases of the Heart. Dallas, American Heart Association, 1999.
12. Guide to Physical Therapist Practice. 2nd ed. Phys Ther 2001;81:9–744.
13. Heart and Stroke Statistical Update. Dallas, American Heart Association, 1998.
14. Hillegass EA, Sadowsky HS: Essentials of Cardiopulmonary Physical Therapy. Philadelphia, WB Saunders, 1994.
15. Hills LD: Manual of Clinical Problems in Cardiology, ed 3. Philadelphia, Little, Brown, 1989.
16. Howell S, Hill J: Acute respiratory care in open heart surgery. Phys Ther 1972;52:253–260.
17. Hurst W: The Heart, Arteries and Veins, ed 9. New York, McGraw-Hill, 1998.
18. Irwin S, Tecklin JS: Cardiopulmonary Physical Therapy, ed 3. St Louis, Mosby–Year Book, 1995.
19. McArdle WD, Katch FI, Katch VL: Exercise Physiology—Energy, Nutrition, and Human Performance, ed 3. Philadelphia, Lea & Febiger, 1991.
20. Minter RA: Chest Imaging: An Integrated Approach. Baltimore, Williams & Wilkins, 1981.
21. Moore L: Clinically Oriented Anatomy, ed 3. Baltimore, Williams & Wilkins, 1999.
22. Phillips RE, Feeney MK: The Cardiac Rhythm, ed 2. Philadelphia, WB Saunders, 1980.
23. Reul GJ: Implantation of a permanent cardiac pacemaker. *In* Cooley DA (ed): Techniques in Cardiac Surgery, ed 2. Philadelphia, WB Saunders, 1984.
24. Rothstein JM, Roy SH, Wolf SL: The Rehabilitation Specialist's Handbook. Philadelphia, FA Davis, 1991.

25. Sanderson RG, Kurth CL: The Cardiac Patient: A Comprehensive Approach, ed 2. Philadelphia, WB Saunders, 1983.
26. Trends in chronic bronchitis and emphysema: Morbidity and mortality. Retrieved from *http://www.lungusa.org/data/copd/copd1.pdf*, American Lung Association, 1999.
27. Van De Graaff KM, Fox SI: Concepts of Human Anatomy and Physiology, ed 2. Dubuque, IA, WC Brown, 1989.
28. Wenger NK, Hellerstein HK: Rehabilitation of the Coronary Patient, ed 3. New York, Churchill Livingstone, 1992.
29. Williams PL, Warwick R, Dyson M, et al: Gray's Anatomy, ed 37. New York, Churchill Livingstone, 1989.
30. Wuff KS: Management of the cardiovascular surgery patient. *In* Brunner LS, Suddarth DS (eds): Textbook of Medical-Surgical Nursing, ed 6. Philadelphia, JB Lippincott, 1987.

Suggested Reading

Frownfelter D, Dean E: Principles and Practice of Cardiopulmonary Physical Therapy, ed 3. St Louis, Mosby–Year Book, 1996.
Practical and readable, this text covers the basics of cardiopulmonary physical therapy. Throughout the text, the theme of oxygen transport is stressed. Features include key terms, review questions, and a glossary. A case studies workbook is also available.

REVIEW QUESTIONS

1. Create a diagram that illustrates the processes of respiration and ventilation.

2. Explain why we look at the cardiovascular and respiratory systems together. Don't they have distinctly different functions?

3. Generate and label a diagram that helps you identify events associated with different components of the heart cycle.

4. Research the use of at least one of the cardiovascular or pulmonary diagnostic tools discussed in this chapter. Prepare a demonstration, especially if you are able to include a visit to a treatment facility as part of your research.

5. Make up a simple description of a patient in need of cardiac rehabilitation. (A paragraph is long enough.) Then create a flow chart of the typical therapy process and the changes made as the patient progresses.

6. Repeat the steps assigned in question 5, but this time apply it to a patient in pulmonary rehabilitation.

9

10

Problems cannot be solved at the same level of awareness that created them.
Albert Einstein

Physical Therapy for Integumentary Conditions

R. Scott Ward

KEY TERMS

arterial insufficiency
chronic inflammation
collagen
dermatitis
dermis
epidermis

233

ground substance
hypertrophic scar
inflammatory phase
inflammatory skin diseases
integument
keloid scar
maturation phase
neoplastic skin diseases

neuropathic (neurotropic) ulcer
pressure ulcer
proliferative phase
scar contraction
scar contracture
total body surface area (TBSA)
Vancouver Burn Scar Scale
venous insufficiency

OBJECTIVES   After reading this chapter, the reader will be able to

- Discuss the structure and function of the skin
- Discuss the process of wound healing, including the three major phases—inflammation, proliferation, and maturation
- Describe common problems associated with the integument (including vascular compromise, trauma, and disease) and the basic examination principles related to those conditions
- Describe basic intervention principles and strategies necessary in complete patient care (including prevention, management, and education)

Various types of integumentary (skin) wounds or impairments in skin integrity, the consequences of these wounds, and any associated effects of the wound such as inflammation, pain, edema, and scar formation can lead to significant functional limitations and disability. Physical therapists and physical therapist assistants must be aware of the importance of the integumentary system in normal human function. They should be able to provide programs or interventions to prevent loss of skin integrity. Furthermore, appropriate management of patients with various impairments of the skin is a critical part of physical therapy practice.

GENERAL DESCRIPTION

The Integument

The **integument**, the largest organ of the body, ranges from about 1 to 4 mm in thickness and consists of two layers—the epidermis and the dermis. The integument is basically a protective organ, but it also serves a role in temperature control and provides important sensory information regarding the environment. Figure 10–1 illustrates the structure of the skin and its appendages.

EPIDERMIS

The **epidermis** is very thin in comparison to the overall thickness of the skin. The thickness of the epidermis generally ranges from about 0.06 to 0.1 mm. It is thicker only on the soles of the feet and the palms of the hand, where the most superficial layer of the epidermis, the stratum corneum, may increase the thickness to 0.6 mm. This thicker stratum corneum is often referred to as

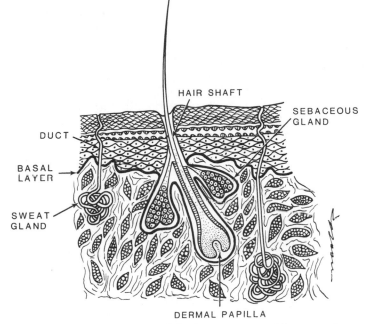

Figure 10–1. The structure of the integument and its appendages.

callus. The preponderance of cells in the epidermis are keratinocytes produced in the basal cell layer. The basal cell layer is also where the epidermis is anchored to the dermis. It takes a minimum of 28 days for keratinocytes to differentiate through their epidermal phases until they are finally sloughed off the most external surface of the stratum corneum. It is the stratum corneum that restricts the loss of fluids from internal tissue and separates this same internal tissue from the external environment.

Other cells that make up the epithelium are Langerhans cells, Merkel cells, and melanocytes. Langerhans cells play a role in the immune response in skin. Merkel cells are acknowledged as sensory receptor cells that provide information about tactile stimuli. Melanocytes (located in the basal cell layer) synthesize melanin, which is a pigment that principally serves as primary protection against harmful ultraviolet radiation. Once produced, melanin is transferred from melanocytes to keratinocytes. Melanocytes are also present in the dermis and hair follicles (as well as other sites such as the retina).

Other components of the epidermis that penetrate into the dermis are hair follicles, sebaceous glands, apocrine glands, and sweat (eccrine) glands. The basal cell layer surrounds each of these structures because of their connection with the epidermis. Hair is formed at the follicle by a process of keratinization that produces three layers of cells. The hair follicle is an invagination of the epidermis. Hair type and amount are dependent on several factors, including hormonal influence, age, and heredity. Sebaceous glands produce a fatty secretion and are found in association with every hair follicle (pilosebaceous glands).

10

Some sebaceous glands not associated with hair follicles are also found in a general distribution over the body with the exception of the soles of the feet, the palms of the hands, and the lower lip. The main function of the sebaceous glands is to keep the skin "moisturized" and pliant and to prevent it from drying and cracking. The apocrine glands begin to secrete a commonly colorless and odorless oily sweat at the onset of puberty. These glands are localized in the anogenital and axillary areas. The odor associated with perspiration in these areas results from bacterial decomposition of the secretions. Sweat is a hypotonic solution that is delivered to the skin surface by sweat glands. Normal function of the sweat glands is critical in temperature regulation.

DERMIS

The **dermis** consists of fibrous and elastic connective tissue encompassed by a ground substance. The dermis varies from 1 to 4 mm in thickness and has two subdivisions—the papillary dermis and the reticular dermis. The papillary dermis, which is composed of a loosely organized collagen matrix and is highly vascular, forms in reflection to the basal cell layer of the epidermis. The junction between these two layers of skin is far from flat. The ridges formed at the dermal-epidermal junction (epidermal ridges and dermal papillae, respectively) provide protection against potentially damaging perturbations such as shearing and deepen the dispersion of the epidermal basal cell layer. The reticular dermis is composed of more densely bundled collagen fibers and less ground substance than the papillary dermis. The ground substance of the dermis is made up of various proteoglycans, glycoproteins, hyaluronic acid, and water. This "gel" forms the interstitial environment that accommodates the composite of dermal elements—fibroelastic collagen, blood vessels, and nerves—along with the epidermal appendages. The fibrous collagen supplies fortification against mechanical stresses on the skin while still allowing the deformation necessary for movement. The elastic connective tissue restores the collagen network to its "resting" arrangement, and the ground substance acts as a "cushion" to protect against many detrimental compression forces.

Blood vessels and nerves are also found within the dermis. The vascular structure in the dermis is vast and allows typically efficient diffusion of gases and nutrients to promote healthy cell function. The vascular system of the dermis additionally participates in the inflammatory response, an important component of wound healing. Along with the sweat glands, the capillaries in the skin also contribute to human thermal regulation. An equally expansive and efficient lymphatic system is associated with the vascular system in the dermis. The dermal nervous network provides the central nervous system with essential sensory information about temperature, pain, and various tactile stimuli (light touch, deep touch, and vibration) singly or in combination to allow for recognition of objects and textures. Efferent nerves innervate the vessels, sweat glands, and arrector pili muscles of the hair follicles.

SUBCUTANEOUS TISSUE

This layer of tissue consists of loose connective tissue, often containing various amounts of adipose tissue. The loose connective tissue binds the skin to the organ immediately below it in a fashion that allows a reasonable amount of movement of the skin over the underlying organ without displacement or damage.

Wound Healing

Wound healing is commonly described in three phases: the inflammatory phase, the proliferative phase, and the remodeling phase. Each of the phases, along with applicable interventions for each phase, will be discussed briefly in this section. It is important that all the phases of wound repair occur simultaneously to some extent. For example, inflammation can occur while the proliferative process is in progress.

Inflammatory Phase. With any injury comes an **inflammatory phase** that initiates repair of the damaged tissue. Local cellular and vascular reactions are included in this wound-healing phase. Initial blood loss is decreased by the immediate vasoconstriction of vessels. This vasoconstrictive response may last about 5 to 10 minutes. This time frame also allows for accumulation of platelets and the formation of temporary "platelet clots" along the damaged endothelial lining of the vessels. Activation of the clotting cascade leading to the eventual formation of fibrin clots begins at this time.

This period of vasoconstriction is followed by an episode of vasodilatation and increased capillary permeability. Leukocytes, which are chemotactically recruited to the wound site, are delivered by the increased flow of blood with vasodilatation. Early battles against infection are waged at this point by neutrophils.[13, 33] Macrophages also migrate to the wound site to phagocytose wound debris and spent cells. Macrophages also release factors important in wound repair, such as cytokines, growth factors, and collagenases.[23, 38] Lymphocytes also follow neutrophils into the wound site. They are important because of their role in the immune response and because they release factors that stimulate macrophages and fibroblasts.[12, 35, 36] The increased capillary permeability during inflammation can lead to the formation of local edema. Edema hinders healing by reducing the local arterial, venous, and lymphatic circulation and increases the chance of infection for the same reasons. Edema may also restrict motion, which increases the possibility of tissue fibrosis.

Exposure of injured nerves and the release of chemical mediators at the wound site can produce pain. Pain often causes a patient to restrict activity because the activity may increase the pain. Decreases in appropriate activity can lead to a reduction in motion and mobility.

The inflammatory phase of healing may normally last about 2 weeks. Longer periods of inflammation are referred to as **chronic inflammation**.

During this phase, appropriate physical therapy interventions might include wound care, edema management, positioning, splinting, cautious passive range-of-motion exercises, active range-of-motion exercises, ambulation, and functional activities such as activities of daily living.

Proliferative Phase. Fibroblasts start converging on the wound site during inflammation, and the **proliferative phase** of wound healing commences with

10

the production of collagen by these cells. Fibroblasts produce a connective tissue scaffold made up of elastin, collagen, and glycosaminoglycans. This process contributes to one of the major events during the proliferative phase of healing—rebuilding and strengthening of the wound site. Elastin is an elastic fibrous protein that provides flexibility to the wound, but it makes up only a small percentage in comparison to collagen.

Collagen is the chief protein produced by fibroblasts.[25] Collagen fibrils formed by fibroblasts combine and form collagen fibers. Collagen fibers supply the preponderance of strength to the wound. The strength lies in the collagen fiber, not in the amount of collagen at the wound site,[16] so a patient does not need a big scar to have a strong and well-healed wound.

Ground substance (glycosaminoglycans, water, and salts) occupies the space in between the elastin, collagen, vascular structures, and other cells in the healing wound. The ground substance allows cell proliferation and migration and provides some cushion for the healing tissue.

Angiogenesis (the formation of new blood vessels) begins during the inflammatory phase of healing, but the majority of regrowth occurs during the proliferative healing phase. Vascular genesis is important for the distribution of nutrients and oxygen to cells at the site of healing.

Wounds that are not deep enough to destroy the epidermal basal cell layer can heal through real epidermal regeneration. In epidermal regeneration, proliferation of both epithelial cells at the margin of a wound and epidermal cells from any existing basal cell (such as those in the dermis that encompass hair follicles or sweat glands) ultimately leads to wound coverage. Deeper wounds that do not have basal cells available may still achieve wound closure with epithelium that migrates from adjacent uninjured skin. This process generally occurs only in smaller wounds.

One other concern associated with the proliferative phase of healing is wound contraction. Wounds begin to contract slightly during inflammation; however, aggressive contraction at the wound commences during the proliferative phase. Fibroblasts, particularly myofibroblasts, have contractile capability.[2, 11, 14, 15] It appears that the physiological function of wound contraction is to decrease the surface area of the wound, but contraction takes place in all sizes of wounds. Although potentially beneficial in small wounds, contraction is more frequently the cause of decreased mobility and cosmetic change, particularly in wounds that are associated with joints.

Physical therapy interventions for this phase of healing may include wound care, edema management, positioning, splinting, cautious passive range-of-motion exercises, active range-of-motion exercises, ambulation, and functional activities such as activities of daily living, similar to interventions during the inflammatory phase. Additionally, active assisted range-of-motion exercises, stretching, strengthening exercises, and endurance exercises may be appropriate. Handling of wounds during this phase must be done carefully because the wound may be at a range of only 15% to 80% of its normal strength.[10, 32]

Maturation Phase. The **maturation phase** of healing is also often referred to as the remodeling phase. During the maturation phase, collagen continues to be actively deposited while it is also going through active lysis. The balance between the amount of collagen deposition by fibroblasts and the magnitude of collagen lysis influences the ultimate appearance of the scar (if scar formation occurs). If deposition exceeds lysis, either a **hypertrophic scar** or a **keloid scar** forms.[20, 28] Keloid scars differ from hypertrophic scars in that they extend beyond the original boundaries of the wound.

During this phase, collagen fibers are deposited in an unorganized fashion. The arrangement of these fibers, however, is influenced by stresses placed on them. For example, stretching an actively forming scar will cause the collagen fibers to align themselves along the length of the stretch and therefore become oriented in an alignment that favors mobility over restriction of movement.

This phase of wound healing may last for several months. While the phase is active, that is, collagen is being produced, the wound continues to contract with varying degrees of vitality. As the phase nears its end, wound contraction tends to diminish. Contraction during this phase is often referred to as **scar contraction.** If scar contraction leads to either a permanent or semifixed positional fault at a joint, it is referred to as a **scar contracture.** Race, family history, depth of the wound, size of the wound, patient age, and location of the wound all appear to be factors affecting scar formation.[7, 8, 21, 29]

All therapeutic interventions listed for the previous two phases may be applied to the maturation phase of healing. However, the physical therapist or physical therapist assistant can generally be more aggressive with manipulation of the wound site. Depending on circumstances, the maturation phase would also be the phase where work-hardening and work-conditioning exercises are energetically pursued. Moreover, depending on the size and location of the scar, scar management techniques should be instituted to control scar formation.

Additional Considerations. The variables of repair and patient response to skin wounds include depth of the damage, location of the injury, size of the wound, healing time, and etiology of the disruption. The depth of injury probably has the greatest impact on repair and eventual healing of a wound. For example, superficial wounds that leave a majority of the epidermal basal cells intact often heal without complication. Deeper skin damage that destroys much if not all the epidermal basal cell layer may take weeks to heal or require surgical intervention to hasten repair. Generally, the deeper the wound, the longer it takes to heal. Figure 10–2 illustrates depths of wounds and the integumentary structures involved at the varying depths.

The location of the injury can affect rehabilitation in many ways. For example, wounds on the feet can affect gait, wounds on hands can affect activities that require hand function, and wounds over any joint can lead to impairment in motion and therefore also lead to changes in strength and activities of daily living. Furthermore, wounds at cosmetic sites such as the face and hands may offer psychological challenges for a patient to overcome.

The size of a wound, often measured as the percentage of **total body surface area (TBSA)** affected, has an effect on the extent of the physiological response. A few of the physiological responses that should be considered include the

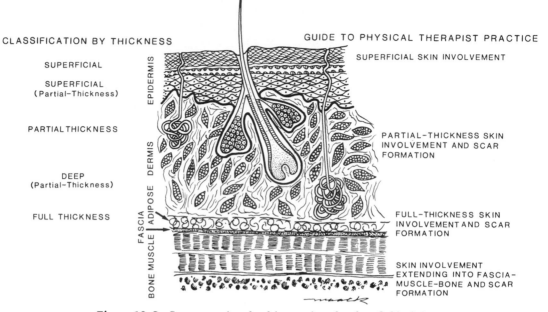

CLASSIFICATION BY THICKNESS

SUPERFICIAL

SUPERFICIAL
(Partial-Thickness)

PARTIAL THICKNESS

DEEP
(Partial-Thickness)

FULL THICKNESS

EPIDERMIS

DERMIS

FASCIA ADIPOSE

BONE MUSCLE

GUIDE TO PHYSICAL THERAPIST PRACTICE

SUPERFICIAL SKIN INVOLVEMENT

PARTIAL-THICKNESS SKIN
INVOLVEMENT AND SCAR
FORMATION

FULL-THICKNESS SKIN
INVOLVEMENT AND SCAR
FORMATION

SKIN INVOLVEMENT
EXTENDING INTO FASCIA-
MUSCLE-BONE AND SCAR
FORMATION

Figure 10–2. Structures involved in varying depths of skin injury.

local inflammatory response, the basal metabolic rate, temperature control, cardiopulmonary stresses, hematopoietic reactions, and pain. For example, a large skin wound (such as an extensive burn injury) may dangerously decrease the ability of a patient to control body temperature. Also, a big wound will lead to an increased basal metabolic rate and impose extra nutritional demands on a patient that need to be met to avert the protein catabolism that could lead to muscle loss. Potential infection is a problem with any open wound, and increased wound size may increase the risk of infection. As wound size increases, so does the magnitude of the physiological response.

Wounds that require a long time to finally heal are associated with two primary problems. The first is that the risk of infection increases the longer that the wound is open. Second, a wound is more likely to scar if it takes longer than 2 to 3 weeks to heal.

COMMON CONDITIONS

Damage to the integument most commonly occurs secondary to vascular compromise or trauma. Vascular deficiencies such as local tissue ischemia (pressure ulcers and arterial disease) and venous insufficiency can create an unhealthy tissue environment that leads to skin breakdown. Wounds from various types of trauma may include cuts, abrasions, and burns.

The etiology of a wound can provide insight into its prognosis. For example, it is expected that patients with wounds secondary to arterial disease will require surgical intervention to improve arterial function and eventually improve healing of the associated skin wound. In addition, electrical injures should lead to suspicion of the potential for injuries that involve tissue damage deeper than the skin.

Vascular Compromise

Wounds caused by **arterial insufficiency** are most commonly situated on the foot or ankle, but they can certainly occur at other locations. These wounds are caused by primary loss of vascular flow to an anatomical site, which leads to tissue death. **Venous insufficiency** (venous stasis) can also lead to ulceration of the skin and generally occurs on the lower part of the legs. Venous stasis may result from venous hypertension, venous thrombosis, varicose (dilated) veins, or obstruction of a portion of the venous system. The precise cause of ulcers caused by venous stasis has not been determined. One theory to explain venous stasis ulceration includes the notion of "fibrin cuff formation," which occurs as a result of an increase in capillary leakage of fibrinogen (as well as other large molecules) secondary to venous hypertension.[4] Fibrin then accumulates in the interstitial space and around capillaries and produces an obstacle to the transportation of oxygen and nutrients to tissue. Another theory regarding venous stasis ulcers is referred to as "white cell trapping." Venous hypertension decreases capillary flow and the subsequent removal of leukocytes. The trapped cells then occlude capillaries, which leads to ischemic damage, and may also release substances that bring about direct local tissue damage.[5]

Pressure on tissue leads to damage secondary to ischemia and to subsequent tissue hypoxia and death and a wound referred to as a **pressure ulcer.**[6, 27] It may take only a few hours of pressure to cause severe tissue injury.[19, 24] Pressure occurs most commonly over areas of bony prominence, such as the sacral/coccygeal area, ischial tuberosity, heel, lateral malleolus, and greater trochanter. Pressure may increase or decrease, depending on the position of the patient.[22] Table 10–1 lists sites at risk for pressure ulcers by position. For example, a person can do damage to the skin simply by being positioned incorrectly in a bed.

Although most pressure ulcers occur at sites of bony prominence, they can develop at any location in which enough pressure is generated to cause ischemia. Inactivity and immobility increase the chance of development of pressure sores.[1] Shearing of the tissue at the site of pressure can further increase the tissue damage. Shearing can occur when a patient is moved from one surface to another or by moving (sliding) on the same surface. This activity causes friction damage to the skin. Friction can denude the epidermal covering and increase the likelihood for pressure ulcer formation. If the skin is exposed to moisture for a certain period, it can become macerated and is more liable to breakdown. Common sources of moisture may include sweat, urine, and feces. Poor nutrition increases the risk for pressure ulcers. Increases in age also amplify the chance of a pressure ulcer's developing. This increased risk is

10

Table 10–1
Body Areas Commonly at Risk for Pressure
Ulcer Development

POSITION	AREAS AT RISK
Supine	Occiput, elbows, scapulae, spinous processes, sacrum, coccyx, heels
Seated	Elbows, spinous processes, sacrum, coccyx, ischial tuberosities, greater trochanters, heels
Side-lying	Ear, shoulder, elbow, greater trochanters, medial and lateral aspects of knees, medial and lateral malleoli, heels
Prone	Forehead, nose, chin, anterior of shoulder, iliac crest, patella, dorsal surface of foot or toes

Data from Kosiak M: Etiology and pathology of ischemic ulcers. Arch Phys Med Rehabil 1981;62:492–498.

secondary to several age-related changes such as a decrease in overall soft tissue mass, which increases the protuberance of bony prominences. Age-related changes in the skin include atrophy of the dermis, decreased vascularization, and impaired sensory perception.

Ischemic injury can take place as a result of loss of sensory feedback. An ulcer secondary to insensitivity is called a **neuropathic (neurotropic) ulcer.** Decreased sensation limits a person from making appropriate adjustments to potentially damaging situations. For example, a patient with sensory loss over the soles of the feet secondary to diabetes mellitus may not notice a tiny pebble in the shoe. Blood flow to the tissue compressed by the pebble decreases as the person continues to bear weight on the stone. Pressure ulcers may also occur with loss of sensory feedback, such as the case of a patient with a spinal cord injury. If the patient does not perform frequent weight shifts, ischemia resulting from pressure secondary to the sensory loss will lead to damage to the integument.

Trauma

Abrasions are integumentary wounds caused by scraping away skin through contact with a rough object or surface. Lacerations are cuts or tears of the integument and may be caused by sharp objects or surfaces. Injuries where much if not all the skin and generally the subcutaneous tissue are separated from the underlying tissue are referred to as avulsion injuries. When an avulsion injury occurs in a hand or a foot, it may be called a degloving injury. A puncture wound is a hole in the skin created by a pointed, generally sharp object. Burn injuries include damage to skin from many possible causes, such as flame, chemicals, scalding, radiation, and electrical current.

As with some cases of ischemic skin damage, trauma can also arise from loss of sensory feedback. Decreased sensation prevents a person from making appropriate adjustments to potentially damaging situations. For example, a patient with decreased sensation in the upper extremities secondary to edema resulting from surgical removal of axillary lymph nodes may not perceive the hazardous temperature of a dish when removing it from the oven or dangerously hot water, either of which could lead to a burn injury.

Disease

The skin can be affected by a number of disorders that may be either benign or life threatening. **Inflammatory skin diseases** are generally patchy sites of acute or chronic inflammation referred to as **dermatitis.** Dermatitis often includes associated symptoms of itching and some scaling of the epidermis. Certain viruses can lead to warts or rashes. Bacteria, foreign bodies, and plugged sebaceous glands are some of the causes that may lead to acne or other skin abscesses.

Neoplastic skin diseases (skin cancer) include basal cell carcinoma, squamous cell carcinoma, and malignant melanoma, which are the three most common types of cancer associated with the integument. Although other causes are possible, extensive exposure to sunlight is the most common etiology for each of these cancers.

PRINCIPLES OF EXAMINATION

Examination of a wound should include a thorough history and physical assessment of the etiology, depth, and size of the wound and signs of infection. Some variations in actual examination procedures may be applicable to different etiologies (see later). The skin adjacent to or otherwise associated with the wound should also be examined to determine whether it has any alteration from normal function (e.g., sensation, temperature, hair growth, mobility, pliability) and appearance (e.g., texture and color [red for inflammation or bluish for cyanosis or poor perfusion]).

All ulcers, regardless of their etiology, should be examined for size and depth. The size of a wound can be charted by using several methods that might include tracing diagrams of the wound, TBSA estimates (see burns), and photography. The depth of a wound can be measured by using known volumes of saline injected into the wound cavity (with the amount of saline left over subtracted from the total to give a volume). Depth may also be measured by using a wound filler (such as dental alginate) that can be transferred to a volumeter to allow for a volumetric measurement of the depth of the wound via displacement of fluid from the volumeter. Depth can be further determined by observation of the tissue that is exposed. For example, a moist pink or red wound that is hypersensitive and on an even plane with adjacent, uninjured skin is probably a partial-thickness wound, whereas deeper wounds often allow identification of subcutaneous adipose tissue or fascia. Wounds that extend beyond defined subcutaneous tissue will provide visualization of muscle, tendon, ligament, bone, and other structures.

10

Besides assessing integrity of the integument, the physical therapist should perform other tests and measures to be fully capable of evaluating the patient. A patient's ability to communicate and comprehend, joint mobility, muscle performance, gait (if applicable), ventilation and circulation, and sensory tests (including assessment of pain) should be part of the physical therapy examination.

Vascular Compromise

Arterial Wounds. Wounds caused by arterial insufficiency are commonly found on the lower part of the leg, including the feet and toes. Minimal, if any, exudate is seen because of the poor circulation to the wound. The shape of these wounds is commonly irregular, and the wounds are often deep with a pale wound base. The diminished circulation also contributes to poor wound healing. The pain associated with arterial wounds is severe and generally increases when the leg is elevated. Skin adjacent to these wounds is characterized by hair loss and pallor on elevation, is cool to the touch, and appears "thin" and shiny. Pulses associated with arterial wounds are very weak or absent.

Venous Ulcers. Wounds caused by venous insufficiency are commonly found on the lower part of the leg. Exudate and edema are present, the shape of these wounds is commonly irregular, and the wounds are generally shallow with a red or pink wound base. Edema is a factor in poor wound healing. Some mild pain is associated with venous ulcers, and the pain can commonly be decreased when the leg is elevated. The skin adjacent to these wounds is characterized by inflammation, dilated veins, abnormal pigmentation, and induration (hardness) and may be dry or scaly. Pulses associated with venous ulcers are present.

Neuropathic Ulcers. Neuropathic ulcers are usually located on the plantar surface of the foot at pressure points or bony prominences. The wound may bleed easily unless the condition is coupled with arterial insufficiency. The shape of these wounds is commonly circular, and the wounds are often deep. Because of the sensory neuropathy that led to the wound, no pain is normally associated with these ulcers. The skin adjacent to these wounds is characterized by sensory deficit but might otherwise appear fairly normal.

Pressure Ulcers. Pressure ulcers may be located at diverse sites on the body, but they are generally found over bony prominences. Besides describing the location, the examiner should document the depth and size, which can vary. A well-accepted method for describing a pressure ulcer is to use a staging system provided by the U.S. Department of Health and Human Services.[3] Staging of the ulcer is based on the characteristics of the wound, mainly the depth. Table 10–2 outlines the criteria for staging pressure ulcers. Once an ulcer is staged, the assigned stage should not change as the wound changes. For example, a stage III ulcer that heals does not progress from a stage III to a stage II and then to a stage I ulcer (referred to as back-staging). Rather, healing of the

Table 10–2
Criteria for Staging Pressure Ulcers

ULCER STAGE	DESCRIPTION OF THE ULCER
I	Nonblanchable erythema of intact skin, the heralding lesion of skin ulceration. In individuals with darker skin, discoloration of the skin, warmth, edema, induration, or hardness may also be indicators
II	Partial-thickness loss involving the epidermis, dermis, or both. The ulcer is superficial and is clinically noticeable as an abrasion, blister, or shallow crater
III	Full-thickness skin loss involving damage or necrosis of subcutaneous tissue, which may extend down to but not through underlying fascia. The ulcer is clinically manifested as a deep crater with or without undermining of adjacent tissue
IV	Full-thickness skin loss with extensive destruction, tissue necrosis, or damage to muscle, bone, or supporting structures (such as tendon, joint capsule). Undermining and sinus tracts may also be associated with stage IV ulcers.

From Bergstrom N, Allman RM, Alvarez OM, et al: Treatment of Pressure Ulcers, Clinical Practice Guideline No 15. Rockville, MD, U.S. Department of Health and Human Services, 1994.

wound is described in terms of changes in size, depth, and other characteristics and, when healed, it would be a healed stage III ulcer.

Trauma

It is recommended that any traumatic wound of concern be initially referred for primary medical intervention. This recommendation would hold true for wounds such as abrasions, lacerations, puncture wounds, avulsion injuries, degloving injuries, and burn injuries, regardless of the cause of the wound.

Burn injuries include damage to skin secondary to one or more of the following sources: flame, chemicals, scalding, radiation, and electrical current. The severity of the burn injury depends on several factors, including percent TBSA affected, location of the burn, depth of the wound, presence of associated trauma (i.e., fracture, nerve injury), and smoke inhalation. Figure 10–3 provides a method for calculating percent TBSA and documenting the location and depth of injury. The size of the wound as reported in percent TBSA affected and the location of the burns are important clues that indicate sites of potential impairment and functional loss. Impairments may be acute secondary to pain or wound contraction in superficial, partial-thickness, and full-thickness burns, whereas wound and scar contracture at a burn site can lead

10

Area	1 year	1–4 years	5–9 Years	10–14 years	15 years	Adult	Partial-thickness	Full-thickness	Total
Head	19	17	13	11	9	7			
Neck	2	2	2	2	2	2			
Ant. trunk	13	13	13	13	13	13			
Post. trunk	13	13	13	13	13	13			
Right buttock	2 1/2	2 1/2	2 1/2	2 1/2	2 1/2	2 1/2			
Left buttock	2 1/2	2 1/2	2 1/2	2 1/2	2 1/2	2 1/2			
Genitalia	1	1	1	1	1	1			
Right upper arm	4	4	4	4	4	4			
Left upper arm	4	4	4	4	4	4			
Right lower arm	3	3	3	3	3	3			
Left lower arm	3	3	3	3	3	3			
Right hand	2 1/2	2 1/2	2 1/2	2 1/2	2 1/2	2 1/2			
Left hand	2 1/2	2 1/2	2 1/2	2 1/2	2 1/2	2 1/2			
Right thigh	5 1/2	6 1/2	8	8 1/2	9	9 1/2			
Left thigh	5 1/2	6 1/2	8	8 1/2	9	9 1/2			
Right leg	5	5	5 1/2	6	6 1/2	7			
Left leg	5	5	5 1/2	6	6 1/2	7			
Right foot	3 1/2	3 1/2	3 1/2	3 1/2	3 1/2	3 1/2			
Left foot	3 1/2	3 1/2	3 1/2	3 1/2	3 1/2	3 1/2			
						Total			

Etiology of injury _____

Date of injury _____

Time of injury _____

Patient age _____

Patient sex _____

Patient weight _____

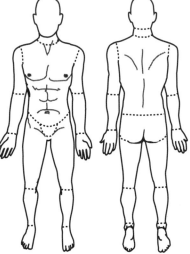

Figure 10–3. Burn diagram used to calculate the size, location, and depth of a burn injury.

to chronic struggles with decreased function and potential disability. The location of the burn may also have cosmetic implications for long-term socialization of a patient with burns. The depth of a wound can be determined by the presence of certain clinical findings.[37] A superficial burn injury is painful and erythematous (like a sunburn), with the possibility of some minor localized swelling. Partial-thickness injuries are typically very painful, red, and weepy. The skin is normally pliable. A blistering wound is also commonly associated with a partial-thickness burn. A full-thickness burn is generally not painful when palpated, may be tan or yellowish brown, and has a leathery, nonpliable texture.

Associated trauma can increase the severity of a burn injury as a result of the increased level of impairment that a patient will experience beyond that caused by the burns. Documentation of any associated trauma is critical to the establishment of a comprehensive plan of care. Smoke inhalation (inhalation injury) may lead to cardiopulmonary impairment. Impaired ventilation, gas exchange, aerobic capacity, and endurance secondary to an inhalation injury may need to be addressed in the plan of care.

Disease

A physician carries out the actual diagnosis and primary treatment of skin disease. However, it is very important that physical therapists and physical therapist assistants be able to recognize the signs and symptoms of skin cancer so that patients can be provided with an appropriate and prompt medical referral. Key warning signs for any skin cancer include a new skin growth, a sore that does not heal within 3 months, or a bump that is getting larger. Detection of melanoma is based on alterations in a growth on the skin or in a mole and may include changes in size, color, shape, elevation, surface appearance, or sensation.

Scar Tissue

As some wounds heal, scar tissue may form. Assessment of the scar tissue may be performed with the **Vancouver Burn Scar Scale**.[34] This scale rates characteristics of scars, including pigmentation, vascularity, pliability, and height (Table 10–3). A higher score on the Vancouver Burn Scar Scale correlates with more scarring. Scars are generally referred to as either hypertrophic scars or keloid scars. Both keloid scars and hypertrophic scars hypertrophy, but as keloid scars grow, they extend beyond the boundaries of the wound whereas hypertrophic scars do not.[30] In addition to examination of the scar itself, the

Table 10–3
The Vancouver Burn Scar Scale

SCORE	PIGMENTATION	VASCULARITY	PLIABILITY	HEIGHT
0	Normal pigmentation, close to the pigment over the rest of the body	Normal	Normal	Flat (normal)
1	Hypopigmentation	Pink	Flexible with minimal resistance	Raised <2 mm
2	Hyperpigmentation	Red	Gives way to pressure	Raised <5 mm
3		Purple	Firm, not easily moved	Raised >5 mm
4			Banding: raised tissue that blanches with stretching of the scar	
5			Contracture: permanent tightening that produces a deformity	

From Sullivan T, Smith J, Kermode J, et al: Rating the burn scar. J Burn Care Rehabil 1990;11:256–260.

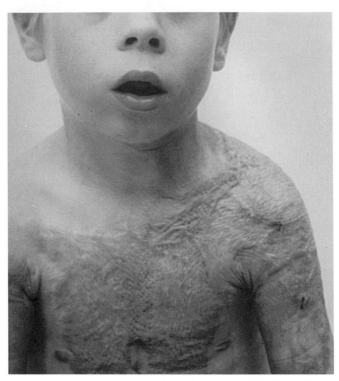

Figure 10–4. Hypertrophic burn scar. (From Carrougher GJ: Burn Care and Therapy. St. Louis, CV Mosby, 1998.)

location of the scar should also be assessed. Scars located over or near joints may impede joint mobility, and scars in areas of cosmetic importance may have a detrimental effect on patient motivation and activity (Fig. 10–4). Scar contraction, which can lead to contracture, is a major contributor to wound-related disability.

PRINCIPLES OF EVALUATION, DIAGNOSIS, AND PROGNOSIS

Evaluation of a patient with a skin wound encompasses the extent of the condition, identification of related impairments, the level of associated loss of function, the patient's basic health condition, and social factors affecting care. The decisions made through an evaluation render a diagnosis about the meaning of a patient's signs and symptoms. The *Guide to Physical Therapist Practice* provides groupings of signs and symptoms in "integumentary patterns" that are readily associated with the various skin conditions presented in this chapter.[17] The practice patterns presented in the *Guide* also provide diagnoses that can be used for patients with integumentary involvement.

The prognosis of a patient with integumentary involvement is related to the diagnosis and will be enhanced by making sure that the wound is stable, clean, healing, or healed. Some indication of the potential for scarring or the course of the scarring should be included in the prognosis because scarring clearly affects the time needed for treatment and follow-up. The prognosis of problems associated with wounds will be influenced by the severity of the problems. For example, severe edema will lead to a poorer prognosis than will a diagnosis of mild edema. Additionally, the presence of any comorbidity, infection, chronicity of the problem, and any number of other physical, psychological, or social factors will affect the prognosis.

PRINCIPLES OF DIRECT INTERVENTION

Proper attention by the physical therapist and physical therapist assistant to the integument ranges from preventing skin breakdown to promoting healing of wounds. Patients must also be educated about possible concerns associated with the wound, including management of the risks and signs of infection, wound care and dressing procedures, and the management of scar tissue. Setting appropriate goals for the interventions is imperative to minimize impairment and functional loss.

This section establishes some basic elements of physical therapy intervention related to the integument. For details about integumentary management, the reader should refer to the Suggested Readings at the end of the chapter and continue to peruse current literature on the topic.

Prevention

When patients are at risk for ulcers (i.e., decreased sensation, decreased vascularity, decreased mobility, poor nutrition, incontinence), it is important to become involved in the prevention element of physical therapy care. Positioning, supports or cushions that reduce pressure, and self-inspection of the skin are important elements of preventing ulcers secondary to decreased mobility, impaired sensation, or lack of circulation. Water-repellant lotions and absorbent products can be used to decrease the damaging effects of incontinence on the skin. Appropriate dressings and proper transfer techniques are important in preventing skin breakdown secondary to shear and friction. When edema is associated with a wound, compression therapies such as intermittent compression pumps and compression garments may be beneficial

Wound Management

Any wound, depending on its depth and other complications, may require surgery such as grafting to achieve closure of the wound. However, many wounds require short- or long-term conservative management with appropriate dressings and possibly with topical agents. As noted in the *Guide to Physical Therapist Practice*, the extent of physical therapy interventions is based on the depth of injury.[17]

Conservative management of arterial wounds and neuropathic ulcers commonly consists of wound care, protection of the wound and surrounding tissue, and possibly bed rest. The wound should be cleansed when dressings are changed. Dressings that maintain or increase moisture at the site of the wound should be used because of the lack of exudate from the wound. Cushions or protective casting (total contact casting) may be useful in preventing further trauma to the wound as it heals. Bed rest may be helpful in protecting the

10

wound, but it must be used with caution to avoid leading to other impairments secondary to disuse.

Venous wounds should be managed by wound care and compression of the affected extremity. Wound care should consist of cleansing the wound and applying a dressing. The dressing used will depend on the amount of exudate at the wound site. Generally, the dressing of choice is a pliable semiabsorbent or gel-type dressing. If a dressing is to be worn during compression therapy, the dressing should not be bulky. Compression of the extremity helps reduce swelling and venous hypertension in the limb. Activity such as ambulation, swimming, or cycling should be encouraged unless a medical contraindication is present.

Pressure ulcers require wound care and pressure relief. Much like venous ulcers, pressure ulcers should be cleansed and dressed in such a way to provide a moist healing environment but still manage any excess exudate. Pressure-relieving devices might include any of the following options. Seat cushions should decrease the likelihood of shear and pressure while also protecting against increases in heat and moisture. Wheelchairs should be also appropriately aligned to minimize the chance of pressure ulcer formation. Foam that is either premanufactured for certain anatomical areas or custom-cut by the therapist can be used to help position patients while they are in bed. Air mattresses and other pressure relief mattresses are available and help decrease the build-up of pressure in any one location on the body. Turning schedules should also be established and followed. A typical turning schedule would ideally have a patient turned every 2 hours with equal time spent supine, prone, lying on the right side, and lying on the left side.

Treatment of burns is generally based on the depth of the wound, with skin grafting being inevitable for full-thickness wounds of any consequential percent TBSA. Wounds of any depth should be carefully cleansed. After cleansing, superficial burns require only a moisturizer to help keep the skin moist, which may provide some pain relief. Partial-thickness burns are commonly covered with a topical agent, either an ointment such as Polysporin or a cream such as silver sulfadiazine. These wounds are then covered with nonadherent gauze and wrapped lightly with a gauze dressing. Full-thickness burns are characteristically treated with a topical silver sulfadiazine cream and wrapped in gauze dressing.

With any of these wounds, appropriate exercises and activities should be prescribed to decrease other impairments. Exercises should emphasize joint mobility, muscle performance, gait (if applicable), ventilation, and circulation.

Scar Management

The major functional problem with scar tissue is the continuous contraction associated with it. Scar hypertrophy may not only contribute to loss of function but also lead to cosmetic defects. Surgery to correct problems associated with scarring may be considered in an attempt to improve specific impairments or particular cosmetic deformities. Nonsurgical management of a scar is accomplished in a variety of ways. Positioning may be used to counter scar contraction by lengthening tissue for a maintained period.[29] Generally, anticontracture positions are positions of extension at each affected joint region, such as elbow extension with supination or a neutral ankle position with no flexion of the toes. Splints may be used as static positioning devices to hold a joint in a certain position.[39] Serial splinting may also be used to progressively increase joint range of motion.[18] Dynamic splints, which apply a gentle stretch to tissue, are used for mobilization or exercise purposes.[9] Some prefabricated splints are available, but most clinicians fabricate custom splints from malleable thermoplastic material. Passive stretching may be used to help gently elongate contracting tissue. Active exercise (including ambulation) is used for the same purpose as passive stretching, but it provides a way to involve patients in their own rehabilitation.[31] With any stretching, passive or active, the patient should feel the tissue stretch and try to "push the stretch" as much as possible (Fig. 10–5). Effective stretching does not require induction of pain in the affected tissue during the stretch or exercise.

Pressure garments are used to decrease hypertrophy of the scar (see Fig. 10–5). These supports also assist in conforming the scar to normal anatomical parameters. Typically, patients are prescribed pressure garments during the maturation phase of healing. The pressure garments can be custom-ordered to fit a patient and can be made for any extremity, the face or head, the hands, the feet, and the torso.

Patient Education

The patient should be the most important member of the rehabilitation team. Those who will be assisting with care of the patient should be included as well in all sessions preparing the patient for discharge. Obvious items that should be taught to the patient and other caregivers include skin care and wound management protocols, positioning techniques, exercise programs, and the application and wearing of pressure garments (if needed). Demonstrating the technique and allowing the patient or caregiver to perform any of the protocols under observation should reinforce all these procedures. It is important to inform the patient about the reasons for the procedures being applied. If patients know what techniques or procedures they must do, how to do them, and the reasons for doing the specific protocols assigned, they will be more apt to comply with their care.[26]

10

Case Studies   *Mrs. George—Venous Insufficiency Causing Ulcer* _____

Mrs. George is a 53-year-old woman in whom venous insufficiency had been diagnosed 5 years earlier. She has managed it well until recently, when a small ulcer developed on the left lateral aspect of the lower part of her leg about 8 cm above her lateral malleolus. The ulcer is approximately 2 by 3 cm in size and is partial to deep partial thickness. A measurable amount of exudate is oozing from the wound. The limb is edematous (in comparison to the contralateral limb). Lower extremity pulses are palpable. The patient complains of mild

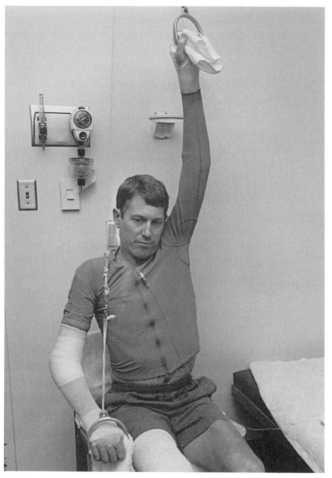

Figure 10–5. Patient using overhead reciprocal pulleys to perform a self-stretch of scar tissue in the axillae and over the elbows. The patient is also wearing pressure garments to help control scar hypertrophy. (From Carrougher GJ: Burn Care and Therapy. St. Louis, CV Mosby, 1998.)

pain at the wound site, but she is otherwise functionally independent in all activities.

Goals. Management goals include a reduction in risk factors for infection, reduced wound size, attainment of wound healing, and a reduction in edema. The patient should understand these goals and what the desired outcomes from intervention are.

Intervention. To decrease the risk for infection, the wound should be selectively débrided to remove nonviable tissue. Appropriate dressings should be applied, including, in this particular case, a semiabsorbent, nonbulky dressing that will maintain a moist wound environment but also absorb some of the exudate from the wound. Intermittent compression with an extremity lymphedema pump may be useful in decreasing edema. A graduated compression stocking should be fitted for this individual. The patient should be encouraged to ambulate and if necessary be prescribed a walking schedule. While seated, she should elevate the limb and perform ankle pumps. Standing for long periods should be discouraged. The patient should be educated and be able to demonstrate how to (1) perform dressing changes, (2) apply and operate the intermittent compression pump (one could be rented for home use), (3) apply and monitor the fit of the graduated compression stocking, and (4) describe the reasoning for the prescribed interventions and the importance of exercise and elevation in preventing further problems related to edema and venous stasis.

Stan—Burn

Stan is 47 years old and was injured in a house fire. He incurred a 14% TBSA burn. Full-thickness injuries totaling 7% TBSA occurred on his right upper extremity and hand. The other 7% TBSA included the upper right portion of his chest and back. The patient is right hand dominant. He was previously healthy and suffered no associated injuries (i.e., smoke inhalation). Stan was employed as a worker in a warehouse and lives at home with his wife and three teenage children. Four days after his admission to the burn center, his right upper extremity and hand burns were skin-grafted.

Goals. Risk factors for infection need to be reduced to enhance partial-thickness wound healing and prepare full-thickness wounds for skin grafting. Joint mobility is to be maintained and soft tissue restriction (wound and scar contraction) reduced. The risk of impairment secondary to scar formation needs to be decreased. Independence in activities of daily living and the ability to perform tasks associated with his work are goals to be regained. The patient should understand these goals and what the desired outcomes from intervention are.

Intervention. When dealing with such a burn, the patient must be treated before any surgery to alleviate and prevent increased impairment and disability. The patient must continue with postsurgical treatment to achieve the final desired outcomes of therapy intervention.

Presurgery. The wounds should be cleansed and dressed twice a day to reduce the risk of infection and promote healing of the partial-thickness wounds and to prepare the full-thickness wounds for skin grafting. Active range-of-motion exercises for the upper extremity and hand will enhance joint mobility and decrease the soft tissue restriction associated with wound contraction. Positioning of the upper extremity will also help prevent decreases in mobility and increases in soft tissue restriction. The patient should also be encouraged to participate in his personal care (i.e., brushing teeth, combing hair, and personal hygiene), which will aid in future independence in activities of daily living.

Postsurgery. Any remaining partial-thickness wounds should be cleansed and dressed twice a day to reduce the risk of infection and promote healing. Active range-of-motion exercises and positioning that began presurgically should be

10

continued after surgery. Passive range of motion or stretching of the upper extremity might be helpful in overcoming any relentless contraction of the scar tissue forming at the sites of skin grafting. The patient should be required to manage his personal care independently. Strengthening exercises and exercises specific to preparation for return to work should also be included as the patient can tolerate them. The patient's upper extremity should be measured for and fitted with a scar control compression garment (specifically, an arm sleeve and a glove). Scar control will help maintain anatomical contours and decrease the risk of soft tissue restriction secondary to scar formation.

The patient should be educated and be able to demonstrate how to (1) assist with dressing changes, (2) perform any of the specifically prescribed exercises, and (3) apply and monitor the fit of the scar control compression garments. The patient should also be able to describe the rationale behind each of the interventions.

Summary

This chapter outlined the many components of integumentary care. The anatomy of the skin and the phases of wound healing are important elements to understand when considering interventions. Common conditions of skin breakdown arise secondary to problems with local circulation, decreased sensation, long-standing pressure, and trauma. Understanding the implications of wound depth, size, and location is critical in developing treatments. Beyond direct management of the wound, interventions that stress prevention of further skin breakdown and decrease impairments related to other systems were discussed. Treatments that enhance wound healing and involve the patient directly as part of the rehabilitation team will be most beneficial in generating optimum patient outcomes.

References

1. Allman RM, Goode PS, Patrick MM, et al: Pressure ulcer risk factors among hospitalized patients with activity limitations. JAMA 1995;273:865–870.
2. Bell E, Iverson B, Merril C: Production of a tissue-like structure by contraction of collagen lattices by human fibroblasts of different proliferative potential in vitro. Proc Natl Acad Sci U S A 1979;76:1274–1278.
3. Bergstrom N, Allman RM, Alvarez OM, et al: Treatment of Pressure Ulcers, Clinical Practice Guideline No. 15. Rockville, MD, U.S. Department of Health and Human Services, 1994.
4. Browse NL, Burnand KG: The cause of venous ulceration. Lancet 1982;2:243–245.
5. Coleridge Smith PD, Thomas P, Scurr JH, et al: Causes of venous ulceration: A new hypothesis. BMJ 1988;296:1726–1727.
6. Daniel RK, Priest DL, Wheatley DC: Etiologic factors in pressure sores: An experimental model. Arch Phys Med Rehabil 1981;62:492–498.
7. Davies DM: Scars, hypertrophic scars and keloids. BMJ 1985;290:1056–1058.
8. Deitch EA, Wheelahan TM, Rose MP: Hypertrophic burn scars: Analysis of variables. J Trauma 1983;23:895–898.
9. Duncan RM: Basic principles of splinting the hand. Phys Ther 1989;69:1104–1116.
10. Dunphy JE, Jackson DS: Practical applications of experimental studies in the care of primarily closed wounds. Am J Surg 1962;104:273–282.
11. Eddy RJ, Petro JA, Tomasek JJ: Evidence for the nonmuscular nature of the "myofibroblast" of granulation tissue and hypertrophic scar: An immunofluorescence study. Am J Pathol 1988;130:252–260.

12. Fishel RS, Barbul A, Beschorner WE, et al: Lymphocyte participation in wound healing. Morphologic assessment using monoclonal antibodies. Ann Surg 1987;206:25–29.
13. Ford-Hutchinson EW, Bray MA, Doig MV, et al: Leukotriene B, a potent chemokinetic and aggregating substance released from polymorphonuclear leukocytes. Nature 1980;286:264–265.
14. Gabbiani G, Hirschel BJ, Ryan GB, et al: Granulation tissue as a contractile organ. A study of structure and function. J Exp Med 1972;135:719–734.
15. Gabbiani G, Ryan G, Majne G: Presence of modified fibroblasts in granulation tissue and their possible role in wound contraction. Experientia 1971;27:549–550.
16. Gogia PP: Clinical Wound Management. Thorofare, NJ, Slack, 1995.
17. Guide to Physical Therapist Practice. 2nd ed. Phys Ther 2001;81:9–744.
18. Hunter JM, Mackin EJ, Callahan AD: Rehabilitation of the Hand, ed 4. St Louis, CV Mosby, 1995.
19. Husain T: An experimental study of some pressure effects on tissues, with reference to the bedsore problem. J Pathol Bacteriol 1953;66:347–358.
20. Ketchum LD: Hypertrophic scars and keloids. Clin Plast Surg 1977;4:301–310.
21. Ketchum LD, Cohen IK, Masters FW: Hypertrophic scars and keloids. Plast Reconstr Surg 1974;53:140–154.
22. Kosiak M: Etiology and pathology of ischemic ulcers. Arch Phys Med Rehabil 1981;62:492–498.
23. Leibovich SJ, Ross R: The role of the macrophage in wound repair: A study with hydrocortisone and antimacrophage serum. Am J Pathol 1975;78:71–100.
24. Lindon O, Greenway RM, Piazza JM: Pressure distributor on the surface of the human body. Arch Phys Med Rehabil 1965;46:378.
25. Peacock EE: Wound Repair, ed 3. Philadelphia, WB Saunders, 1984.
26. Peloquin SM: Linking purpose to procedure during interactions with patients. Am J Occup Ther 1988;42:775–781.
27. Reuler JB, Cooney TG: The pressure sore: Pathophysiology and principles of management. Ann Intern Med 1981;94:661.
28. Rockwell WB, Cohen IK, Erlich JP: Keloids and hypertrophic scars: A comprehensive report. Plast Reconstr Surg 1989;84:827–837.
29. Rudolf R: Construction and the control of contraction. World J Surg 1980;4:279–287.
30. Rudolf R: Wide spread scars, hypertrophic scars and keloids. Clin Plast Surg 1987;14:253–260.
31. Schnebly WA, Ward RS, Warden GD, et al: A nonsplinting approach to the care of the thermally injured patient. J Burn Care Rehabil 1989;10:263–266.
32. Schumann D: The nature of wound healing. AORN J 1982;35:1068–1077.
33. Simpson DM, Ross R: The neutrophilic leukocyte in wound repair: A study with antineutrophil serum. J Clin Invest 1972;51:2009–2023.
34. Sullivan T, Smith J, Kermode J, et al: Rating the burn scar. J Burn Care Rehabil 1990;11:256–260.
35. Wahl LM, Wahl SM: Lymphokine modulation of connective tissue metabolism. Ann N Y Acad Sci 1979;332:411–422.
36. Wahl SM, Wahl LM, McCarthy JB: Lymphocyte-mediated activation of fibroblast proliferation and collagen production. J Immunol 1978;121:942–946.
37. Ward RS: The rehabilitation of burn patients. CRC Crit Rev Phys Med Rehabil 1991;2:121–138.
38. Ward RS, et al: Evaluation of therapeutic ultrasound to improve response to physical therapy and lessen scar contracture after burn injury. J Burn Care Rehabil 1994;15:74–79.
39. Waymack JP, Fidler J, Warden GD: Surgical correction of burn scar contractures of the foot in children. Burns 1988;14:156–160.

10

Suggested Readings

Carrougher GJ: Burn Care and Therapy. St Louis, CV Mosby, 1998.

This nicely written textbook covers broad issues in burn care from both a nursing and a therapy perspective.

Guide to Physical Therapist Practice. Alexandria, VA, American Physical Therapy Association, July 1999.

This text presents critical descriptions of practice patterns and guidelines related to care of the integument.

McCulloch JM, Kloth LC, Feedar JA: Wound Healing: Alternatives in Management. Philadelphia, FA Davis, 1995.

A very useful textbook that reviews wound healing and management of wounds.

Richard RL, Staley MJ: Burn Care and Rehabilitation: Principles and Practice. Philadelphia, FA Davis, 1994.

This excellent textbook provides the essential information one requires to understand and treat patients with burn injuries and selected serious skin diseases.

Sussman C, Bates-Jensen BM: Wound Care: A Collaborative Practice Manual for Physical Therapists and Nurses. Gaithersburg, MD, Aspen, 1998.

A well-written textbook that focuses on clinical examination and management of many common wounds.

REVIEW QUESTIONS

1. Describe the three phases of wound healing and develop a rationale for physical therapy involvement in each phase.

2. List the variables that should be identified during your examination of a patient to determine the etiology and seriousness of the wound. How might these variables affect your intervention?

3. What characteristics differentiate a venous ulcer from an arterial ulcer, as well as these ulcers from a pressure ulcer?

4. Explain the differences involved in treating a superficial wound versus a deep wound.

5. How might an increased understanding of integumentary wounds and wound healing help you better understand injuries to tissues that you cannot visualize (i.e., soft tissue injury, fracture, tissue necrosis).

6. Why is it important for physical therapists to be aware of scar formation?

What path will we take? Let us not take one that others have made. . . . Instead, let us make our own path.
Ruth Wood, PT, FAPTA

Physical Therapy for Pediatric Conditions

Angela Easley Rosenberg

KEY TERMS

cerebral palsy (CP)

clubfoot

congenital dislocation of the hip (CDH)

cystic fibrosis (CF)

developmental delay

developmental milestone

disablement process

Down syndrome

Duchenne muscular dystrophy (DMD)

eclectic approach

enablement process

family assessment

fetal alcohol syndrome (FAS)

goal-directed movement approach

Individualized Education Plan (IEP)

Individualized Family Service Plan (IFSP)

juvenile rheumatoid arthritis (JRA)

meningocele

meningomyelocele

normal developmental theory

osteogenesis imperfecta (OI)

prenatal cocaine exposure

scoliosis

secondary condition

sensory integration (SI)

spina bifida

spina bifida occulta

spinal muscular atrophy (SMA)

standardized testing

OBJECTIVES   After reading this chapter, the reader will be able to

- Describe the enablement and disablement processes as presented by the World Health Organization
- Describe the impact of federal legislation on the delivery of physical therapy services to children
- Describe the general features of common pediatric conditions seen by a physical therapist or physical therapist assistant
- Describe aspects of the patient/client examination that are unique to pediatric clients
- Describe the general features of four physical therapy treatment approaches for pediatric clients

Children will be children, first and foremost. They are not merely scaled-down versions of adults; rather, they progress through unique age-related movement stages, or developmental milestones. Pediatric physical therapists will observe these milestones to determine whether discrepancies exist between the child's chronological and neurological (or developmental) ages. If so, evaluation and subsequent intervention may be appropriate. More important, pediatric physical therapists must assess each child's ability to meet the task-related challenges of that child's daily environment. This type of assessment and intervention planning require thoughtful, structured strategies that often involve a constellation of players, including the child's family, caregivers, teachers, and community professionals. This chapter describes the examination and intervention techniques used by pediatric physical therapists. It includes common conditions seen and two case studies to illustrate a variety of approaches for the management of pediatric clients.

The primary focus for pediatric therapists is to observe children as they portray their individual strengths and abilities and to promote a functional, optimal developmental process. By acquiring knowledge of normal development through observation of movement patterns and transitions, the therapist can more accurately detect abnormal movements. The challenge is differentiating normal delays from those that signal potential developmental problems.[22] For example, observations of generations of children tell us that walking is initiated at approximately 10 to 13 months, yet some infants may take their first steps as early as 8 months or as late as 18 months. This type of variation occurs at all stages of child development and requires pediatric therapists to examine and provide interventions to children on a constantly changing developmental base.[16] Pediatric therapists play a crucial role in determining the absence of movement components that may impede the accomplishment of **developmental milestones** or functional goals for a child. In addition to child development, pediatric practice requires the therapist to acquire specific knowledge in basic areas ranging from child psychology to motor learning. The cognitive strategies and learning methods of adults are generally functionally oriented toward work, leisure, or daily living activities, whereas children learn from a different point of view—play. The pediatric physical therapist is often found in what might be called compromising situations—hopping, rolling, tumbling—in order to engage and invite the child to participate in therapeutic activities.

Play is the medium most used to promote therapeutic activities in a young child, whereas in an adolescent, therapy goals may be structured around social situations.[57] The primary goal is to identify meaningful activities that correspond to the learning style of each pediatric client, given the age, culture, and most natural social and physical environments (Fig. 11–1).

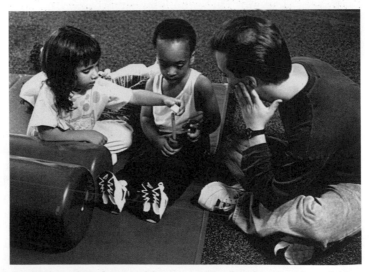

Figure 11–1. Cooperative play provides an avenue for therapeutic activities. (Courtesy of Bruce Wang.)

11

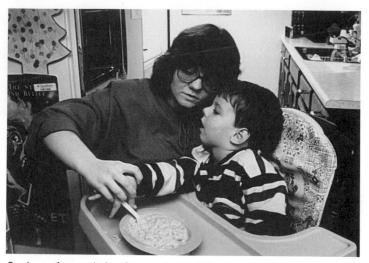

Figure 11–2. A mother assisting her son's special motor needs at dinnertime. (Courtesy of Bruce Wang.)

Children who have health problems that require specialty or subspecialty care are often referred to as "children with special health care needs."[91] Pediatric therapists may provide direct or consultative therapy to these children over long periods, depending on the child's changing needs. When caring for children with special needs, physical therapists collaborate closely with the family and other health professionals in designing a long-term, family-centered plan of care (Fig. 11–2). This plan includes a full range of services—prevention, early identification, evaluation, diagnostics, treatment, habilitation, and rehabilitation.[66] Throughout service provision, emphasis is placed on recognizing each child as part of a family system, with unique cultural characteristics that must be considered when designing treatment goals.

GENERAL DESCRIPTION

If the physical therapist focuses solely on the child's motor strengths and needs while neglecting the cultural impact of family and community factors on that child, a successful treatment outcome is unlikely. The World Health Organization (WHO) has acknowledged this focus by viewing a *process of enablement and disablement* on several levels: impairment, activity/functional limitations, and disability/participation restriction (Fig. 11–3 and Table 11–1).[42, 52] **Enablement processes** and **disablement processes** represent the dynamic, interactive relationships that a child has within different environmental contexts. Through this model it becomes evident that in the disease process, physical impairment (e.g., central nervous system abnormality) directly affects the child in several realms, including the physical, all of which must be considered when designing a plan of care. The child's functional limitations or manifestation of the impairment (e.g., inability to speak or walk) is influenced by the degree of impairment, as well as other factors, including the child's motivational level and course of rehabilitation. In turn, the child's functional limitations may have an impact on the family system (e.g., interaction style) and peer relation-

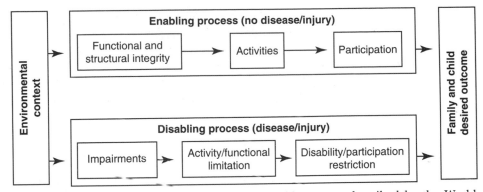

Figure 11–3. The process of enablement and disablement as described by the World Health Organization. (Adapted from the International Classification of Impairments, Activities and Participation [ICIDH-2], A Manual of Dimensions of Disablement and Functioning, Beta-1 Draft for Field Trials. Geneva, 1997, World Health Organization.)

ships. Finally, disability, or the influence of social or environmental restrictions on participation (e.g., access to schools, sports), is a result of the culture, society, and environment in which the child lives. (See Chapter 1 for further description of the disablement model.)

When the child is cared for using the WHO model as a guide, all these

TABLE 11–1
Classification of Disablement

DISABLEMENT CLASSIFICATION	CHARACTERISTICS	INTERACTION LEVEL
Impairment	Reflex development	Child
	Joint motion	
	Muscle length/strength	
	Respiratory status	
	Postural stability	
Activity/functional limitations	Locomotion	Child/daily environment
	Communication	
	Oral motor function	
	Social/emotional	
Disability/participation restriction	Community recreation	Child/community and society
	School participation	
	Employment	
	Access to facilities	

Adapted from International Classification of Impairments, Activities and Participation (ICIDH-2), A Manual of Dimensions of Disablement and Functioning, Beta-1 Draft for Field Trials. Geneva, World Health Organization, 1997.

11

factors are considered equal elements in designing a plan of care. It is important to note that the WHO framework is consistent with the American Physical Therapy Association's *Guide to Physical Therapist Practice*[43] and the practice model adopted by the National Center for Medical Rehabilitation Research.[64] Throughout each of these frameworks the physical therapist addresses impairments, functional limitations, and disability as a result of disease or injury. It is also important to note that the physical therapist can advance a child through an enabling process by addressing the body's structural integrity so that age-appropriate movement and interactive activities can occur. In a climate of radical health care reform and shifting venues for pediatric practice, a practitioner's understanding of the interdependence of all levels of the WHO model is germane to treatment success.

Impact of Federal Legislation

The scope of pediatric specialization within the field of physical therapy is rapidly evolving as a result of a variety of factors that directly affect the care of children: public policy, family-centered care, and environments for practice. These elements, although seemingly unrelated, have become entwined through passage of federal legislation unique to the practice of pediatrics.

The Education of All Handicapped Children Act (EHCA), Public Law 94-142, passed in 1975, was landmark legislation that has continued to shape and evolve the nature of pediatric practice for all professional disciplines.[28] The main premise of the EHCA was that all children from ages 6 to 21 years, regardless of disability, were entitled to free and appropriate public education. This premise set the basic framework for policy and standards, which were amended in 1986 with passage of Public Law 99-457 (Amendments to the EHCA) and again in 1991 with reauthorization as the Individuals with Disabilities Education Act.[50] These amendments provide distinct policy for children from birth until 3 years and from 3 through 5 years of age.[30] Embedded within the amendments is specific language that stipulates the concept of parent/professional collaboration and a family-centered focus throughout the process of pediatric examination, intervention, and care coordination. In addition, this legislation set forth policy guidelines requiring that children be cared for in their "least restrictive" environment or in "natural" environments ranging from home to daycare centers as optimal sites for physical therapy intervention (Fig. 11–4).[50, 86]

The focus on the family system, family-centered care, individualized child and family plans, and natural environments is now commonplace in pediatric practice. This focus on family and community in essence speaks to the evolving societal and cultural contexts in which pediatric physical therapists collaborate in the care of children with special needs.

COMMON CONDITIONS

It is impractical to list the full range of pediatric diagnostic conditions in this chapter. Children, like adults, have conditions that require expertise in all specialty areas. Many children are seen for acute, short-term orthopaedic needs, such as an adolescent who sprains an ankle while playing soccer. The majority

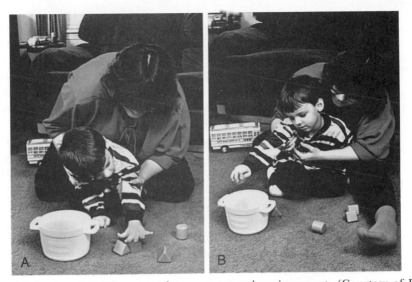

Figure 11–4. *A* and *B*, Therapy at home—a natural environment. (Courtesy of Bruce Wang.)

of these pediatric clients are seen in physical therapy outpatient orthopaedic clinics or by sports physical therapy specialists.

Another subset of pediatric clients and the group most associated with pediatric practice are children with developmental delays and disabilities. A child with a **developmental delay** has not attained predictable movement patterns or behavior associated with children of a similar chronological age. In the course of fetal development, a multitude of risk factors have the potential to cause a developmental problem. These factors, such as genetic and chromosomal anomalies or environmental toxins, may cause impairment in the central or peripheral nervous system that results in immediate or eventual developmental delays or potential disability. These children generally require some combination of short- and long-term therapies that continually shift given each child's changing physical, cognitive, and emotional abilities.

The remainder of this section consists of brief descriptions of selected pediatric conditions that are categorized as orthopaedic, genetic, or environmental. Later in the chapter, two of these conditions will be described through case studies of children to provide the reader with snapshots of the many "faces" of pediatric practice.

Orthopaedic Disorders

Children may be born with or acquire problems with bones, muscles, fascia, and joints. Some of the more common disorders are discussed in the following sections.

Juvenile Rheumatoid Arthritis. One of many rheumatic diseases, **juvenile rheumatoid arthritis (JRA)** is characterized by inflammation of connective tissue manifested as a painful inflamed joint (arthritis). The actual cause of JRA is unknown, with possibilities ranging from a viral onset to genetic predisposition.[20, 81] JRA may be manifested in several distinct forms or subtypes, each with different characteristics. These subtypes vary in the number of joints affected, age at onset, male-to-female ratio, clinical findings, and prognosis. Signs and symptoms usually include joint pain, swelling, decreased motion, stiffness, and muscle atrophy. The majority of children in whom JRA is diagnosed lead active lives with the assistance of medications, therapeutic exercise, and specialized care programs. It is generally believed that an interdisciplinary team including parents, a pediatric rheumatologist, nurse, psychologist, physical therapist, and occupational therapist is best for total care coordination.

The primary role of the physical therapist is to assist in the prevention of deformity and improvement in the overall quality of life for the child. The primary focus is generally the musculoskeletal needs of the child with a special emphasis on needs that affect function. Individualized goals are collaboratively formed to address posture, strength, mobility, and joint motion within the child's daily functional routine. Parent and child collaboration, education, and instruction are vital because the home is where the majority of the child's goals will be reinforced.[81]

Clubfoot. The term **clubfoot** is derived from the position of the affected foot, which is turned inward and slanted upward. Because of this position, certain muscles become shortened and cause the foot to remain in a fixed position. Treatment includes progressive and prolonged casting, as well as manual correction immediately after birth.

Scoliosis. **Scoliosis** is characterized by a lateral curvature of the spine. The curve may vary in severity from mild to severe. Scoliosis may be idiopathic (of unknown origin), neuromuscular, or congenital (present at birth). Scoliosis is now detected more frequently because of school-based screening programs and is noted by asymmetry of the shoulders, breasts, and pelvis, among other factors. Treatment involves a wide range of external or internal fixations and, in select cases, electrical stimulation, depending on the degree of development of the curve. Exercise assists in reducing back pain and improving range of motion.

Congenital Dislocation of the Hip. **Congenital dislocation of the hip (CDH)** results from abnormal development of some of the structures surrounding the hip joint, such that the head of the femur (thigh bone) can move into and out of the hip socket. The cause of CDH is unknown, but the disorder is thought to be related to a number of factors such as maternal hormonal changes during pregnancy, birth trauma, or improper positioning after birth. Treatment involves manually or surgically returning the femoral head to the hip socket and stabilizing it with splints or casts, depending on the degree of impairment and age of the child. Intensive exercise protocols are required postsurgically to regain full range of joint motion, muscle strength, and function. Children with spina bifida and certain forms of cerebral palsy (CP) are more prone to CDH and are monitored through regular physical examinations.

Osteogenesis Imperfecta. A common and severe bone disorder of genetic origin, **osteogenesis imperfecta (OI)** affects the formation of collagen during bone development, with the subsequent development of frequent fractures during the fetal or newborn period. The fetal form of OI is associated with high mortality, whereas the infantile form is less severe, with increased vulnerability to frequent fractures of the long bones in early childhood. Children with OI are identified through characteristic limb deformities, dental abnormalities, stunted growth, scoliosis, loose ligaments, and an unusually shaped skull. Treatment of fractures and prevention of deformity are the major focus of intervention, as well as gentle exercise after postsurgical healing.

Genetic Disorders

Duchenne Muscular Dystrophy. In **Duchenne muscular dystrophy (DMD)**, females do not manifest symptoms but are carriers of the disease, whereas males do manifest symptoms. Boys with DMD usually develop normally until 6 to 9 years of age, when progressive pelvic muscle weakness and wasting become apparent and are combined with enlarged yet weak thigh muscles and tight heel cords. Associated complications include muscle contractures, spinal curvature (scoliosis), and wheelchair dependence at 10 to 12 years of age. Progressive weakness, pneumonia, and cardiac abnormalities eventually reduce the life span of persons with DMD.[6] Developmentally, a child with this type of muscular dystrophy may have mild mental retardation or learning disabilities, low muscle tone, and delays in attainment of motor milestones.[49]

Spinal Muscular Atrophy. Symptoms of **spinal muscular atrophy (SMA)** include severe muscle weakness in infancy and progressive respiratory failure. Developmentally, children with the infantile form of SMA have a decreased life span, whereas children with the juvenile form have a longer (but less than normal) life span and require aggressive physical therapy and orthopaedic management.[93]

Spina Bifida. **Spina bifida** is a prenatal disorder involving orthopaedic malformations in its mild form and neurological malformations in its severe form (Fig. 11–5). Although its etiology is unknown, the neurological impairment appears to be a result of faulty closure of the neural groove in the first month of pregnancy. Recent hypotheses suggest that this impairment may be a result of genetic expression in combination with factors in the fetal (maternal) environment.[58] Environmental factors such as organic solvents, ethanol, and valproic acid have been suggested, and most recently, maternal folate deficiency has been determined to exert a strong influence.[56, 60, 63] In fact, studies have shown that daily folic acid supplementation can reduce the incidence of new cases of neural tube defects by at least 50%.[92]

The following are several types of neural tube defects that differ in level of severity, depending on the degree of vertebral closure and spinal cord exposure.

Spina Bifida Occulta. A common impairment of a vertebra (separation of the spinous process) that is not associated with disability, **spina bifida occulta** may be discovered only through diagnostic tests such as radiographic studies.

11

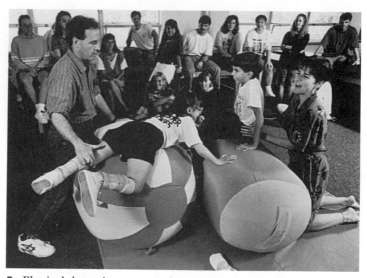

Figure 11–5. Physical therapists promote interactive play to assist the movement patterns of two children with spina bifida. (Courtesy of Bruce Wang.)

Meningocele. A benign herniation of the meninges manifesting as a soft tissue cyst or lump that surrounds a normal spinal cord, **meningocele** does not result in any neurological deficits.

Meningomyelocele. **Meningomyelocele** is an open lesion with minimal to no skin protection covering the deeper nerve roots. This condition is the most severe of the closure defects, with the potential for leakage of spinal fluid and infection before surgical intervention and healing. Because this impairment is usually at the lower end of the spine, loss of motor function and sensation of the lower part of the body often results, including problems with bowel and bladder function.

Chromosomal Disorders

Cystic Fibrosis. The pulmonary disorder **cystic fibrosis (CF)** is the most common inherited chronic disease in white children. CF is characterized by the production of thick mucus with progressive lung damage, and children with CF require frequent hospitalization for acute respiratory attacks. A variety of medications and therapies can assist in decreasing the side effects of this disease. Genetic research has resulted in isolation of the defective gene for CF.[75]

Down Syndrome. **Down syndrome** is a congenital developmental disability caused by a defect in chromosome 21; it is sometimes called trisomy 21. A child with Down syndrome is characterized by low muscle tone, a flat facial profile, upwardly slanted eyes, short stature, mental retardation, slowed growth and development, a small nose with a low nasal bridge, and congenital heart disease.[7, 74, 85] Associated complications may include instability of the first and second vertebrae, lax ligaments, seizures, leukemia, and premature senility.[2, 5, 73] The combination of these features is often manifested as deficiencies in balance, stability, and agility across many tasks and environmental contexts. Developmentally, a child with Down syndrome has decreased muscle tone, which improves with age. This abnormality is offset by loose ligaments that result in increased range of joint motion. The level of mental retardation varies, and the rate of developmental progress decreases with age.[24, 73]

Environmentally Related Disorders

A variety of risk factors affecting the health of either the mother or the fetus may present a risk to the newborn infant's health. Some of these factors include maternal health and nutrition (e.g., vitamin deficiency), radiation, drugs, infections, environmental toxins (e.g., lead), prelabor or postlabor infant hypoxia (lack of oxygen), and birth trauma. Depending on the nature and timing of appearance of the risk factor during the pregnancy, the newborn may have a variety of developmental disabilities ranging from mild to severe.

Cerebral Palsy. **Cerebral palsy** is a group of conditions, rather than a disease, and is caused by a nonprogressive lesion on the brain. Most often, CP occurs during gestation (before birth), at birth, or immediately after birth from interruption of oxygen to the brain of the fetus or newborn.[77] A variety of environmental toxins, maternal or infant infections, or early childhood trauma can cause this condition. The core problem with CP is an inability of the brain to control nerve and muscle activity. Manifestations of CP depend on the cause, timing (age of the fetus or child), and location and extent of the original impairment to the brain. Often, early signs of CP include poor sucking, irritability, stiff muscles (hypertonia), or floppy muscles (hypotonia). Later manifestations may include delayed motor milestones, poor coordination, involuntary movements (dyskinesia), writhing movements (athetosis), poor visual tracking (ability of the eyes to follow a moving object), and language delay.[1] Approximately 60% to 70% of all children with CP are mentally retarded.[9] Management emphasis is on attaining optimal growth and development. A variety of specialists may be involved in caring for a child with CP, including physical therapists, occupational therapists, and speech-language pathologists. In many cases, neurosurgical intervention, orthotic devices, adaptive equipment, or pharmacological intervention is required to ameliorate or correct deformities (Fig. 11–6).[89]

Fetal Alcohol Syndrome. The most severe condition in a continuum of alcohol-induced disabilities,[61, 65] **fetal alcohol syndrome (FAS)** is related to a presumed history of a significant level of maternal alcohol consumption during pregnancy.[51] It is the leading known cause of mental retardation, even surpassing Down syndrome and spina bifida. Children are generally born at term (on their due date) but are smaller than normal in weight and height. Children with FAS have distinct physical features that assist in identifying their condition. Complications are widespread and include an increased incidence of congenital

11

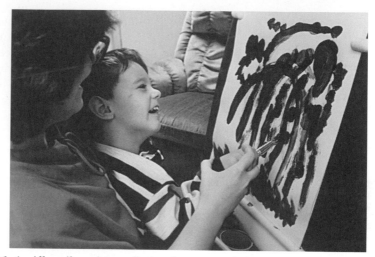

Figure 11–6. All smiles when painting is a part of therapy for a child with cerebral palsy. (Courtesy of Bruce Wang.)

heart defects, joint contractures, visual and auditory impairments, and hip dislocation.[41, 87] Developmentally, a child with FAS may experience a range of delays in the areas of language, fine motor control, eye-hand coordination, speech, IQ, and psychosocial behavior.[87, 88]

Prenatal Cocaine Exposure. **Prenatal cocaine exposure** is related to fetal exposure to cocaine in utero from maternal cocaine use during pregnancy.[21, 80] Infants often have clinical signs of exposure after birth, including hyperirritability, poor feeding patterns, high respiratory and heart rates, increased tremulousness, and irregular sleeping patterns.[67] Developmentally, a child with prenatal cocaine exposure may experience abnormalities in muscle tone, reflexes, movement, and attention that may continue many months after birth.[27, 79] If these problems persist, including increased muscle tone or tremors, other developmental milestones may be delayed.[78] Research on the long-term effects of fetal cocaine exposure are currently being conducted nationwide. While several studies have reported neurobehavioral and neuromotor dysfunction in infants exposed to cocaine, the findings have neither been consistently replicated nor been found to predict long-term sequelae.[10]

PRINCIPLES OF EXAMINATION

The process of examination and evaluation of children involves measures to determine whether a child is in need of physical therapy intervention, in addition to monitoring the child's progress after physical therapy has been initiated. If a child is suspected of having or is at risk for a developmental disability, an examination is initiated that involves the history, a systems review, screening, and tests and measures. After the examination, the physical therapist performs an evaluation in which clinical judgment is used to synthesize the clinical and social information gathered during the examination. During the evaluation, a prognosis is determined, as well as a plan of care, including the child's goals and objectives and any intervention strategies, if indicated.

Initial information about a child, the history, is generally obtained through a review of medical records and discussions with family members. For a child up to 5 years of age, the discussion may take the form of a **family assessment.**[4] Family assessment is an essential part of the examination because the child will be treated in the context of that family system.[33] Family assessment may take the form of an interview, discussion, or standardized survey and is often initiated by the team member who will be the primary coordinator of care for the family. Regardless of the format, the purpose of family assessment is to obtain the family's insights regarding the child, including the family history, relationships, satisfactions, concerns, needs, and resources. The history has a direct impact on planning services for each child. As children get older, they may become more directly involved and state their own opinions and thoughts, thus providing vital information about their condition and areas of satisfaction or concern with their care coordination.

The administration of tests and measures, an initial and continuing part of any pediatric examination, primarily consists of two components: screening and assessment. Each component has a distinct purpose in determining a child's prognosis and ultimate plan of care (Table 11–2).

TABLE 11–2
Components of Tests and Measures in Pediatric Physical Therapy

COMPONENT	DESCRIPTION	EXAMPLE
Screening	Short, inexpensive tests used to distinguish children with behavior different from that of other children of the same age; may indicate a need for further evaluation	Denver II Developmental Screening Test[34]
Assessment	Instruments used to gain a comprehensive profile of a child's physical, cognitive, social, emotional, communication, and adaptive abilities to assist in determining therapeutic service needs, as well as act as a guide for initial frequency and duration of service	Bayley II Scales of Infant Development,[8] Gross Motor Function Measure,[76] Peabody Developmental Motor Scales[32]
	Assessment also involves the use of measures to determine the need for disability-related adapted equipment, as well as activity preferences addressed by the child and/or family	Pediatric Evaluation of Disability Inventory,[44] Canadian Occupational Performance Measure[54]

11

Depending on the availability and type of diagnosis at the time of referral, screening may or may not be required as an initial measurement. Screening is usually indicated when a child is at risk for developmental delay or disability and is a quick way to determine whether the child is in need of further diagnostic services.

If a child has a definite diagnosis, screening is generally bypassed and a comprehensive assessment is recommended. Assessment measures are used to gain more in-depth information regarding the child's strengths and needs in all developmental domains. In the case of an orthopaedic condition, assessment may entail an examination of posture or movement, as well as special diagnostic tests such as radiographs. Assessment measures for a child with a developmental disability are generally obtained through **standardized testing**, which refers to a type of formal test in which the procedures remain the same when administered by different therapists and at variable test locations. A large variety and number of standardized measures are available for pediatric testing, and these measures are targeted according to the specific purpose of the assessment (Fig. 11–7).

In addition to choosing an assessment tool that meets the needs of the child being tested, it is also imperative to review each measure for (1) validity, or the ability of the test to measure the content area or areas that it claims to measure (e.g., evaluation of mobility); (2) reliability, or the consistency of the test between separate administrations or examiners; and (3) the appropriateness of the instrument for the individual disability or culture of the child being assessed (normative group). An equally important element of objective measurement is the information provided through observation of a child's caregivers in a variety of natural environments (home, daycare, school).

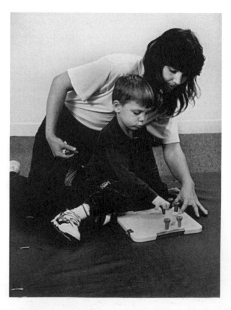

Figure 11–7. Standardized testing: assessment of eye-hand coordination and fine motor skills. (Courtesy of Bruce Wang.)

PRINCIPLES OF EVALUATION, DIAGNOSIS, AND PROGNOSIS

The results of tests and measures performed during the examination are used in the evaluation process to confirm, revise, or establish a diagnosis, prognosis, and plan of care. The evaluation can be vital for the child, family, and medical professionals. In many cases, the diagnosis and corresponding prognosis provide a mechanism by which physical therapists can determine treatment prerogatives and design the plan of care. With certain conditions that have defined physical manifestations, initial therapy can be planned to counteract negative physical outcomes, or **secondary conditions** of disability (e.g., muscle contractures). Diagnosis is also important for determining clinical conditions that pose contraindications to specific treatment regimens. Several positive outcomes are associated with establishing a clinical diagnosis, as are negative outcomes, many of which have psychological and social ramifications (Table 11–3). In all children, their families, and friends, the impact of childhood disablement is multifaceted, and all those who are touched by it continually experience the many phases of grief and acceptance.

During the evaluation, individualized goals and objectives are developed from the information derived from the examination (family assessment, child observations, and standardized assessment measures). The SOAP note format is rarely used as a documentation method for pediatric patients, with the possible exception of specific hospital or rehabilitation settings (see Chapters 2 and 7 regarding the SOAP note). Instead, the necessary information is contained in an **Individualized Family Service Plan (IFSP)** or an **Individualized Education Plan (IEP)** developed for each child. These plans are reviewed on a regular basis as the framework for treatment and serve as a baseline by which progress is monitored.

TABLE 11–3
Outcomes of Establishing a Diagnosis for a Pediatric Patient

POSITIVE OUTCOMES	NEGATIVE OUTCOMES
Ability to establish a prognosis (future)	May lead to a negative stereotype (label)
Validates the need for services/supports	May disenfranchise the child from obtaining certain services
May indicate a need for genetic counseling	May cause a state of depression or denial
Assists in possible prevention of secondary disabilities	A false-positive diagnosis has negative immediate consequences for both the child and family
Knowledge may assist the family with coping mechanisms	A false-negative diagnosis will have long-term consequences for both the child and family
Aids research efforts targeted to specific conditions	

11

As the name implies, the IFSP describes in detail the total plan of care for the child in the context of the family unit.[26, 59] This type of plan, designed for children from birth to 3 years of age, is always determined in collaboration with the family, and therapeutic needs are intertwined with family needs and priorities. This strategy recognizes that the family unit must remain healthy to provide optimum care for the child. The IFSP might include services such as special baby-sitting assistance, transportation provisions, or specialized medical care at home. The IFSP also includes the different therapeutic services that the child will receive, the specific duration and frequency of these services, and location of the intervention.

On entry into the school system, physical therapy objectives shift to interface with an educational service delivery system and become part of the IEP. Through this model, therapists often interface with the family, educators, and other health team members to provide direct intervention in the classroom setting.[36, 47] The physical therapist may work individually with the child, may work in a group setting, or may serve as a consultant to direct care providers. In the latter case, the physical therapist instructs persons who directly care for the child. Instruction may include certain positioning or movement techniques to provide therapeutic benefit throughout the day. Regardless of the environment, treatment should be provided in a context in which activities can be targeted to achieve the manner or quality of movement desired.

Young children may be seen by a physical therapist at a variety of locations with different therapist-child ratios, depending on the particular objectives of therapy. Generally, the site of choice is the child's most natural environment, which may be the home, school, or a daycare setting. Therapists may choose to work with a child in a 1:1 ratio, in a group with other children, or with the parents. Often, some mixture of formats and environments provides treatment variety and the greatest benefit for the child.

It is important to remember that the initiation of therapy does not signal the end of examination. Examination is an ongoing process that begins with the history and continues throughout each therapy session. It includes assessment of each child's strengths and needs and evolves as the child, family, and therapist continue to determine appropriate therapeutic activities. Annual or biannual re-examination is extremely important for monitoring the child's progress and redirecting intervention if necessary. By applying the results of the examination and subsequent evaluation, the health care team and family work in a partnership to determine a well-coordinated plan of care for each child.

PRINCIPLES OF DIRECT INTERVENTION

Intervention in pediatric physical therapy involves helping each child gain abilities to assist in meeting the daily challenges of the most natural environments. As mentioned earlier, the initial task of the therapist, in collaboration with the family, is an examination of the child's individual strengths and needs. With this information, a unique plan of care is developed that supports the child's strengths while facilitating skills in needed areas. Depending on the child's needs or diagnosis, intervention may involve a variety of approaches.

Box 11–1

Knowledge Base for Pediatric Orthopaedic Assessment and Treatment

- Normal pediatric biomechanical alignment
- Specific orthopaedic assessment procedures
- Pre-surgical evaluation of posture and movement
- Post-operative management of specialized surgical interventions
- Rationale and indications/contraindications for using manual therapy
- Use of casts and orthotics for correction or management of musculoskeletal malalignment
- Appropriate use of modalities and exercise protocols for children

From Pediatric Orthopedics. Alexandria, VA, American Physical Therapy Association, 1992.

The following will detail several methods used to provide services to children with common orthopaedic and neurological conditions.

To initiate therapy with pediatric orthopaedic patients, it is useful to have specific knowledge in the area of pediatric orthopaedics (Box 11–1).[72] Orthopaedic examination and intervention will vary by condition, but certain procedures are common to all orthopaedic clients, such as measurement of range of motion, muscle and sensory testing, gait assessment, and postural evaluation. (See Chapter 7 for a further description of these procedures.) Children may require specialized orthopaedic management for acute and long-term orthopaedic conditions, as well as for neuromuscular diseases. Intervention in both cases requires knowledge of the specific diagnoses, as well as of protocols for management. For example, specialized surgical procedures often require the therapist to know specific postoperative management protocols (e.g., positioning) in order to maintain the surgical correction. Often, physical therapists are requested to fabricate splints or casts for a pediatric patient to assist in muscle lengthening or joint stabilization (Fig. 11–8).

In addition to orthopaedic techniques, physical therapists use a range of therapeutic techniques to further enhance the rehabilitation process. A variety of neuromotor approaches are used to treat a child with neurological and orthopaedic disabilities. These approaches were primarily developed between 1950 and 1980 and were based on the theory, literature, and patient observations current at that time. These approaches are now being reviewed and adapted in light of current nervous system theories.[62, 90] A primary task for both new and veteran pediatric physical therapists is to continue to research the effectiveness of each approach and assess the use of these approaches in a variety of settings and their ability to facilitate the neuromotor changes that they purport. It is also imperative that physical therapists evaluate the effectiveness of each approach in facilitating the child's achievement of targeted goals.

Most pediatric physical therapists continue to rely on an "eclectic," or multiple-method, approach when providing therapy. An **eclectic approach** in-

11

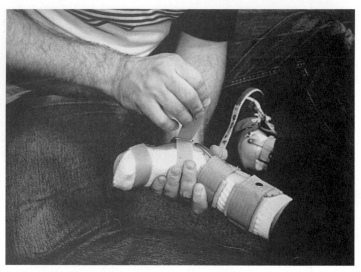

Figure 11–8. An ankle-foot orthosis is used to assist the orthopaedic needs of a child. (Courtesy of Bruce Wang.)

cludes some combination of therapeutic strategies used by the physical therapist that are thought to be helpful in the treatment of a given client.[18] Although the common use of eclectic practice has made it difficult to isolate and study the effectiveness of each specific approach, numerous published articles have discussed both the controversial nature and the effectiveness of a variety of neuromotor approaches.[25, 38–40, 45, 46, 68–70] Additional clinical research is necessary to achieve a sound basis of support for the continued use of many therapeutic approaches.

At present, a variety of approaches continue to be used in an effort to habilitate and rehabilitate the pediatric client. The following brief descriptions provide an objective overview of the more common neuromotor approaches currently in use.

Neurodevelopmental Treatment Approach

The neurodevelopmental treatment (NDT) approach was originated by Berta and Karel Bobath in England almost 50 years ago to both analyze and treat neurological disorders of posture and movement.[12–14] Through the use of a motivating environment and a child's active participation, manual facilitation and inhibition techniques are used by the therapist to present the child with a "normal" sensory experience and thereby encourage facilitation of a more functional motor response.[11, 13, 15] Continued active repetition of normal developmental skills is theorized to assist the child in establishing more coordinated, efficient movement patterns.[11, 14, 15] The primary emphasis of the NDT approach is on movement quality, and parent/provider training is stressed for the purpose of incorporating movement concepts into the child's functional daily routines. Pediatric therapists using this approach should realize that although some studies have demonstrated the efficacy of NDT,[37] a number of studies do not provide support for its usefulness as a treatment approach.[70] Despite the controversy, NDT continues to be one of the most widely used and documented therapeutic approaches in the United States for the treatment of upper motor neuron lesions such as CP (Fig. 11–9).[23, 29]

Sensory Integration Theory

This technique is based on the theory that poor integration of the use of sensory information (e.g., tactile or visual feedback) prevents the organization of resultant motor behavior (e.g., walking or jumping). The **sensory integration (SI)** approach assesses the child's sensory systems through clinical observations and tests before initiation of therapy. The provision of controlled vestibular and somatosensory experiences within meaningful environments is believed to enable the child to integrate the sensory information and evoke a spontaneous functional response (Fig. 11–10).[3, 31, 68]

Normal Developmental Theory

Therapy goals and objectives are designed to follow the progression of normal motor development (developmental milestones), as well as developmental theory (e.g., development proceeds in a proximal-to-distal direction). This **normal developmental theory** approach is based on a model of higher-level cortical control that dictates the maturation process. The theory assumes that children with central nervous system damage will acquire motor skills in a similar fashion as children with normally developing nervous systems.[18] Many of the

11

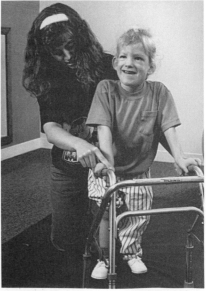

Figure 11–9. A child ambulates with facilitation from the therapist. (Courtesy of Bruce Wang.)

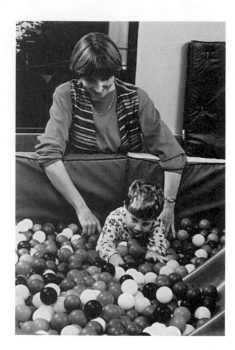

Figure 11–10. Sensory integration can be fun. (Courtesy of Bruce Wang.)

neuromotor therapies used today were originally based on this theoretical foundation.[19]

Task-Oriented Movement Model

Based on the work of Gentile,[35] a **goal-directed movement approach** to intervention has been established by Carr and Shepard[83] and by others,[84] who were seeking to use environmental task conditions as an impetus for improved motor control and motor learning. In Gentile's paradigm, goal-directed movements include both the investigative and the adaptive behaviors resulting from a child's interactions with the environment. In observing such behavior, the pediatric physical therapist can orient therapy so that it focuses on the child's impairments, on task reorganization, and/or on environmental modifications that may serve to promote improved child outcomes. Therapy is environment specific and task specific and is designed to promote a child's development of solutions to movement problems.

Conclusion

Regardless of the type of intervention, pediatric therapy should pave a pathway for a healthy, high-quality life for each child. Campbell outlined a checklist, or "defining strategy," for the evaluation of pediatric interventions.[17] The questions she poses can be used to evaluate intervention collaborations in the home, school, or other community-based venues:

1. Does the intervention encourage the child to initiate a program of lifelong fitness activities, including proper nutrition, exercise, weight control, and stress management?

2. Does the intervention encourage the child to assume responsibility for personal health, including knowledge of the condition? Is the child encouraged to become personally involved in decisions on rehabilitation?
3. Does the intervention motivate the child and foster self-esteem?
4. Does the intervention promote meaningful pursuits that will foster the prevention of secondary conditions and thereby lead to lifelong musculoskeletal health and improved cardiovascular fitness?

The answers to these questions provide the litmus test for successful pediatric intervention.

Case Studies

Matthew—Down Syndrome ___ _____

Matthew is 3 years old and one of many preschoolers at Rosedale Preschool. He has Down syndrome.

Matthew attends preschool with other infants and toddlers. He plays with balls and puzzles and loves to swim. Administration of a formal evaluation revealed that Matthew has many strengths as well as needs in the gross and fine motor domains. Matthew is severely hypotonic (low muscle tone) and has difficulty running without falling. This problem was noted on the formal examination as well as in observations by Matthew's parents and preschool teacher. It was also noted that his automatic reactions to disturbances in balance (righting reactions and protective responses) were delayed, especially when moving into and out of various positions (transitions). Matthew was able to grasp objects in a manner appropriate for other 3-year-olds and enjoys drawing and playing with building blocks. He continues to exhibit needs in feeding skills because of the low muscle tone in muscles used for chewing and mouth closure. His medical history reveals that Matthew has a congenital heart problem, as well as several other distinguishing features associated with Down syndrome.

Researchers have attempted to determine appropriate physical therapy interventions for children with Down syndrome.[82] Conclusions drawn from this research indicate that it appears most important to provide a child with Down syndrome opportunities to explore a variety of environments requiring different postural adjustments or movement patterns in response to changing task conditions. In accordance with this research, the therapist must observe the individual motor learning style of each child and respond by creating motivating and challenging learning situations.

In Matthew's case, the physical therapist will provide therapy in the school as designed in his IEP and collaborate with his preschool staff by instructing them to carry out physical therapy goals throughout his daily school routine. An inclusion program, such as the one at Rosedale Preschool, maintains a philosophy that children with a variety of developmental abilities should play and learn together in an atmosphere that fosters a sense of belonging and personal growth for all its members. This type of environment is naturally where a child who is as special as Matthew belongs.

Matthew's Individualized Education Plan. Because of Matthew's diagnosis of congenital heart disease, it is important that he avoid excessive exertion and

11

Box 11-2

Example of a Goal and Criterion for Matthew

Goal: Matthew will run across a level (hard) mat surface without falling when prompted with his favorite toy.
Criterion: Three to four times during four play sessions.

fatigue. Activities that involve impact to the cervical vertebrae should also be avoided because of his vertebral instability. In designing a plan for Matthew, consideration is placed primarily on family goals and Matthew's current interests. Several pediatric assessment tools can assist in identifying and prioritizing Matthew's therapy goals. The Canadian Occupational Performance Measure is one measure designed specifically to identify and determine the importance of the child's and family's goals for therapy.[55] It is from this frame of reference that therapeutic goals and objectives will be designed. Specific objectives might involve achieving a task that is appropriate for Matthew's developmental abilities, as well as his functional level. Most objectives target a particular skill, the manner of performance or assistance, and the criterion to be met (Box 11–2).

The same skill can also be scaled[71] so that Matthew will always achieve different measures of success and his individual progress can be monitored over time (Box 11–3). Initial therapeutic goals are vital for assessing his response to intervention, as well as for maintaining treatment consistency. Through the ongoing assessment process Matthew's progress will be monitored, with alterations made to his care plan if warranted.

Intervention. Physical therapy intervention may first involve assisting Matthew in developing a relationship with his environment. Matthew may initially move

Box 11-3

Goal Attainment Scaling

−2   Matthew will walk across a level mat surface without falling when prompted with his favorite toy.
−1   Matthew will run across a level mat surface with one stop to regain his balance (hands down on mat) when prompted with his favorite toy.
 0   Matthew will run across a level mat surface without falling when prompted with his favorite toy.
+1   Matthew will run across a mat angled 10 degrees with one stop to regain his balance (hands down on mat) when prompted with his favorite toy.
+1   Matthew will run across a mat raised by a 10-degree angle without a stop or fall when prompted with his favorite toy.

too quickly or slowly, take steps that are too large or uneven, or resist the challenge to ambulate altogether. During an activity, the therapist may use NDT techniques such as guided handling to assist with movement. Another strategy may involve Matthew's active participation through the use of cognitive and verbal reinforcement during a motivating recreational activity to reinforce learning. As mentioned previously, some combination of techniques may best accomplish the task (see the section Principles of Direct Intervention). If each of Matthew's goals can be designed according to his motivations (e.g., eating, play, recreation), the inclusion of therapeutic approaches and techniques becomes more functional and likely to meet with success.

Emmie—Spina Bifida

Emmie began her life in the neonatal intensive care unit of Eastern Shore Memorial Hospital. Her first experiences were the sounds of the slow beeps and hums of the infant monitors. Her first visions were obstructed by glass, and her human touch limited to persons performing routine checks of her medical status. Unlike other newborn infants who experience the sounds of home and arms of friends or siblings, Emmie will have to wait until she has surgery because she was born with spina bifida (meningomyelocele). Children with spina bifida and their families have no choice but to begin their lives in the hospital environment. Despite diligent efforts, which have improved the comfort and familiarity of hospital neonatal intensive care and pediatric units, they continue to be a threatening, imposing environment for families.

Management. The general goals of physical therapy management for Emmie and other children with spina bifida are (1) to prevent physiological impairment from causing functional limitations, which are a potential consequence of an impairment (e.g., "can't crawl"), and (2) to improve the quality of life for each child and family by preventing functional limitations from becoming a disability, as manifested through decreased participation in daily activities and social events (e.g., "can't go to the school dance").[48] Accomplishing these goals requires a collaborative approach involving the child, the family, and the health care team. Physical therapy examination should be comprehensive and interface closely with the observations and examinations of other health care team and family members. Evaluation and continued follow-up (monitoring) should include the following specific objectives:

- General multidomain screening and evaluation of developmental level
- Neurological examination, including monitoring for signs of increased intracranial pressure
- Orthopaedic examination for joint range and mobility, kyphosis, scoliosis, or dislocations
- Examination of bowel and bladder function
- Examination of skin integrity
- Activities of daily living
- Examination of mobility
- Promotion of recreational activities

11

Emmie's Individualized Family Service Plan. Activities are generally centered on the goals and objectives indicated in each child's individualized plan. For a child of Emmie's age, the format would probably be an IFSP. A child with spina bifida often has a range of cognitive delays and skills in the psychosocial area. Consideration of these abilities, as well as physical and environmental factors, is essential when designing a plan of care. During the first few years of life, Emmie will develop a sense of her autonomy and self-esteem, so physical therapy will focus on her ability to explore her environment.

Depending on each child's abilities, the physical therapist will explore options to accomplish mobility goals. Many children with spina bifida use orthoses or braces to assist in locomotion. A popular choice for a young child is a parapodium. This upright brace places the child in a standing position on a flat swivel base with unencumbered arms and hands, thereby allowing the child freedom to explore the environment.[58] Therapy goals may also focus on other functional activities, such as position transitions, muscle strengthening, and self-care activities. Assistive technology devices such as an adapted computer keyboard will be especially useful in creating a more accessible environment for Emmie as she enters school.[53] As Emmie reaches adolescence, she will probably choose to use a wheelchair, which allows greater speed and efficiency for daily living. The team should encourage Emmie to explore a variety of recreational activities that are motivating and will improve general fitness and quality of life. She may continue to be seen on a periodic basis through the hospital's outpatient clinic or opt for private outpatient care. Therapy will continue only on an "as-needed" basis to assist with problems that arise during transitional developmental phases.

Summary

Physical therapists who work with pediatric patients focus on child development, psychology, and learning. They may provide services to the patient for a long period, for a short time, or on a consultant basis. Intervention is family centered and usually incorporates activities adapted to play. Physical therapy is frequently rendered in the school setting as directed by federal entitlement programs.

Common conditions seen by pediatric physical therapists are generally classified as orthopaedic, genetic, chromosomal, or environmentally related disorders. Screening, evaluation, and assessment techniques are used to establish functional goals and objectives, which are incorporated into an IFSP or IEP. Intervention is often eclectic, that is, it combines components from a variety of approaches, including neurodevelopmental treatment, sensory integration, normal developmental theory, and a task-oriented model. Early and continuing intervention programs for children are designed to incorporate a child's motivation and desire to play or participate in community-based recreation and leisure activities. Parents can become partners in assessing their child's individual motivation and help design the environments that will support therapy goals while matching the child's interests. With careful observation and the use of environmental adaptations and assistive devices, community activities (e.g., soccer, art class) can be modified to embrace a child with special needs.

Pediatric physical therapy is challenging and rewarding. Research, legislation, and new techniques create a changing practice environment to enhance the quality of care. The result is an exciting specialty in physical therapy.

References

1. Allen MC, Capute AJ: Neonatal neurodevelopmental examination as a predictor of neuromotor outcome in premature infants. Pediatrics 1989;83:498–506.
2. American Academy of Pediatrics. Committee on Sports Medicine. Atlantoaxial instability in Down syndrome. Pediatrics 1984;74:152–154.
3. Ayres AJ: Sensory Integration and Learning Disorders. Los Angeles, Western Psychological Services, 1972.
4. Bailey D, Simeonsson R (eds): Family Assessment in Early Intervention: Rationale and Model for Family Assessment in Early Intervention. Columbus, OH, Merrill, 1988.
5. Barden HS: Growth and development of selected hard tissues in Down's syndrome: A review. Hum Biol 1983;55:539–576.
6. Batshaw M, Perret Y: Bones, joints, and muscles: Support and movement. *In* Batshaw M, Perret Y (eds): Children with Disabilities: A Medical Primer, ed 4. Baltimore, Brookes, 1997.
7. Batshaw M, Perret Y, Shapiro B: Normal and abnormal development. *In* Batshaw M, Perret Y (eds): Children with Disabilities: A Medical Primer, ed 4. Baltimore, Brookes, 1997.
8. Bayley N: Bayley Scales of Infant Development. New York, Psychological Corporation, 1969.
9. Blackman JA: Medical Aspects of Developmental Disabilities in Children Birth to Three, ed 2. Rockville, MD, Aspen, 1990.
10. Blanchard Y: Neurobehavioral and neuromotor long-term sequelae of prenatal exposure to cocaine and other drugs: An unresolved issue. Pediatr Phys Ther 1999;11(3):140–146.
11. Bly A: Historical and current view of the basis of NDT. Pediatr Phys Ther 1991;3:131–135.
12. Bobath B: A neurodevelopmental treatment of cerebral palsy. Physiotherapy 1963;49:242–244.
13. Bobath B, Bobath K: The neuro-developmental treatment. *In* Sutton D (ed): Management of Motor Disorders in Children with Cerebral Palsy. Philadelphia, JB Lippincott, 1984.
14. Bobath K: A Neurophysiological Basis for the Treatment of Cerebral Palsy. Philadelphia, JB Lippincott, 1980.
15. Bobath K, Bobath B: Facilitation of normal postural reactions and movement in the treatment of cerebral palsy. Physiotherapy 1964;50:246–262.
16. Bottos M, Dalla Barba B, Stefani D, et al: Locomotor strategies preceding independent walking: Prospective study of neurological and language development in 424 cases. Dev Med Child Neurol 1989;31:25–34.
17. Campbell S: Physical therapy programs that last a lifetime. Phys Occup Ther Pediatr 1997;17(1):1–15.
18. Campbell PH: Posture and movement. *In* Tingey C (ed): Implementing Early Intervention. Baltimore, Brookes, 1989.
19. Campbell PH, Finn D: Programming to influence acquisition of motor abilities in infants and young children. Pediatr Phys Ther 1991;3(4):200–205.
20. Cassidy JT, Petty RE: Textbook of Pediatric Rheumatology, ed 2. New York, Churchill Livingstone, 1990.
21. Chasnoff IJ, Burns KA, Burns WJ: Cocaine use in pregnancy: Perinatal morbidity and mortality. Neurotoxicol Teratol 1987;9:291–293.
22. Cherry DB: Pediatric physical therapy: Philosophy, science and techniques. Pediatr Phys Ther 1991;3(2):70–76.
23. Conner F, Williamson G, Sieff JA: Programming for the Infants and Toddlers with Neuromotor and other Developmental Disabilities. New York, Teachers College Press, 1978.
24. Cooley WC, Graham JM Jr: Common syndromes and management issues for primary care physicians: Down's syndrome: An update and review for the primary pediatrician. Clin Pediatr (Phila) 1991;30:233–253.
25. Cotton E: Improvement of motor function with the use of conductive education. Dev Med Child Neurol 1974;16:637–643.
26. Deal A, Dunst C: A flexible and functional approach to developing individualized family support plans. Infants Young Children 1989;1(4):32–43.
27. Doberczak TM, Shanzer S, Senie RT, et al: Neonatal neurologic and electroencephalographic effects of intrauterine cocaine exposure. J Pediatr 1988;113:354–358.
28. Education of All Handicapped Children Act of 1975. Public Law 94-142, 20 USC 1401, 1975.

11

29. Finnie N: Handling Your Young Cerebral Palsied Child at Home. New York, Dutton, 1975.
30. Fischer J: Physical therapy in education environments: Moving through time with reflections and visions. Pediatr Phys Ther 1994;6(3):144–147.
31. Fisher AG, Bundy AC: Sensory integration theory. Med Sport Sci 1992;36:16.
32. Folio R, Fewell R, DuBose RF: Peabody Developmental Motor Scales. Toronto, Teaching Resources, 1983.
33. Foster M, Phillips W: Family systems theory as a framework for problem solving in pediatric physical therapy. Pediatr Phys Ther 1992;4(2):70–73.
34. Frankenburg WK: Denver Developmental Screening Test Manual. Denver, LADOCA Project & Publishing Foundation, 1973.
35. Gentile AM: Skill acquisition: Action, movement, and neuromotor processes. *In* Carr JA, Shepherd RB (eds): Movement Science: Foundations for Physical Therapy in Rehabilitation. Rockville, MD, Aspen, 1987.
36. Giangreco M: Delivery of therapeutic services in special education programs for learners with severe handicaps. Phys Occup Ther Pediatr 1986;6(2):5–15.
37. Girolami GL, Campbell SK: Efficacy of a neuro-developmental treatment program to improve motor control in infants born prematurely. Pediatr Phys Ther 1994;6(4):175–184.
38. Golden GS: Nonstandard therapies in the developmental disabilities. Am J Dis Child 1980;134:487–491.
39. Golden GS: Controversial therapies in developmental disabilities. *In* Gottlieb MI, Williams JE (eds): Developmental Behavioral Disorders: Selected Topics, vol 3. New York, Plenum, 1990.
40. Goodgold-Edwards SA: Principles for guiding action during motor learning: A critical evaluation of neurodevelopmental treatment. Phys Ther Pract 1993;2(4):30–39.
41. Graham JM: Independent dysmorphology evaluations at birth and 4 years of age for children exposed to varying amounts of alcohol in utero. Pediatrics 1988;81:772–778.
42. Guccione A: Physical therapy diagnosis and the relationship between impairments and function. Phys Ther 1991;71:499–503.
43. Guide to Physical Therapist Practice. 2nd ed. Phys Ther 2001;81:9–744.
44. Haley SM, Coster WJ, Ludlow LH, et al: Pediatric Evaluation of Disability Inventory (PEDI): Development, Standardization and Administration Manual. Boston, New England Medical Center Hospitals and PEDI Research Group, 1992.
45. Harris S: Early intervention: Does developmental therapy make a difference? Topics Early Child Special Educ 1988;7:20–32.
46. Harris SR, Atwater SE, Crowe TK: Accepted and controversial neuromotor therapies for infants at high risk for cerebral palsy. J Perinatol 1988;8:3–13.
47. Henry B: The role of physical therapists in development of individualized educational plans. Totline 1986;12:13–15.
48. Hirst M: Patterns of impairment and disability related to social handicap in young people with cerebral palsy and spina bifida J Biosoc Sci 1989;21:1–12.
49. Hyser CL, Mendell JR: Recent advances in Duchenne and Becker muscular dystrophy. Neurol Clin 1988;6:429–453.
50. Individuals with Disabilities Education Act Amendments of 1991. Public Law 102–119, 105 STAT.587, 1991.
51. Institute of Medicine (IOM), Stratton KR, How CJ, Battaglia FC (eds): Fetal Alcohol Syndrome: Diagnosis, Epidemiology, Prevention and Treatment. Washington, DC, National Academy Press, 1996.
52. International Classification of Impairments, Activities and Participation (ICIDH-2), A Manual of Dimensions of Disablement and Functioning, Beta-1 Draft for Field Trials. Geneva, World Health Organization, 1997.
53. Langone J, Malone MD, Kinsley T: Technology solutions for young children with developmental concerns. Infants Young Children 1999;11(4):65–78.
54. Law M, Baptiste S, McColl M, et al: The Canadian occupational performance measure: An outcome measure for occupational therapy. Can J Occup Ther 1990;57(2):82–87.
55. Law M, Narrah J, Pollock N, et al: Family-centered functional therapy for children with cerebral palsy: An emerging practice model. Phys Occup Ther Pediatr 1998;18(1):83–102.
56. Lawrence KM: Neural tube defects: A two-pronged approach to primary prevention. Pediatrics 1982;70:648–650.
57. Linder TW: Transdisciplinary Play-Based Assessment: A Functional Approach to Working with Young Children. Baltimore, Brookes, 1990.
58. Liptak G: Spina bifida. *In* Hoekelman RA (ed): Primary Pediatric Care. St Louis, Mosby–Year Book, 1992.

59. McGonigel M, Garland C: The individualized family service plan and the early intervention team: Team and family issues and recommended practices. Infants Young Children 1988;1(1):10–21.
60. Mills JL: The absence of a relation between the periconceptional use of vitamins and neural-tube defects. N Engl J Med 1989;321:430–435.
61. Mills JL, Graubard BI: Is moderate drinking during pregnancy associated with an increased risk of malformations? Pediatrics 1987;80:309–314.
62. Montgomery P: Neurodevelopmental treatment and sensory integrative theory. *In* Lister MJ (ed): Contemporary Management and Motor Control Problems: Proceedings from the II Step Conference. Alexandria, VA, Foundation for Physical Therapy, 1991.
63. MRC Vitamin Study Research Group: Prevention of neural tube defects: Results of the medical research council vitamin study. Lancet 1991;338:131–137.
64. National Advisory Board of Medical Rehabilitation Research: Research Plan for the National Center for Medical Rehabilitation. Bethesda, MD, National Institute of Child Health and Human Development, National Institutes of Health, 1993.
65. National Institute on Alcohol Abuse and Alcoholism (NIAA): Sixth Special Report to the U.S. Congress on Alcohol and Health. Washington, DC, U.S. Department of Health and Human Services, 1987.
66. National Maternal & Child Health Resource Center: Community-Based Service Systems for Children with Special Health Care Needs and Their Families. Washington, DC, U.S. Surgeon General's Conference Campaign '88, September 1988.
67. Newald J: Cocaine infants: A new arrival at hospital's step? Hospitals 60(7):96, 1986.
68. Ottenbacher K: Sensory integration therapy: Affect or effect. Am J Occup Ther 1982;36:571–578.
69. Ottenbacher KJ, Biocca Z, DeCremer G, et al: Quantitative analysis of the effectiveness of pediatric therapy. Emphasis on the neurodevelopmental treatment approach. Phys Ther 1986;66:1095–1101.
70. Palisano R: Research on the effectiveness of neurodevelopmental treatment. Pediatr Phys Ther 1991;3(3):143–148.
71. Palisano R, Haley SM, Brown DA: Goal attainment scaling as a measure of change in infants with motor delays. Phys Ther 1992;72:432–437.
72. Pediatric Orthopedics. Alexandria, VA, American Physical Therapy Association, 1992.
73. Pueschel SM: Clinical aspects of Down's syndrome from infancy to adulthood. Am J Med Genet 1990;7(suppl):52–56.
74. Roche AF: The cranium in mongolism. Acta Neurol 1966;42:62–78.
75. Rommens JM, Iannuzzi MC, Kerem B, et al: Identification of the cystic fibrosis gene: Chromosome walking and jumping. Science 1989;245:1059–1065.
76. Russell D, Rosenbaum PL, Cadman DT, et al: The gross motor function measure: A means to evaluate the effects of physical therapy. Dev Med Child Neurol 1989,31:341–352.
77. Scher MS, Belfar H, Martin J, et al: Destructive brain lesions of presumed fetal onset: Antepartum causes of cerebral palsy. Pediatrics 1991;88:898–906.
78. Schneider JW: Motor assessment and parent education beyond the newborn period. *In* Chasnoff IJ (ed): Drugs, Alcohol, Pregnancy and Parenting. Lancaster, UK, Kluwer, 1988.
79. Schneider JW, Chasnoff IJ: Cocaine abuse during pregnancy: Its effects on infant motor development—a clinical perspective. Topics Acute Care Trauma Rehabil 1987;2:59–69.
80. Schneider JW, Griffith DR, Chasnoff IJ: Infants exposed to cocaine in utero: Implications for developmental assessment and intervention. Infants Young Children 1989;2(1):25–36.
81. Scull S: Juvenile rheumatoid arthritis. *In* Tecklin JS (ed): Pediatric Physical Therapy. Philadelphia, JB Lippincott, 1998.
82. Shea AM: Motor attainments in Down's syndrome. *In* Lister MJ (ed): Contemporary Management of Motor Control Problems: Proceedings of the II Step Conference. Alexandria, VA, Foundation for Physical Therapy, 1991.
83. Shepherd RB: Training motor control and optimizing motor learning. *In* Shepherd RB (ed): Physiotherapy in Paediatrics, ed 3. Oxford, Butterworth-Heinemann, 1995.
84. Shumway-Cook A, Woollacott M: Motor Control: Theory and Practical Applications. Baltimore, Williams & Wilkins, 1995.
85. Spicer RL: Cardiovascular disease in Down's syndrome. Pediatr Clin North Am 1984;31:1331–1343.
86. Strain P: LRE for preschool children with handicaps: What we know, what we should be doing. J Early Intervent 1990;14:291–296.
87. Streissguth A: Fetal Alcohol Syndrome: A Guide for Families and Communities. Baltimore, Brookes, 1997.

11

88. Streissguth AP, Barr HM, Sampson PD, et al: Attention, distraction and reaction time at age 7 years and prenatal alcohol exposure. Neurobehav Toxicol Teratol 1986,8:717–725.

89. Styer-Acevedo J: Physical therapy for the child with cerebral palsy. *In* Tecklin JS (ed): Pediatric Physical Therapy. Philadelphia, JB Lippincott, 1994.

90. Umphred D: Merging neurophysiologic approaches with contemporary theories. *In* Lister MJ (ed): Contemporary Management of Motor Control Problems: Proceedings from the II Step Conference. Alexandria, VA, Foundation for Physical Therapy, 1991.

91. US Department of Health and Human Services, Public Health Service: US Surgeon General's Report, Children with Special Health Care Needs, Campaign '87, June 1987.

92. Werler MM, Shapiro S, Mitchell AA: Periconceptional folic acid exposure and risk of occurrent neural tube defects. JAMA 1993;269:1257–1261.

93. Wessel HB: Spinal muscular atrophy. Pediatric Ann 1989;18:421–427.

REVIEW QUESTIONS

1. Distinguish the components of the WHO enablement/disablement model. Create scenarios to demonstrate examples of the disabling/enabling process.

2. Suggest practice approaches that would be in violation of Public Law 99-457 (e.g., activities that would not support the family-centered and environmental aspects of treatment).

3. Describe what is meant by a developmental delay and identify fetal risk factors.

4. Define juvenile rheumatoid arthritis and describe how distinct subtypes might vary. Speculate on how these variations might affect treatment approaches, and then create a brief scenario to illustrate your point.

5. Create a list of tests and measures and identify them as either *screening* or *assessment* tools.

6. Describe the kinds of questions you might raise in determining whether a selected test or measure would be the best one for a given client.

7. Identify the positive and negative outcomes of a clinical diagnosis and then apply them to a specific example.

8. Differentiate among the several therapeutic approaches discussed in this chapter and describe the key elements of each approach.

It is always the season for the old to learn.
Aeschylus, 500 BC

PHYSICAL THERAPY FOR THE OLDER ADULT

Jennifer E. Collins

KEY TERMS

activities of daily living (ADLs)

adaptive equipment

assistive device

dynamic balance

frail elderly

functional reach test

hypokinesis

instrumental activities of daily living (IADLs)

osteoarthritis

osteoporosis

presbycusis

rheumatoid arthritis

static balance

well elderly

OBJECTIVES   After reading this chapter, the reader will be able to

- Identify three specific reasons why a physical therapist would modify an intervention for an older person
- Differentiate between static and dynamic balance
- Describe the primary role for the physical therapist in each of the common conditions discussed in this chapter
- Explain why an interdisciplinary approach is important when developing a plan of care for an older person

Geriatrics, elderly, senior citizen, older American—what kind of individual comes to mind when one sees or hears these words? Is it a white-haired gentleman struggling to move a walker through long hallways? Is it a silver-haired woman swimming laps at the community pool? Both of them should come to mind, as well as countless other descriptions of appearance, abilities, and challenges. In health care, professionals tend to think first of the multiple medical problems many older people have. However, because physical therapists and physical therapist assistants have roles in prevention as well as treatment, one may be as likely to intervene with an 85-year-old athlete as with a 70-year-old person who has had a stroke. So as the words *senior, elderly,* and *older person* are used for this population group, consider the wide variation of functional abilities that may be present. While keeping this individual variation in mind, also recognize the commonality that we are all part of the aging population.

**GENERAL
DESCRIPTION**

Demographics

Physical therapists have provided services to individuals with conditions common to people older than 65 years for many decades. However, only in the last decade have physical therapists and physical therapist assistants worked with older persons in such large (and growing) numbers. Current trends in health care and life expectancy have rapidly increased the numbers of older adults requiring some type of physical therapy services, whether rehabilitative or preventive. To illustrate, in the year 1990, the population 65 years and older accounted for 12.5% of the U.S. population.[2] This figure represents a threefold increase since 1900, with the trend expected to continue. For an individual born in 1997, the life expectancy is 76.5 years, the highest life expectancy that the United States has ever experienced.[20]

As people live longer, they tend to have more physical and medical conditions that require a physical therapist's assistance in maintaining or regaining skills necessary for maximum function in their daily activities. While each individual requiring physical therapy will benefit from specific, unique interventions, the goals for most people will include skills to independently perform such activities as bathing, cooking, dressing, and shopping. Such activities are described as **activities of daily living (ADLs)**; more complex activities necessary for community living are called **instrumental activities of daily living (IADLs)**.

These are skills that allow an older person to be less dependent on caregivers. For instance, shopping is a difficult skill for many older adults with physical impairments. If physical therapists assist older adults in improving balance and provide an appropriate assistive device, more individuals may be able to complete shopping trips with less assistance.

Figure 12–1 presents data on ADLs and IADLs of persons 70 years of age and over who are noninstitutionalized.[19] The data indicate that nearly 97% of these individuals have difficulty in performing one or more of the activities. The percentage increases with age and is higher for women in all categories. This information confirms that physical therapists have an important role in improving functional performance.

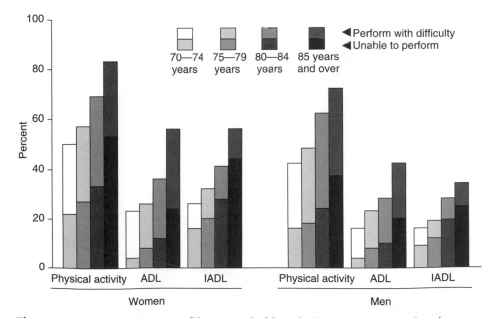

Figure 12–1. Percent of persons 70 years and older who have difficulty performing one or more physical activity, activities of daily living (ADL), and instrumental activities of daily living (IADL), by age and sex: United States, 1995. (From National Center for Health Statistics. Health, United States, 1999 With Health and Aging Chartbook. Hyattsville, MD, 1999.)

12

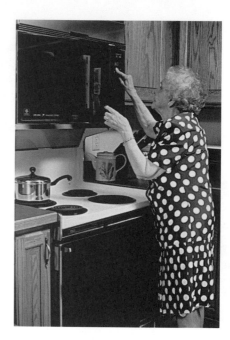

Figure 12–2. As an example of the "well elderly," this 86-year-old woman continues to function independently at home. (Courtesy of Bruce Wang.)

While individual differences exist, the aging process includes changes that are common in older persons. Sometimes, professionals find it useful to differentiate between "well elderly" and "frail elderly" because people in each group have needs quite distinct from those of people in the other group. **Well elderly** refers to people 65 years and older who are not experiencing physical limitations or who have age-related changes that are not significant enough to affect function. The 86-year-old woman in Figure 12–2 is a good example of a person described as one of the "well elderly." While she has minor medical problems, these problems do not significantly affect her daily activities. In contrast, the term **frail elderly** is used to describe people older than 65 with conditions that significantly impair their daily function or require frequent medical intervention.

Settings

Because the abilities and disabilities of older adults are very diverse, so are the environments in which these individuals live. Physical therapists and physical therapist assistants may work with older individuals in a wide variety of settings. People with acute medical conditions such as pneumonia, cardiovascular dysfunction, or hip fractures will be treated in hospitals. Older people with conditions such as cerebral vascular accident (stroke), Parkinson's disease, or amputation may be seen for physical therapy in rehabilitation centers once they are medically stable. A variety of long-term care centers (skilled nursing facilities, extended care facilities, and others) provide services to older people who are not acutely ill but who require nursing care or assistance with functional activities. Physical therapists and physical therapist assistants in long-term care settings generally provide two types of services. Rehabilitative services improve skills so that people may return to their own homes or are less dependent on caregivers in the long-term care facility. Functional maintenance programs assist older adults in maintaining the skills they currently possess and in preventing further limitations or disability.

Many older people with functional limitations are healthy enough to live at home independently or have family members who are able to care for them. Depending on the medical condition of the individual and the availability of appropriate transportation, older people living at home who require physical therapy may receive these services at an adult daycare facility, at an outpatient clinic, or through a home health care agency.

Healthy older people who want to maintain their optimum physical status may attend exercise classes at senior centers or those sponsored by such groups as the Arthritis Foundation. Traditional or aquatic exercise programs may be conducted, supervised, or developed by physical therapists. The common purpose for physical therapy in all these settings is to assist the individual in achieving the highest attainable level of independent function.

Roles for Physical Therapists with Older Adults

It is easy to envision the physical therapist as a clinician who provides hands-on services (direct intervention) to older adults. However, in each of the settings just described, physical therapists are also educators. With valuable knowledge of the physiological aging process, physical therapists are the ideal professionals to educate patients, family members, and other professionals in preventing and minimizing functional limitations and disability. Armed with facts, older people will be better able to exercise appropriately and maintain or regain skills. For example, the woman in Figure 12–3 is being taught how

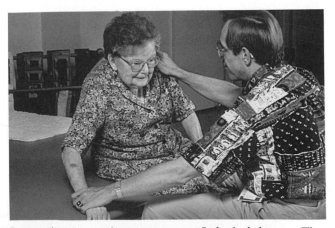

Figure 12–3. Instruction is a major component of physical therapy. The woman in the photo is being taught how to use her arms to sit up from a reclined position. (Courtesy of Bruce Wang.)

12

to use her arms to more easily get up from a reclining position. A physical therapist is in an excellent position to teach an older person that strength and endurance can be increased with properly designed programs.

Physical therapists may act as consultants to individuals and programs. They can be effective advocates for older people in developing appropriate activity programs and ensuring accessibility to all environments. For an individual, the physical therapist provides the knowledge necessary to acquire appropriate adaptive equipment or assistive devices that provide for both safety and convenience. **Adaptive equipment** allows an individual to perform a functional task with increased ease or independence. An **assistive device** provides the individual with assistance during periods of mobility. For example, a cane (an assistive device) may assist an individual in climbing stairs safely, or a bath chair (adaptive equipment) may allow someone to take a bath without supervision. As a program consultant, the physical therapist makes recommendations for group activities to maintain strength and endurance. The physical therapist acts as a resource for other staff members to determine how to incorporate goals related to mobility into other components of the day program.

Other roles that physical therapists may assume with respect to older adults are those of manager and researcher. Physical therapists are prepared to assume such roles as managers of rehabilitation services or case managers. In each of these positions, physical therapists' educational background in managing resources allows them to combine their knowledge of aging issues and management skills to take on additional responsibilities to serve clients. Research related to the aging process, to prevention of disability associated with aging, and to effective intervention for older adults is a priority in the health care field. Physical therapists can contribute to interdisciplinary studies to expand the knowledge of all health care professionals related to aging.

Aging-Related Changes

Physical therapists and physical therapist assistants must be familiar with the changes that occur in "normal" aging and be able to distinguish them from changes that are pathological. These changes, which vary with each individual, should be considered when conducting evaluations, designing programs, and setting goals for people older than 65 years. While certain biological changes are associated with aging, many changes once thought to be an inevitable part of aging are now considered to be related to the reduced activity and sedentary lifestyle experienced by many elders. The physical therapist, along with the health care team, has an important role in evaluating older adults to determine what impairments and limitations can be addressed through physical therapy. Changes that are not amenable to improvement may be addressed through accommodation or compensation.

The physical changes observed in older adults that affect the musculoskeletal system (bones, muscles, and connective tissue) often result in decreased strength, decreased flexibility, and poor posture. Decreased strength is frequently related to the **hypokinesis** (decreased activity or movement) and decreased muscle mass typically seen in older people. Muscle mass is reduced as a result of a decrease in the number of muscle fibers.[15] This reduction in fibers is related to loss of motor neurons (nerves innervating muscles) and active motor units (single motor neurons and all muscle fibers that they innervate).[3]

Changes in flexibility with age are related to both hypokinesis and biological changes in connective tissue. Connective tissue tends to become less hydrated and stiffer in older persons. As older people move less and become more sedentary, the muscles are not required to lengthen and actually become shorter over time. As muscles shorten, individuals display more flexed positions that lead to postural changes.

Bone also undergoes changes with age. In studies of vertebral bodies, bone mass was shown to decrease by 35% to 40% between the age of 20 and 80 years,[18] which means that bones are weaker in older people. This change may eventually advance to a condition known as osteoporosis (see Common Conditions).

The central nervous system shows a reduction in conduction velocity that is associated with age.[14] This reduced velocity affects the ability of the nerve to transmit impulses. Such change tends to make movement responses slower in older persons and may explain the slowed gait pattern often seen in later life.

Several of the sensory systems display changes that significantly affect mobility—specifically, changes in the ability to move safely in one's environment. The visual system is important in providing older people accurate information regarding the environment. The lens becomes less elastic and the muscles around the lens decrease in their ability to rapidly accommodate from seeing far to near distance.[13] Visual acuity is also reduced. These changes make lighting and contrasting colors important in offering the older person more cues about objects or surfaces that might interfere with safe mobility.

Older people display a group of characteristics titled **presbycusis** ("old people's hearing"). This term refers to a decreased ability to perceive higher pitches and distinguish between similar sounds.[25] Auditory acuity is also reduced. These changes are extremely important to consider when giving instructions or teaching an older person.

The tactile system is another sensory system whose changes may affect mobility. The tactile system provides important information regarding the texture and changes in the walking surface. Age-related changes reduce the amount of information that the individual receives regarding the environment. If an older person does not receive accurate information about the surface underfoot, ambulation may become altered.

Age-related changes in the cardiovascular system are complicated by the characteristic cardiovascular diseases of old age. For example, 64% of people between the ages of 65 and 74 display hypertension (high blood pressure).[28] It appears that whereas overall cardiac performance at rest is not altered by age in healthy people, the cardiac response to stress does differ. This aging change is demonstrated by a decrease in maximum cardiopulmonary function and work capacity.[24] Increased stiffness in the chest wall has an impact on the

12

respiratory system, which in turn further reduces the effectiveness of cardiopulmonary function. These changes need to be considered carefully when designing exercise programs for individuals older than 65 years.

Balance is a skill essential for daily function. Limitation in balance and an increase in the risk of falling are common problems in older adults. More than 35% of people older than 75 years have been reported to have experienced a fall.[30] Static and dynamic balance is the result of a complex interaction of the systems subject to potential age-related change mentioned before. If any of these systems undergoes change, balance could be affected as well. A fall from a loss of balance can expose an elder to a multitude of subsequent impairments such as fracture or other trauma, pneumonia, decubitus ulcers, and loss of strength or range of motion. Additionally, the psychosocial sequelae of falling may be numerous. Problems such as fear, isolation, and loss of an independent living situation are common consequences of a fall for an elderly individual.

For many years, one of the most common myths of aging was that cognitive function always significantly decreases with advanced age. In fact, people seemed to assume that dementia was inevitable. It is now known that the deterioration in cognitive function characterized as dementia is related to Alzheimer's disease or some other pathological condition, not to aging itself. Reports indicate that 10% of the general population older than 65 years display dementia.[5] The prevalence of dementia increases to 20% in people older than 85. Health professionals serving older people should be aware of dementia and techniques for interacting with people with dementia. However, the characteristics of dementia are not displayed universally in people older than 65 or even those older than 85.

Significant cognitive changes that fall into the category of normal aging occur in memory and conceptualization (tasks requiring abstract thinking).[23] Specifically, a change occurs in the manner in which new information is stored (encoded) in memory. This change leads to difficulty in retrieval of newer information. However, recent studies seem to show that training in memory techniques, such as list organization, can improve recall in older persons.[21]

Finally, people in older population groups may have psychosocial changes. These changes vary widely, depending on the individual, family, environment, and presence of other alterations or actual pathology. What is important for the physical therapist to remember is that psychosocial issues are extremely important to the success of any rehabilitation program. Social considerations such as adjustment to retirement, loss of lifetime roles (worker, parent, homeowner, athlete, etc.), living environment, and the presence or absence of health insurance have tremendous impact on an elder's life. Psychologically, older persons may be required to adjust to the loss of a spouse, friends, and siblings. The presence of psychiatric disorders such as depression, dysthymia (disorder of mood), and anxiety is higher in homebound older people than those who are able to be out in the community.[1] The physical therapist or physical therapist assistant has a responsibility to bring signs of psychological problems to the attention of other members of the health care team.

**COMMON
CONDITIONS**

Many impairments more prevalent in older people will benefit from physical therapy intervention. Individuals with the following common conditions are frequently seen by physical therapists and physical therapist assistants. (See also Parkinson's disease and stroke in Chapter 8.)

Arthritis

By far the most common problem in older people is one of the joint diseases described as arthritis. In 1984, nearly 50% of people in the United States older than 65 reported physician-diagnosed arthritis.[2] Two primary types of arthritis are recognized. **Osteoarthritis** is characterized by degeneration of cartilage. The hands, spine, knees, and hips are the most commonly affected areas. Osteoarthritis occurs when the cartilage deteriorates as a result of many years of use. This disease causes pain on movement. It is important for a person with osteoarthritis to maintain at least a moderate activity level while protecting the joints. Physical therapists can teach older adults appropriate exercise routines to maintain flexibility without excessively stressing the joints.

In contrast to osteoarthritis, **rheumatoid arthritis**, a disease of the immune system, is a chronic inflammation of the joints. It is more common in women than men, and the peak incidence is between 40 and 60 years of age.[26] It is characterized by enlarged joints that are often reddened and warm to the touch. The affected joints are stiff and painful, usually more so in the morning or after extended periods of inactivity. This disease process leads to limited range of motion, joint deformity, and eventually, progressive joint destruction. Typical physical therapy goals for a person with arthritis are pain relief, increased joint movement, assistive devices, and rehabilitation when joint surgery is required.

Pain relief may be provided by heat modalities such as hot packs or paraffin baths. The physical therapist may teach the individual positioning principles for pain relief when in resting postures. Active range-of-motion exercises will be developed. Provision of assistive devices such as canes or walkers may reduce pain in the affected joints during ambulation.

Total joint replacements of the hip and knee are common surgeries in older adults that are undertaken to decrease the pain associated with arthritis and to improve function. If joint replacements are performed for a person with arthritis, the physical therapist will be involved with the patient or client before surgery, as well as during the rehabilitation process. Before surgery, the physical therapist can teach an older person strengthening and flexibility exercises in order to go to surgery in optimal condition. The therapist can also teach the individual important guidelines to follow after surgery, order assistive devices, and reinforce the importance of exercise and rehabilitation after surgery. After joint replacement, the physical therapist will provide intervention to regain muscle strength, joint motion, and ADLs.

Osteoporosis

Osteoporosis, another extremely common disease in older people, is characterized by decreased mineralization of bones as a result of decreased production

12

of new bone cells and increased resorption of bone. Osteoporosis is more common in women than men. Other factors that predispose people to osteoporosis are postmenopausal status, family history, little physical activity, smoking, diet, and certain medications.[26] The most important problem related to osteoporosis is bone fracture. Wrist and hip fractures occur most often in the older population. The physical therapist's primary role in osteoporosis is prevention. This role is discussed in the next section, which addresses hip fracture.

Hip Fracture

The combination of osteoporosis and accidental falls has made hip fracture one of the most important health care issues for older people. More than 300,000 hospitalizations among people older than 65 were due to hip fractures in 1996 in the United States.[19] As larger proportions of the population enter the older-than-65 age group, these numbers are likely to increase. Hip fracture is considered by many to be a major public health problem. A study conducted in Boston illustrates the significant impact that hip fracture has on the functional skills that an elderly person may hope to regain after surgery to repair the hip. Only 33% of the people in that study regained their prefracture status in five basic ADLs 1 year after the fracture.[11] Another study showed that 2 months after hospital discharge, about 40% had regained ADLs but that only 18% had returned to previous levels of IADLs.[17]

Physical therapists are active in the rehabilitation of patients after hip fracture. In the hospital, transfer skills, ambulation, and the use of assistive devices are taught. These skills are continued at a rehabilitation center, skilled nursing facility, or the person's home (Fig. 12–4). As these basic skills are attained, physical therapists will then train the person to regain functional skills within the setting in which the individual will be living.

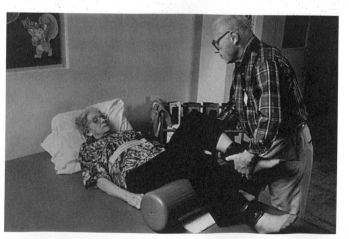

Figure 12–4. After instruction by the physical therapist, a volunteer provides assistance in an exercise program to regain hip and knee strength after surgery to repair a hip fracture. (Courtesy of Bruce Wang.)

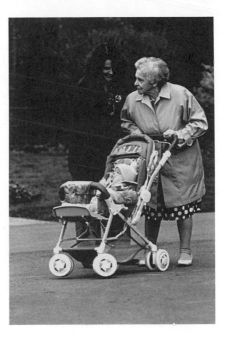

Figure 12–5. The home care physical therapist uses another family member (child) as a meaningful approach to increasing the strength and endurance of an older individual. (Courtesy of Bruce Wang.)

Physical therapists play an important role in the prevention of both osteoporosis and hip fracture. The most beneficial programs are directed at maintenance of activity levels, preservation of weight-bearing abilities and flexibility, strengthening, and education regarding a safe physical environment. Prevention of falls requires input from the entire health care team.[12] Falls may be related to any of several medical conditions, musculoskeletal or neurological changes, side effects of medication, cognitive status, the environment, or any combination of these factors. The health care team needs to be alert to these issues and teach older people and family members the importance of prevention. Routine opportunities for weight bearing and walking are important as prevention strategies (Fig. 12–5).

Diabetes

Diabetes mellitus affects 10% to 20% of Americans older than 60 years[16] and is a chronic disorder with effects on many body systems. It is a disease of insufficient insulin action that affects the efficient transport of glucose into muscle, adipose tissue, and liver cells. Glucose is not transported into these cells and accumulates in the blood. Some of the common complications of diabetes include the following: renal failure, neurological lesions (termed diabetic neuropathies), neuropathic skin ulceration, atherosclerotic vascular disease (which makes heart attacks and stroke more common in people with diabetes), and retinopathy, which may culminate in blindness. Many of these complications lead to specific problems for which physical therapy may benefit a person with diabetes. For instance, common physical therapy interventions for foot ulcers

12

are hydrotherapy, débridement, other wound care techniques, and the provision of adaptive footwear. When not responsive to treatment, foot ulcers may lead to the development of gangrene and often amputation. The rehabilitation process after an amputation requires physical therapy for care of the residual limb, prosthetic training, and gait training.

For people with non–insulin-dependent diabetes, management of the disease through diet and exercise is important. Physical therapists play an important role in developing exercise programs that take into consideration the problems associated with diabetes.

PRINCIPLES OF EXAMINATION

Physical therapy for an older adult begins with examination and evaluation. The physical therapist's examination is only one component of a team evaluation, and it is necessary for professionals from a variety of disciplines to critically examine an older person. If they all effectively share their findings, each will be able to better serve the individual.

As pointed out earlier, older people constantly undergo a wide variety of changes after receiving services from a myriad of providers. Only if all these changes are considered and all providers are aware of the others' interventions will the health care be of optimum benefit. However, many settings may not have every health care discipline available to its clients. In these situations, the physical therapist should be able to make observations about the individual that include not only musculoskeletal and neurological status but also basic information regarding the person's cognitive status, social situation, and communication abilities. Table 12–1 lists the components of a physical therapy examination with examples of possible sources of data and information.[8] It should be noted that only a sampling of tests and measures is listed and that the array of tests and measures will vary substantially from one individual to the next.

Examination and evaluation should be specifically oriented to the skills and capabilities that are necessary for maximum independence. These capabilities will differ for each older person. For example, a 70-year-old who has been inactive and sedentary since retirement at age 55 will have very different needs for rehabilitation than will a 78-year-old who walks 2 miles every day and continues to work 4 hours a day as a volunteer in a recreation program. In each case, the health care team must consider the individual's function before the condition requiring therapy. A thorough examination will include information related to the person's typical daily function.

History

The aforementioned information is often obtained through the patient and family interview as part of the process of obtaining the patient/client history. When interviewing the individual, the physical therapist should seek out information about how that older person views the current problem. A person's perceptions of the seriousness of the problem and expectations regarding therapy are important to consider when developing a plan of care and interven-

Table 12–1
Physical Therapy Examination for an Older Person

COMPONENTS OF EXAMINATION	SOURCES OF INFORMATION
History	Patient/client interview
	Family interview
	Caregiver interview
	Medical chart
	Referral information
System review	Limited examination of
	Cardiopulmonary status
	Integumentary status
	Musculoskeletal status
	Neuromuscular status
	Communication ability
	Affect
	Cognition
Tests and measures*	Aerobic capacity/endurance
	Human body measurements
	Arousal
	Assistive devices, orthoses, prostheses
	ADL/IADL
	Gait and balance
	Joint integrity and mobility/ROM
	Motor function
	Muscle performance
	Neuromotor status
	Pain
	Posture
	Sensation
	Ventilation/respiration

*This entry is a sampling of possible tests and measures and should not be considered comprehensive.

ADL, activities of daily living; IADL, instrumental ADL; ROM, range of motion.

Data from Guide to Physical Therapist Practice. 2nd ed. Phys Ther 2001;81:9–744.

12

tions. It is also important to obtain information from the person regarding any culturally based beliefs about illness, disability, and health. An older person may have very long held beliefs that the physical therapist should consider.

Interviewing an older person will also give the physical therapist some general impressions of cognitive function to help determine whether a more formal examination of cognition is necessary. The individual should be able to give the physical therapist information about family support, typical activity level, occupation or former occupation, and the living environment.

Input from family members and other caregivers is an important component of the history. This information is very useful in determining the amount of assistance that a person may need from other sources. In some circumstances, these individuals will also be able to verify information for the practitioner. Another component of the history comes from the chart review. Objective information is gained from reports, records, and patient charts. The chart and other documents provide information such as medical diagnosis, dates of hospitalization, laboratory reports, and other documented facts about the present illness or complaint, as well as past problems that may influence the plan of care for the current problem.

Systems Review

The examination often begins with a systems review, which entails a brief examination of the individual's systems to provide the physical therapist information regarding the older adult's general health. Data from the brief examination help the physical therapist select the most appropriate tests and measures for the individual.

Tests and Measures

Examination of an older person will proceed much like the physical therapist's examination of any individual, except that the physical therapist will be especially alert to the common problems of this age group. The physical therapist may adapt some examination procedures to be more appropriate to the older individual. Tasks that are requested of the individual should be explained as they relate to function. For example, an older adult may resist an examination activity such as creeping or kneeling on the floor. The person may be afraid of the positions or feel foolish. However, if the physical therapist explains that the activity is necessary to determine whether the person could get up from the floor if a fall occurred, the person may be more willing to cooperate.

In examining the musculoskeletal system of an older person, the physical therapist should keep in mind the potential for the age-related changes described earlier. The therapist needs to examine strength in terms of what activities the individual wants or needs to be able to perform. In other words, strength may need to be expressed in terms of function. Norms for range of motion in people older than 65 years have not been scientifically established, nor are there any that are commonly used. Depending on the person's activity level, some deficits may be expected. The therapist and the older person should determine how much limitation of movement at the joints is acceptable. Posture can be examined in an older adult by using the same means as with other patient groups. The physical therapist should determine whether the observed posture is due to actual structural changes or whether it is a result of habit or functional issues. If the changes are not structural, education and exercise may bring significant improvement to abnormal postural findings.

The neurological examination of an older person is similar to that of any individual. Some slowed responses may be noted, as described earlier but it is a matter of determining what impact, if any, these slowed responses have on the person's quality of life. The neurological examination should include specific sensory testing. Such testing might include two-point discrimination, proprioception, and visual and auditory testing performed by other members of the health care team. Sensory deficits may significantly affect functional tasks such as balance. As noted earlier, balance is a complex interaction of visual, perceptual, and motor skills. The physical therapist needs to examine each of these systems individually to determine which may be contributing to a balance problem.

Both static (while standing still) and dynamic (while moving) balance should be examined. Tests and measures for examining **static balance** include such tests as observing the person standing with eyes open and eyes closed, timing of standing on one foot, and the degree of postural sway. A specific balance test that can predict the likelihood of falling is the **functional reach test.**[4] In this test, a simple measure of how far the person can reach in front of the body gives an indication of the likelihood of falls.

Dynamic balance is assessed in a number of ways. Gait is an important aspect of dynamic balance, as is functional mobility. The physical therapist may measure how long it takes an older person to walk a set distance (timed walk). Other tests include the Tinnetti Scale for Balance and Gait.[29] The Gait Abnormality Rating Scale looks at several components of gait and relates them to balance.[31] These scales are just two examples of the many tools available to assess balance. Gait examination should always include the use of any required assistive device and a description or consideration of the type of footwear that the person uses. The type of sole or the weight of the shoe will affect the way someone ambulates. In Figure 12–6, the physical therapist is performing an initial gait examination of a man approximately 1 month after hospital discharge following a stroke. A quadruped cane is needed at this time to assist with dynamic balance.

Information regarding balance and the potential for falling is very useful to the entire interdisciplinary team working with the older person. The team will be able to develop strategies in fall prevention that range from exercise and environmental modification to teaching fall prevention skills to the older person.

Standard tests of cardiopulmonary function may be used in older persons. Older people receiving physical therapy often fatigue easily and have reduced endurance. Physical therapists examine and evaluate these individuals to determine whether modifications in exercise programs are necessary. Measurements of cardiopulmonary function will also help the physical therapist determine whether goals to increase endurance are realistic and appropriate (see also Chapter 9).

Another important part of the examination process in an older person is to determine whether the individual is experiencing pain related to movement. It is important to obtain a description of pain location and intensity and circum-

12

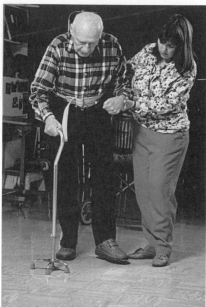

Figure 12–6. Gait assessment using a quadruped cane after a stroke. (Courtesy of Bruce Wang.)

stances that elicit the pain or alleviate it. It should be noted whether the pain is acute or chronic and whether it increases or decreases from one session to the next. Because pain is perceived differently from one individual to the next, it is important to assess how much discomfort the person is willing to tolerate to maintain independent function.

One simple means of measuring pain is on a visual analog rating scale.[27] The individual indicates the amount of pain being experienced along a 10-cm scale (see Fig. 7–2). If such an objective pain index is used, decreasing pain from one measurable point to another on the scale may be an appropriate goal for an older adult. Another approach is to set a goal for a specific functional task to be performed with a tolerable level of pain.

The tests and measures just described relate to specific impairments or function. It is also important for the physical therapist to examine an older adult's overall function. For many years physical therapists have used checklists to indicate whether a patient or client can perform particular tasks. More recently, several standardized measures have been developed. Standardized measures allow health care professionals to measure change by comparing a person's scores. Such comparisons might occur between particular points in time or when the person relocates from one setting to another. Examples of standardized self-report measures include the Functional Status Questionnaire[10] and the Functional Status Index,[9] in which the older person or the caregiver reports the older person's ability to perform functional activities. Others tests may also be performed, such as the Physical Performance Test, in which the therapist observes the older person performing tasks and scores the person's performance according to the instructions for the particular tool.[22]

Information about the environment in which the older person lives is essential. Whether the individual is in a nursing home, living in a relative's house, or living alone, several aspects of the environment must be considered. The physical layout of the living area, access to and from the residence, and access from the home to outside services are important. Ideally, the physical therapist should visit the residence rather than rely on reports from others.

The physical therapist will need to investigate access to and from the residence in light of the individual's specific abilities and limitations. The following items are of importance in determining how much assistance an older person may require to be as independent in the living environment as possible:

- Ground surfaces—gravel, pavement, grass, sidewalks
- Curbs and curb cuts
- Ramps or steps outside the home
- Stairways within the home
- Presence or absence of handrails
- Size of door openings
- Door handles, latches
- Furnishings and floor coverings
- Arrangement of the kitchen and bathroom fixtures

In addition to the aforementioned, a thorough examination should include such items as lighting, doorways, floor plans, furniture, and adequate space for adaptive equipment. Because so many items must be considered, it is most efficient for the clinician to use some type of checklist for this assessment with space for individual notation.

An environmental examination is equally important whether the older person is in a private home or a long-term care facility. According to regulations promulgated by the Health Care Financing Administration, long-term care facilities receiving federal reimbursement (such as Medicare or Medicaid) are obligated to ensure that residents are as free from the use of restraints as practical. Items such as seat belts in wheelchairs, chest or hand straps in beds, and bedrails are to be used as infrequently as possible. Physical therapists in these settings are obligated to assess mobility skills and safety and make recommendations to the interdisciplinary team regarding the need, if any, for these devices. The team must first attempt to modify the physical environment to meet individual needs for safety before using restraints. Only when other options have been exhausted should the team recommend the use of such supports.

As described earlier, few cognitive changes are solely a result of aging in a healthy older person. However, many conditions common in the elderly do have the potential for the development of dementia. For this reason, the physical therapist should either obtain information from other health care professionals or make observations during the physical therapy evaluation regarding cognitive function. Cognitive abilities have a great influence on how the physical therapist should provide instructions, the amount of repetition required when demonstrating tasks, and how much practice will be required

12

when teaching a new skill. Standard, quick cognitive assessment tools, such as the Mini-Mental State Examination, can easily be used by physical therapists without obtaining extensive training.[7]

As with all patients, it is essential that the physical therapist include psychosocial information as part of the complete evaluation of an older person. It is important to know how the person is adjusting to the present disability. This knowledge will help the therapist determine the individual's level of motivation and whether special strategies are necessary to increase that level. An older person may see a problem such as stroke or heart attack as "the beginning of the end" and may be depressed. The therapist will benefit from knowing who the significant people are in the patient's life—spouse, family, friends, or caregivers.

It is also extremely important to know the setting to which the person will return so that the available social support can be determined. Social workers or case managers are able to provide the physical therapist with pertinent details regarding each patient's specific health insurance coverage and financial status so that the impact on rehabilitation services can be considered. The health care team will need to plan and prioritize interventions for each individual based not only on the findings of the examination but also on social support.

PRINCIPLES OF EVALUATION, DIAGNOSIS, AND PROGNOSIS

Once information about the patient or client has been obtained, the next step in providing physical therapy intervention for an older adult is to evaluate the findings of the examination. From this evaluation, the physical therapist then determines a diagnosis that will direct the course of rehabilitation. The diagnosis is a label or classification assigned to the cluster of findings related to the individual. It is important to remember that older adults frequently have multiple medical diagnoses. The physical therapist's role is to consider these medical conditions, impairments, and functional limitations and evaluate how they affect the individual's ability to function. The physical therapy diagnosis reflects the result of this evaluation process.

Similarly, all these variables must be weighed to arrive at a prognosis that will direct the planning and goal-setting process for the older adult. Two 80-year-old individuals with identical medical conditions will not necessarily have the same prognosis or subsequent plans for physical therapy. Social support, environmental factors, internal factors such as cognitive level, and other variables all contribute to an appropriate prognosis.

PRINCIPLES OF DIRECT INTERVENTION

The individual's diagnosis and prognosis form the basis of the plan for physical therapy intervention. Physical therapy for any patient should focus on the problems identified from the evaluation; however, care for an older person requires emphasis on certain aspects of intervention, including (1) direct intervention techniques with the expectation of improved function, (2) instruction, (3) modification of accepted intervention techniques as necessary for the effects of aging, (4) recommendations for environmental modification, (5) training in the use of appropriate adaptive equipment, and (6) setting.

Direct Intervention

The first consideration when establishing goals for direct intervention in an older person is to be sure to set goals that are meaningful for the individual and address daily function. In other words, a goal to have the person reach full or normal shoulder flexion (arm up over head to 180 degrees) may not be meaningful if the person does not have any need to reach straight up overhead. If the highest cupboards in the house require only partial flexion and the person does not put any clothing on over the head, perhaps valuable time for direct intervention should be spent on other activities. However, if this older adult continues to work part-time and must reach overhead to do so, full shoulder flexion is very important.

To set goals that are meaningful and functional, the older person needs to be involved throughout the process. Such involvement may require some encouragement from the professional, especially if the person believes that the role of the health care professional is to issue direction and wait for patient compliance. Many older people feel that it is not the role of the patient to determine treatment. The professional should be prepared to help older adults be more involved in decision making regarding care.

The interdisciplinary approach mentioned throughout this chapter is also important when setting goals. The individual may have multiple medical and rehabilitative needs. The team, including the patient and family, should examine all those needs and prioritize which should be addressed initially and which are more long term.

Instruction

Instruction of an older person should be both general and specific. General, factual information about the effects of aging on the various body systems will give an older person a good background and model from which to judge the changes that that individual may experience. This information will help an older person appreciate the importance of achieving or maintaining an active lifestyle to prevent those changes that are linked to being inactive. More specific information pertaining to the particular problem that an older adult is experiencing is also important. A basic understanding of the disablement process, including the relationships among pathology, impairment, function, and disability, may help an older person understand why the physical therapist is selecting particular interventions. Such topics as the typical course of the disorder, expected type and length of treatment, expectations for the home program, and impact on function should be clearly outlined.

Education plays a role in motivating older adults; however, other techniques can help with motivation as well. Often, older people will enjoy therapy if social interaction can be built into the process. Establishing a group of people with similar abilities for exercise may be very beneficial and fun. Designing interventions in such a way that the person is competing, either with results of the last session or with peers, may also serve to increase motivation to perform.

For some individuals, motivation will not be an issue at all. These people

12

may be very motivated, but not confident in their own abilities to carry out a program when the therapist works with another person or when the individual performs the program at home. Such items as lists of activities, diagrams, charts with spaces to check off, or a notebook may be very valuable in assisting this type of person to take control of the routine.

Modification

Intervention for an older adult should focus on improving the individual's function. It is important to develop programs that incorporate movement patterns that normally occur during the person's routine. For example, treatment of balance problems is most beneficial if it includes such activities as balance during transitional movements (up and down from chairs, in and out of bed) and on uneven surfaces. On the other hand, one-legged standing is probably not meaningful for most older persons. In most cases, direct intervention need not be modified solely based on aging factors. Healthy older persons can increase strength, range of motion, endurance, and overall performance with traditional approaches. For example, it has been demonstrated that 86- to 96-year-old nursing home residents who participated in exercise (resistance training) programs were able to increase quadriceps strength.[6] In Figure 12–7, the woman is engaged in resistive exercise to increase strength in her hip and knee musculature. Modification may be necessary, however, depending on the presence of medical conditions. Cardiovascular and cardiopulmonary conditions, arthritis, and diabetes are examples of conditions common in older

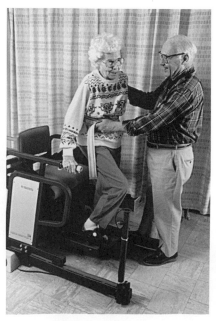

Figure 12–7. Resistive exercises to increase strength, in this case in the hip and knee musculature, are effective in the elderly. (Courtesy of Bruce Wang.)

individuals for which modifications of accepted approaches might be necessary. Physical therapists and physical therapist assistants working with the elderly should be alert to these conditions and be prepared to modify the program accordingly.

Physical therapists must also recognize that some medications taken by older individuals may necessitate modification of the intervention. Some medications affect the ability to perform physical activity. Frequently, older people take multiple medications, both prescribed and over-the-counter medications. The physical therapist should be aware of the medications being taken by the individual, possible drug interactions, and side effects of the medication. For example, many drugs have dizziness as a side effect. If the physical therapist is working with someone on activities such as getting out of bed, getting up from the floor, or more advanced balance activities, it is essential that the therapist be alert to any signs of dizziness. If the person is taking medication that may increase dizziness, it may be necessary for the physical therapist to take increased safety precautions during performance of these activities. For information related to medical conditions and medications, the physical therapist should remain in close contact with the physician and other team members.

Environmental Modification/Adaptive Equipment

When providing services to an older person, the physical therapist should keep the need for environmental modification and adaptive equipment in mind. Simple changes in the environment (improved lighting, removal of throw rugs, or furniture rearrangement) may make the individual more functional and safe in the living environment. Appropriate adaptive equipment and training in its use may enable an older person to be more independent. Training in adaptive equipment should include demonstration and repeated opportunities to practice.

Setting

A final consideration in determining the most appropriate intervention for an older person relates to the setting. In a physical therapy department within a health care facility, multiple pieces of equipment are usually available to help achieve improved strength and mobility or to decrease pain. However, in this setting, the physical therapist may have to be creative to ensure that enhanced performance on objective tests will actually translate into improvement in daily function in more home-like environments. Physical therapy provided in the home setting provides the opposite challenge. There will be many opportunities in a home to improve functional skills, but it may be difficult to increase strength or endurance over long distances. The therapist must keep these advantages and limitations in mind when planning programs for intervention. In Figure 12–8, parallel bars are used to assist the woman in gait training. When she is ready to return to a home environment, another device such as a walker may be necessary to increase the distance that she is able to walk.

12

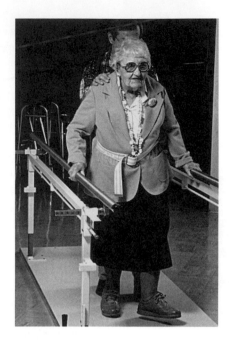

Figure 12–8. Gait training is enhanced by using parallel bars in a clinical setting. (Courtesy of Bruce Wang.)

Case Study

This example is provided with the intent of demonstrating the complex medical, cognitive, psychosocial, and ethical issues that face health care practitioners who work with older people and their families.

Margaret Evans is an 81-year-old woman who has been hospitalized for 7 days after a total hip replacement. She has the multiple diagnoses of rheumatoid arthritis, osteoporosis, and hypertension. She is also hearing impaired. The arthritis causes her almost constant pain in her hips, knees, and hands. The surgery was performed to relieve pain in her right hip, which was the side displaying more severe pain. Mrs. Evans lives alone in her home, where she has resided for 40 years. Payment on her home mortgage was completed 6 years ago. Her husband is deceased, her son lives 250 miles away, and her daughter lives with her family about 10 miles away. Mrs. Evans has a limited income (Social Security), and her medical coverage is Medicare.

Mrs. Evans is considered medically ready for discharge from the hospital. She has been receiving physical therapy once a day consisting of the following: (1) range-of-motion therapy for all extremities that is focused on the hip and knee musculature, (2) transfer training (moving from wheelchair to toilet, bed to standing, etc.), and (3) gait training with a walker. The physical therapist made a home visit and noted the following: (1) four steps must be climbed to get into the house, (2) the bedroom that Mrs. Evans uses is upstairs (13 steps), (3) many throw rugs are arranged on the hardwood floors, (4) both bathrooms have tubs with showers, and (5) the laundry facilities are in the basement.

Mrs. Evans wants to go home as soon as possible. She has never been away from her home more than 3 days and has been very lonely for her neighbors while in the hospital. She sometimes awakens at night disoriented and confused about where she is. Her daughter, who works full-time, is concerned about her mother's safety at home and is not sure whether her mother is ready to go home alone. She has also stated that she wants to be sure that her mother has every opportunity for full rehabilitation and is advocating for daily physical therapy.

The team, including Mrs. Evans and her daughter, meets to discuss a discharge plan. A short-term placement is proposed. In this plan, Mrs. Evans would be discharged to a skilled nursing facility where daily physical therapy could be provided. Mrs. Evans is opposed to that move, although her daughter tries to convince her that it is a good proposal. The social worker suggests discharge to home and asks the team what other support services are necessary to ensure her success at home. The physical therapist indicates that Mrs. Evans should learn to navigate stairs safely with crutches, obtain adaptive equipment such as a bathing chair and a raised toilet seat, and modify the home environment to be successful at home. Physical therapy services could be provided two to three times weekly through a home health care agency. The social worker suggests that a home health aide would be appropriate to assist Mrs. Evans with personal care, housework, and laundry.

Mrs. Evans is pleased, but her daughter is still concerned for the safety of her mother. The rehabilitation nurse suggests an emergency call button for Mrs. Evans to obtain assistance if she falls or experiences any other urgent situation. A bedroom will be set up for her on the first floor to avoid excessive stair climbing. The team agrees to the plan, and the social worker will monitor the services on a weekly basis.

Summary

As we move into the 21st century, the proportion of our population older than 65 and especially older than 85 will continue to grow. Physical therapists and physical therapist assistants are serving older adults in every type of setting, not solely in long-term care facilities. Certainly, some therapists will select people older than 65 years as a preferred population in which to specialize, but almost all therapists and assistants will have contact with patients in this age group at one point or another. To provide quality services to the older population, physical therapists should recognize the similarities and differences between the older person and any other individual in need of physical therapy. The physical therapist should be ready to modify interventions as needed to address documented age-related changes. The physical therapist should be able to educate an older person requiring services and all significant others regarding methods for the person to enhance function. Finally, the physical therapist must be able to communicate and cooperate with older individuals, their families, and team members to develop a meaningful and successful plan for intervention.

12

The author wishes to acknowledge the staff and members of The Friendly Home in Rochester, New York, for their assistance.

References

1. Bruce ML, McNamara R: Psychiatric status among the homebound elderly: An epidemiological perspective. Am Geriatr Soc 1992;40:561–566.
2. Chartbook on Health Data on Older Americans, Series 3, No. 29. Baltimore, National Center for Health Statistics, US Department of Health and Human Services, Public Health Service, US Government Printing Office, 1993.
3. Doherty TJ, Vandervoort AA, Taylor AW, et al: Effects of motor unit losses on strength in older men and woman. J Appl Physiol 1993;74:868–874.
4. Duncan PW, Weiner DK, Chandler J, et al: Functional reach: A new clinical measure of balance. J Gerontol 1990;45(6):M192–M197.
5. Evans DA, Funkenstein HH, Albert MS, et al: Prevalence of Alzheimer's disease in a community population of older persons. Higher than previously reported. JAMA 1989;262:2551–2556.
6. Fiatarone MA, Marks EC, Ryan ND, et al: High intensity strength training on nonagenerians. Effects on skeletal muscle. JAMA 1990;263:3029–3034.
7. Folstein MF, Folstein SE, McHugh PR: "Mini-mental state." A practical method for grading the cognitive state of patients for the clinician. J Psychiatr Res 1975;12(3):189–198.
8. Guide to Physical Therapist Practice. 2nd ed. Phys Ther 2001;81:9–744.
9. Jette AM: The Functional Status Index: Reliability and validity of a self-report functional disability measure. J Rheumatol 1987;14(suppl 15):15–19.
10. Jette AM, Davies AR, Cleary PD, et al: The Functional Status Questionnaire: Reliability and validity when used in primary care. J Gen Intern Med 1986;1:143–149.
11. Jette AM, Harris BA, Cleary PD, et al: Functional recovery after hip fracture. Arch Phys Med Rehabil 1987;68:735–740.
12. Kalchthaler J, Bascon R, Quintos V: Falls in the institutionalized elderly. J Am Geriatr Soc 1978;26:424.
13. Lewis CB: Aging: The Health Care Challenge, ed 3. Philadelphia, FA Davis, 1996.
14. Lewis C, Bottomly J: Geriatric Physical Therapy. E Norwalk, CT, Appleton & Lange, 1991.
15. Lexell J, Taylor CC, Sjostrom L: What is the cause of the aging atrophy? J Neurol Sci 1988;84:275–294.
16. Lipson LG: Diabetes in the elderly: Diagnosis, pathogenesis, and therapy. Am J Med 1986;80(suppl 5A):10–21.
17. Magaziner J, Simonsick EM, Kashner TM, et al: Predictors of functional recovery one year following hospital discharge for hip fracture: A prospective study. J Gerontol 1990;45(3):M101–M107.
18. Mosekilde L: Normal age-related changes in bone mass, structure, and strength—consequences of the remodeling process. Dan Med Bull 1993;40:65–83.
19. National Center for Health Statistics. Health, United States, 1999 With Health and Aging Chartbook. Hyattsville, MD, 1999.
20. National Vital Statistics Report—Preliminary Data. National Center for Health Statistics, vol 47, No. 4, 1997.
21. Norris MP, West RL: Activity memory and aging: The role of motor retrieval and strategic processing. Psychol Aging 1993;8:81–86.
22. Reuben DB, Sui AL: An objective measure of physical function of elderly outpatients: The Physical Performance Test. J Am Geriatr Soc 1990;38:1105–1112.
23. Salthouse TA: Age related changes in basic cognitive processes. *In* Storundt M, VandeBos G (eds): The Adult Years: Continuity and Change. Washington, DC, American Psychiatric Association, 1989.
24. Schneider EL, Rowe JW (eds): Handbook of the Biology of Aging. New York, Academic, 1990.
25. Schaknecht HF: Pathology of the Ear. Philadelphia, Lea & Febiger, 1993.
26. Schumacher HR: Primer on the Rheumatic Diseases. Atlanta, Arthritis Foundation, 1988.
27. Scott J, Huskisson EC: Graphic representation of pain. Pain 1976;2:175–184.
28. Subcommittee on Definition and Prevalence of the 1984 Joint National Committee: Hypertension prevalence and the status of awareness, treatment, and control in the United States. Hypertension 1985;7:457–468.
29. Tinnetti M: Performance oriented assessment of mobility problems in elderly patients. J Am Geriatr Soc 1986;3:119–126.
30. Tinnetti ME, Speechly M, Ginter SF: Risk factors for falls among elderly persons living in the community. N Engl J Med 1985;319:1701–1707.
31. Wolfson L, Whipple R, Amerman P, et al: Gait assessment in the elderly: A gait abnormality rating scale and its relation to falls. J Gerontol 1990;45(1):M12–M19.

Suggested Readings

Bonder BR, Wagner, MB: Functional Performance in Older Adults. Philadelphia, FA Davis, 1994.

This book presents an interdisciplinary perspective to suggest approaches for the improvement of function in older adults. It emphasizes that aging is more than just a biological process, but rather a complex set of interactions resulting in a unique experience for each individual.

Goldstein TS: Geriatric Orthopaedics. Gaithersburg, MD, Aspen, 1991.

Musculoskeletal problems of older individuals are addressed in depth. Clinical management of these problems is described with an emphasis on exercise suggestions. The information is organized according to the involved joint.

Guccione AA: Geriatric Physical Therapy, ed 2. St Louis, Mosby–Year Book, 2000.

This textbook, aimed at the entry-level physical therapy student, provides information necessary to guide professionals in the treatment of older patients. It addresses assessment methods and modification of these methods for people in the older age range. Common problems such as posture, falls, pain management, and wound care are examined. In addition, special population groups within the aging category are included.

Lorig K, Fries JF: The Arthritis Helpbook. Reading, MA, Addison-Wesley, 1990.

The authors define and describe arthritis. However, the focus is on exercise and self-help hints. An inexpensive resource for people with arthritis.

May BJ: Home Health and Rehabilitation. Philadelphia, FA Davis, 1993.

While not written specifically for rehabilitation of older people, this book is a good source for understanding the framework of home health care. Since more patients are receiving health care in their own homes, this information is useful in developing an awareness for this aspect of the continuum of care available to aging individuals.

Schneider EL, Rowe J: Handbook of the Biology of Aging. New York, Academic, 1990.

This textbook takes a scientific look at the biomedical aspects of aging. It reviews human aging research in many areas, including cellular aging, the physiology of aging, disorders in aging, and exercise in older individuals. Information is at a sophisticated level. Chapters include extensive references.

12

REVIEW QUESTIONS

1. If accessible, visit both a long-term care facility and a daycare facility for elders and observe how many kinds of adaptive equipment you can see being used.

2. Explain why it is sometimes difficult for health care practitioners to determine whether health changes are due to (1) the normal aging process, (2) reduced activity, or (3) a specific disease process. Do a little research to come up with at least two specific examples.

3. Challenge yourself to describe a hypothetical case in which an elderly person comes to a physical therapy clinic to be treated for problems resulting from a common condition such as arthritis, osteoporosis, hip fracture, or diabetes. Exchange "cases" with a fellow student and write about special considerations when the patient is an older person.

4. Mr. Jamison comes to you for physical therapy that is related, he says, to his arthritis, but when you try to determine what particular problem he is here for, he is very vague, only pointing out all the joints in which he "has pain off and on." What might you investigate to find more specifics on his immediate needs?

5. Write two brief case scenarios that illustrate very different reasons why it would be necessary to modify intervention because of an age-related consideration.

Glossary

accessory motion: Ability of the joint surfaces to glide, roll, and spin on each other.

active assisted range of motion: Joint movement in which the patient may be assisted either manually or mechanically through an arc of movement.

active free range of motion: Joint movement in which the patient does not receive any support or resistance through an arc of movement.

active member: Membership category in the APTA for the physical therapist.

active range of motion (AROM): Ability of the patient to voluntarily move a limb through an arc of movement.

active resisted exercise: Joint movement in which an external force resists the movement.

activities of daily living (ADLs): Activities that individuals participate in daily to meet their basic needs. Examples include bathing, dressing, using the toilet, and eating.

adaptive equipment: Pieces of equipment that allow individuals to perform functional tasks with increased ease or independence.

aerobics training: Exercise program that uses oxygen as the major energy source.

Affiliate Assembly: Past component of the APTA that represented and was composed of PTAs; precursor to National Assembly.

affiliate member: Membership category in the APTA for the physical therapist assistant.

Affiliate Special Interest Group: Past component of the APTA that served the interests of the PTA; precursor to Affiliate Assembly.

akinesia: Poverty of movements.

alliance: Collaboration of several health care facilities and practices.

ambulatory center: Any facility in which health care is provided on an

311

outpatient basis; the patient is able to walk into the facility, receive care, and walk out of the facility the same day.

American Board of Physical Therapy Specialties (ABPTS):   Unit created by the House of Delegates to provide a formal mechanism for recognizing physical therapists with advanced knowledge, skills, and experience in a special area of practice.

American Physical Therapy Association (APTA):   National organization that represents and promotes the profession of physical therapy.

American Physiotherapy Association (APA):   Organization (formerly called American Women's Physical Therapeutic Association) responsible for maintaining high standards and educational programs for physiotherapists; precursor to APTA.

American Women's Physical Therapeutic Association: First national organization representing "physical therapeutics." Established in 1921 to maintain high standards and provide a mechanism to share information.

amyotrophic lateral sclerosis (ALS):   Also known as Lou Gehrig's disease; rapidly progressive neurological disorder associated with a degeneration of the motor nerve cells.

angina: Condition in which chest pain occurs from ischemia.

angiography: Technique in which radiopaque material is injected into the blood vessels to better visualize and identify problems such as occlusion (blockage) of blood vessels, aneurysms, and vascular malformations.

angioplasty: Process of mechanically dilating a blood vessel.

annual conference and exposition: Yearly (June) meeting of the APTA, held in accordance with the Bylaws, and including an extensive program of educational presentations, meetings, and activities.

aquatic physical therapy: Therapeutic use of water for rehabilitation or prevention of injury.

arterial insufficiency: Deficiency or occlusion of blood flow through an artery.

arteriosclerosis: Hardening of the arteries.

assembly: Component of APTA whose purpose is to provide a means by which members of the same class may meet, confer, and promote the interest of the respective membership class.

assessment: Measurement or assigned value by which physical therapists make a clinical judgment.

assistive device: Device that provides individuals with assistance to perform tasks or during periods of mobility. Examples include canes, walkers, and adapted keyboards.

Bad Ragaz method: Aquatic therapy technique using proprioceptive neuromuscular facilitation techniques while the patient is suspended by rings in the water.

Balanced Budget Act of 1997 (BBA):   Federal legislation passed by the Senate and Congress and signed by President Clinton that cut health care expenditures for Medicare and other government sponsored programs to achieve a balanced budget.

blood gas analysis: Assessment of blood (usually arterial) to determine the concentration of oxygen and carbon dioxide.

Board of Directors (BOD):   APTA unit consisting of six APTA officers and nine directors, whose duty is to carry out the mandates and policies established by the HOD.

bradykinesia: Slowness of movements.

Brunnstrom's approach: Neurological technique based on the natural sequence of recovery following stroke.

bursitis: Inflammation of bursae, fluid-filled sacs located throughout the body that serve to decrease the friction between two structures.

cardiac catheterization: Passage of a catheter (a flexible tube) into an artery in the arm or leg, then along the artery to reach the heart to measure pressure, inject dye, or take a sample of tissue.

cardiac muscle dysfunction: Various pathologies associated with heart failure.

cardiac pacemaker: Electronic device that produces a pulse that controls heart depolarization.

career ladder: Employer's structure, creating levels within a specific field or position to enable promotion of employees in that category.

cerebral palsy (CP):   Group of conditions caused by a nonprogressive lesion on the brain. Most often CP occurs during gestation (before birth), at birth, or immediately after birth, owing to an interruption of oxygen to the brain of the fetus or newborn.

certification: Process by which a state legally regulates the use of a professional title without creating a separate scope of practice. State law will not permit use of the title unless state standards are met. This differs from the private certification offered by private organizations for meeting the standards of that organization.

chapter: Organizational unit of the APTA that is defined by specific legally constituted boundaries such as a state, territory, or commonwealth of the United States or the District of Columbia. Membership is automatic and is based on location of residence or employment, education, or greatest active participation.

chronic inflammation: A low-grade, protracted inflammatory process.

chronic obstructive pulmonary disease (COPD):   Group of disorders that produce certain specific physical symptoms, including chronic productive cough, excessive mucus production, changes in the sound produced when air passes through the bronchial tubes, and shortness of breath (dyspnea).

civil law: Law of a jurisdiction concerned with private rights and remedies; the administration of justice involving the violation of private duties owed by individuals.

client: An individual who seeks the services of a physical therapist to maintain health or a business that hires a physical therapist as a consultant.

closed-chain exercise/kinetic-chain exercise: Exercise incorporating several muscle groups through the use of several joints with the end segment fixed.

clubfoot: Disorder in which the foot is turned inward and slanted upward.

Code of Ethics: Principles set forth for the physical therapy profession by the APTA for maintaining and promoting ethical practice.

collagen: A supportive, strong, and fibrous connective tissue protein that is found in the dermis, tendon, cartilage, fascia, ligament, and bone.

Combined Sections Meeting: Early February meeting of APTA sections' members to provide an opportunity for sharing information.

Commission on Accreditation in Physical Therapy Education (CAPTE):   Unit responsible for evaluating and accrediting professional (entry-level) physical therapy and physical therapist assistant education programs.

common law: Law created by court decision rather than by legislative action.

components: Organizational units within the APTA currently limited to chapters, sections, and assemblies as established by APTA Bylaws.

computed (axial) tomography (CAT or CT):   Computer synthesis of x-rays transmitted through a specific plane of the body.

conducting airways: Passageways and tubes that allow air to pass into or out of the lungs.

congenital dislocation of the hip (CDH):   Dislocation resulting from the abnormal development of some of the structures surrounding the hip joint, allowing the head of the femur (thigh bone) to move in and out of the hip socket; cause is unknown.

congestive heart failure (CHF):   Condition in which the heart muscle is compromised to the point that it cannot move blood volume effectively.

continuous quality improvement/total quality management (CQI/TQM):   Method of examining and improving processes using data management tools.

continuum of care: health care provided within a system that meets all levels of need (e.g., from acute care, to inpatient medical rehabilitation or inpatient subacute rehabilitation, to home care, to outpatient care).

contract: An agreement between two or more persons that creates a legal obligation to do, or not do, a particular thing.

coronary artery bypass grafting (CABG): Grafting (attaching) a small artery or a leg vein to a point beyond the blockage or plaque. This bypasses the blockage, re-establishing blood flow to the heart.

coronary heart disease (CHD): Arteriosclerosis, or a hardening of the arteries, affecting the coronary vessels.

criminal law: Administration of justice, through the enforcement of the criminal code of a state or of the United States; involves violations of duties owed to society at large.

critical pathways: Guidelines for patient hospital care using "milestones" to monitor progress; based on consensus, including only those aspects of care provided to affect patient outcomes.

cross-training: Training health care professionals in treatment skills from a variety of professions to provide a multidisciplinary team in a patient-focused care (PFC) model.

cryotherapy: Application of cold agents to cause a decrease in blood flow and decreased metabolism, which result in a decrease in swelling and pain.

customer satisfaction: satisfaction of the consumer receiving health care with the care and how it was provided.

cystic fibrosis (CF): Most common inherited chronic pulmonary disease among white children, characterized by the production of thick mucus with progressive lung damage.

dermatitis: Inflammation of the skin indicated by any one or all of the following: redness, rash, itching, irritation, and possible skin lesions.

dermis: Portion of the skin directly under the dermis; made up of fibrous connective tissue and supports sweat glands, sebaceous glands, nerves and nerve endings, blood and lymph vessels, hair follicles and their allied smooth muscle.

developmental delay: Failure to attain predictable movement patterns or behaviors associated with children of a similar chronological age.

developmental milestone: Movement pattern that appears at a certain stage of growth and development.

diagnosis: Final interpretation of findings based on examinations; in physical therapy the diagnosis must be made in accordance with a policy adopted by the APTA House of Delegates.

Diagnostic Related Groups (DRGs):   Classification scheme developed by the federal government as a means to establish uniform reimbursement for a variety of diagnostic conditions.

direct access: Availability of the physical therapist to anyone seeking physical therapy services without stipulation of a referral by another health care provider.

disability: Inability to perform a task in a particular context or environment.

disablement model: Conceptual approach to health care based on the functional abilities of the patient/client that result from a medical condition. As applied to physical therapy, includes impairment, functional limitation, and disability.

disablement process: Examination process that focuses on the individual's impairments, functional limitations, disability, and resultant restrictions in activities.

district: Most local organizational unit in the structure of the APTA. Membership is automatic and may be based on location of residence or employment, as provided in the Bylaws of the APTA.

doctor of physical therapy (DPT):   Entry-level professional degree in physical therapy at the clinical doctorate level.

Down syndrome: Congenital developmental disability caused by a defect of chromosome 21; sometimes called trisomy 21.

Duchenne muscular dystrophy (DMD):   Progressive pelvic muscle weakness and wasting in the male child, combined with enlarged, yet weak, thigh muscles and tight heel cords.

dynamic balance: Balance maintained with the body in motion.

dysfunction: Any functional disability.

dyspnea: Shortness of breath.

echocardiography: Technique using high-frequency ultrasound to assess the size of the heart chambers, the thickness of the chamber walls, and the motion of the chamber walls and heart valves.

eclectic approach: Combination of therapeutic approaches used by the physical therapist and thought to be useful for treatment of a given client.

electrical stimulation: Application of electricity at specified locations to stimulate nerves, muscles, and other soft tissues to reduce pain and swelling, to increase strength and range of motion, and to facilitate wound healing.

electrocardiogram (ECG):   Readout produced by placing electrodes on the anterior chest wall to record depolarization or contraction of the heart muscle; assesses the heart's rate and rhythm.

electroencephalography (EEG):   Technique for recording the electrical potential/activity in the brain by placing electrodes on the scalp.

electromyography (EMG):   Technique for recording the electrical activity in the muscle during a state of rest and during voluntary contraction.

embolus: Clot formed by a substance detached from elsewhere.

enablement process: Examination process that focuses on the individual's structural body and concurrent abilities while addressing age-appropriate movement patterns and activities.

encroachment: Situation occurring in health care, in which one health care provider performs the skills and techniques of another health care provider.

epidermis: Outer layer of the skin.

ergonomics: Relationship between the worker, tasks, and work environment.

evaluation: Judgment based on an examination.

Evaluative Criteria for Accreditation of Education Programs for the Preparation of Physical Therapists: Standards and criteria approved by the House of Delegates to ensure quality and consistency in physical therapy education programs.

Evaluative Criteria for Accreditation of Education Programs for the Preparation of Physical Therapist Assistants: Standards and criteria approved by the House of Delegates to ensure quality and consistency in physical therapist assistant education programs.

evidence-based practice: Interventions used in physical therapy based on research that demonstrates the reliability and validity of the procedures.

examination: Process of gathering information about the past and current status of the patient/client.

exercise stress testing: Noninvasive method of determining how the cardiovascular and pulmonary systems respond to controlled increases in activity; most frequently used to diagnose or assess suspected or established cardiovascular disease.

expiration: Breathing out.

expressive aphasia: Impaired ability to express oneself.

family assessment: Family interview, survey, or discussion used to obtain the family's insights regarding a patient, especially a child; includes family history, relationships, concerns, needs, and resources.

Federation of State Boards of Physical Therapy (FSBPT):   National organization through which member state boards work together to promote and protect the health, welfare, and safety of the American public by identifying and promoting desirable and reasonable uniformity in physical therapy regulatory standards and practices.

fetal alcohol syndrome (FAS):   Most severe condition in a continuum of alcohol-induced disabilities related to high levels of maternal alcohol consumption during pregnancy.

flexibility: Ability to move a limb segment through a range of motion.

flexibility exercise: Exercise performed over time, using stress, to change the length and elasticity of soft tissue such as muscle; usually performed for postural or ROM enhancement.

fluidotherapy: Use of a self-contained unit filled with sawdust-type particles heated to the desired temperature and circulated by air pressure around the involved body part.

Foundation for Physical Therapy: Organization, separate from the APTA, that promotes and provides financial support for scientific research, clinical research, and health services research in physical therapy.

fracture: Break in a bone.

frail elderly: People over 65 with conditions that significantly impair their daily function.

functional capacity evaluation: Examination of a worker's physical abilities to perform required tasks.

functional exercise: Exercise that mimics functional movements and activities. Functional movements incorporate strength, flexibility, balance, and coordination.

functional limitation: Decreased ability of a person to perform a task, without regard to the context or environment.

functional reach test: Specific balance test that can predict the likelihood of falling.

gatekeeper: Health care provider who provides the consumer with access to the health care system. Historically, this has been the primary care physician.

goal-directed movement approach: A treatment approach that emphasizes the importance of both task and environmental features as a primary impetus for movement.

goals: Measurable, functional objectives that are linked to a problem identified in a patient evaluation.

goniometer: Instrument used to measure and document ROM.

goniometry: Methods to measure and document ROM.

ground substance: Supportive, amorphous gel-like substance secreted by fibroblasts; fills space between connective tissue fibers and cells.

Halliwick method: quatic therapy technique using a preswim stroke instruction and musculoskeletal rehabilitation.

Health Care Financing Administration (HCFA): Federal agency responsible for Medicare, the reimbursement system for individuals over 65 years of age.

health maintenance organization (HMO): Prepaid health insurance that may provide all health care services needed within one facility.

heart failure: Decrease in the pumping capability of the heart muscle.

history: Description of the past and current health status of the patient/ client.

hot pack: Pouch filled with silica gel and soaked in thermostatically controlled water.

House of Delegates (HOD): Highest policymaking body of the APTA, consisting of voting chapter delegates and nonvoting section and assembly delegates and members of the Board of Directors.

hydrotherapy: Use of the therapeutic effects of water by immersing the body part or entire body into a tank of water.

hypermobile joint: Joint with excessive motion.

hypertonia: High tone.

hypertrophic scar: Excess of amount of collagen deposited at the site of a healing or healed wound that is noticeably different from the normal skin; scar remains within the boundaries of the original wound.

hypokinesis: State of decreased activity or movement.

hypomobile joint: Joint with less motion than is considered functional.

hypotonia: Low tone.

impairment: Loss or abnormality in a function at the cellular, tissue, organ, or system level.

Individualized Education Plan (IEP): Model using collaboration of therapists, family, educators, and other health care team members to provide direct intervention in the classroom setting.

Individualized Family Service Plan (IFSP): Detailed total plan of care for the child in the context of the family unit.

inflammatory phase: Phase of wound healing encompassing vascular reactions that decrease blood loss and initiate vessel repair, and cellular responses that moderate blood loss, fight infection, and provide nutrition and oxygen to initiate and sustain tissue repair.

inflammatory skin diseases: Diseases of the skin whose etiologies invoke an inflammatory response (etiologies for these diseases commonly include immune reactions and contact irritants or allergens).

informed consent: Client-granted permission to treat, required in accordance with the Standards of Practice approved by the APTA; obtained by the physical therapist before rendering physical therapy.

infrared: Radiation used to warm the superficial tissue and create a general feeling of relaxation and pain relief.

inspiration: Contraction of the muscles of respiration, resulting in an increase in the space contained within the thoracic cavity. This expansion causes the air pressure to drop inside the lungs, resulting in movement of air into the lungs.

instrumental activities of daily living (IADLs):   Activities that individuals must perform to function in the community. Examples include shopping, driving, and paying bills.

integument: Skin.

intervention: Procedure conducted with the patient/client to achieve the desired outcomes.

ischemia: Insufficient oxygenation of tissues owing to a blocked blood vessel.

joint mobilization: Technique used when a patient's dysfunction is the result of joint stiffness or hypomobility (loss of motion); applies to a joint specific passive movements, either oscillatory (rapid, repeated movements) or sustained.

juvenile rheumatoid arthritis (JRA):   One of the many rheumatic diseases characterized by an inflammation of the connective tissue that manifests as a painful inflamed joint (arthritis); begins in childhood.

keloid scar: An excess of amount of collagen deposited at the site of a healing or healed wound that is noticeably different from the normal skin; scar commonly extends beyond the boundaries of the original wound.

law: Formal rule having binding legal force laid down, ordained, or established by a governing body.

licensure: Process by which the state grants to an individual who has met state standards permission to practice a profession and grants legal recognition to a particular scope of practice.

lumbar puncture: Injection of a hypodermic needle into the lumbar subarachnoid space.

magnetic resonance imaging (MRI): Creation of a computer image by placing the body part in a magnetic field.

malpractice: Failure to do (or avoid doing) something that a reasonably prudent member of the profession would have done (or would not have done), with subsequent injury to a patient/client.

managed care: Arrangement in which an insurance company contracts with health care providers to provide health care to the consumers who subscribe to the insurance plan.

managed care network: Group of health care providers who form a professional cooperative relationship for the purpose of referring individuals to health care providers within the network.

manual muscle testing (MMT): Test allowing the therapist to assign a specific grade to a muscle, based on whether the patient can hold the limb against gravity, how much manual resistance can be tolerated, and whether there is full range of motion at a joint.

massage: Systematic use of various manual strokes designed to produce certain physiological, mechanical, and psychological effects.

maturation phase: Phase of wound healing that includes collagen synthesis and lysis, and reorientation of the collagen fibers that remain at the wound site; this phase may also be referred to as the remodeling phase.

Medicaid: Reimbursement system established at the state level to provide health care for those with limited financial means.

Medicare: Reimbursement system established at the federal level for individuals over 65 years of age.

meningocele: Benign herniation of the meninges presenting as a soft tissue cyst or lump that surrounds a normal spinal cord and produces no neurological deficits.

meningomyelocele: Open congenital spinal cord lesion with minimal to no skin protection covering the deeper nerve roots.

Minimum Data Set (MDS): A specified collection of data that is documented and used to measure the amount of care provided to a patient at a skilled nursing facility

motor control: Ability to manipulate movement and nonmovement of the body's musculoskeletal components.

motor development: Age-related processes of change in motor behavior.

motor learning: Body's mechanism for acquiring or learning voluntary motor control.

multiple sclerosis (MS):   Disease in which patches of demyelination occur in the nervous system, leading to disturbances in conduction of messages along the nerves.

muscle endurance: Ability to produce and sustain tension over a prolonged period of time.

muscular strength: Maximal amount of tension an individual can produce in one repetition.

myocardial infarction: Heart attack, resulting from blockage by an embolus (clot) of one of the coronary arteries.

myofascial release: Manual stretching of the layers of the body's fascia (connective tissue that surrounds muscle and other soft tissues in the body).

National Assembly of Physical Therapist Assistants (National Assembly):   Component of the APTA that consists of all affiliate (physical therapist assistant) and life affiliate (retired) members. Includes officers and regional directors who represent the interests of its members.

National Foundation for Infantile Paralysis (Foundation):   Foundation established in 1938 in response to repeated polio epidemics. Established to provide research, education, and patient services.

negligence: Failure to do something that a reasonably prudent person would do, or behavior that would normally not be done under similar circumstances.

neoplastic skin diseases: Cancers affecting the skin.

nerve conduction velocity (NCV) study: Study that records the rate at which electrical signals are transmitted along peripheral nerves.

nerve entrapment: Pressure on a nerve.

neurodevelopmental treatment (NDT):   Approach to both analyze and treat neurological disorders of posture and movement. Through the use of a motivating environment and a patient's active participation, manual facilitation and inhibition techniques are employed by the therapist to present the patient with a "normal" sensory experience, thereby encouraging facilitation of a more functional motor response.

neuropathic (neurotropic) ulcer: Skin lesion caused by a decreased cutaneous sensation that disallows protective responses such as weight transfer; these ulcers are commonly associated with diabetes mellitus.

normal developmental theory: Model asserting that therapy goals and objectives are designed to follow the progression of normal motor development. Assumes that children with central nervous system damage will acquire motor skills in a similar fashion to children with normally developing nervous systems.

A Normative Model of Physical Therapist Assistant Education: Approved by the House of Delegates, this document is a means to guide physical therapist assistant education programs to ensure that the academic program meets the quality and comprehensiveness established by the members of the profession.

A Normative Model of Physical Therapist Professional Education: Approved by the House of Delegates, this document is a means to guide physical therapy education programs to ensure that the academic program meets the quality and comprehensiveness established by the members of the profession.

objective examination: Quantitative or qualitative measurements that are taken by the PT or PTA or by use of a mechanical device.

obstructive lung disease: Pathological abnormality in airflow through the bronchial tubes.

open-chain exercise/joint isolation exercise: Exercise in which the end limb segment is free.

osteoarthritis: Condition characterized by degeneration of cartilage as a result of many years of use. Hands, spine, knees, and hips are most commonly affected.

osteogenesis imperfecta (OI): Common and severe bone impairment of genetic origin. Affects the formation of collagen during bone development, resulting in frequent fractures during the fetal or newborn period.

osteoporosis: Decreased mineralization of the bones caused by a decreased production of new bone cells and an increased resorption of bone.

paraffin treatment: Use of a mixture of melted paraffin wax and mineral oil maintained at a specific temperature to promote relaxation and pain relief and allow greater comfort during range-of-motion exercises.

paraplegia: Spinal cord damage and resultant loss of sensory or motor function affecting the lower trunk and legs.

Parkinson's disease: Progressive condition, also referred to as paralysis agitans and idiopathic parkinsonism, characterized by a classic triad of symptoms: tremor, rigidity, and bradykinesia/akinesia.

passive range of motion (PROM): Amount of movement at a joint that is obtained by the therapist's moving the segment without assistance from the patient.

patient: Individual who has a disorder that requires interventions to improve function.

patient-focused care (PFC): Patient-care model in which all departments in a hospital are decentralized, and professional staff are assigned to work on multidisciplinary teams; usually involves cross-training of health care professionals.

perception: Ability to integrate various simultaneous sensory inputs and to respond appropriately.

physiatrist: Title given to physicians who specialize in physical medicine.

physical therapist: Professional who works to evaluate, treat, and/or prevent physical disability, movement dysfunction, and pain resulting from injury, disability, disease, or other health-related conditions.

physical therapist assistant (PTA):   Health care provider who assists the PT in the provision of physical therapy and has graduated from an accredited physical therapist assistant associate degree program.

physical therapy: Assessment, evaluation, treatment, and prevention of physical disability, movement dysfunctions, and pain resulting from injury, disease, disability, or other health-related conditions.

physical therapy aide: Support personnel who perform designated tasks that do not require the clinical decision making of the physical therapist or the clinical problem solving of the physical therapist assistant.

physician-owned physical therapy service (POPTS):   Physical therapy services owned or invested in by a physician.

physiotherapist: Synonym for physical therapist, commonly used outside the United States.

physiotherapy: Synonym for physical therapy, commonly used outside the United States; used by the first national organization, American Women's Physical Therapeutic Association.

plan of care: Goals, interventions (including duration and frequency), desired outcomes, and criteria for discharge.

policy: Plan or course of action designed to influence and determine decisions. APTA further defines this as "a decision which obligates actions or subsequent decisions on similar matters."

postprofessional education: Advanced education of a licensed physical therapist, either at the certificate, master's, or doctorate level.

postural drainage: Utilization of gravity through appropriate positioning and chest wall percussion to promote removal of excessive secretions from the tracheobronchial tree.

practice act: state's official statement or document of definition and regulation of a specific profession, setting down guidelines for those practicing the profession within its jurisdiction.

preferred provider: Provider (e.g., physical therapist) in a managed care setting who has contracted with a specific insurance company to provide health care to the consumers who subscribe to the specified insurance plan.

prenatal cocaine exposure: Fetal exposure to cocaine in utero owing to maternal cocaine use during pregnancy. Infants often present with clinical signs of exposure after birth such as hyperirritability, poor feeding patterns, high respiratory and heart rates, increased tremulousness, and irregular sleeping patterns.

presbycusis: Decreased ability to perceive higher pitches and to distinguish between similar sounds.

pressure ulcer: Skin lesion caused by ischemia of the integument secondary to pressure; these ulcers are generally located at bony prominences.

prevention: Services designed to avoid the occurrence pain and dysfunction or limit/reduce those that exist.

primary care: Level of health care delivered by a member of the health care system who is responsible for the majority of the health care needs of the individual.

profession: Career or means of employment demonstrating five characteristics: commitment to field, a representative organization, knowledge in a specific area, social service, and recognized autonomy.

professional misconduct: Violation of the state statutes and/or regulations that define competent professional practice by those professionals regulated by the state.

professional physical therapy education: All academic programs that prepare students for *entry* into the field of physical therapy, regardless of the degree.

prognosis: Prediction of the level of improvement and time necessary to reach that level.

proliferative phase: Phase of wound healing that involves increased activity of fibroblasts, instigation of aggressive wound contraction, and epithelialization.

proprioception: One's awareness of position and movement.

proprioceptive neuromuscular facilitation (PNF):   Technique used to enhance movement and motor control, emphasizing proprioceptive (joint and position sense) stimuli but also using tactile, visual, and auditory stimuli.

proprioceptors: Receptors found in the skin and joints that respond to stimuli such as pressure, stretch, and position.

Prospective Payment System (PPS):   Establishment of a reimbursement rate to be paid in advance of the delivery of care. It is often based on the diagnosis and level of care needed.

pulmonary function test: Assessment of the effectiveness of the respiratory musculature and the integrity of the airways and lung tissues to help classify lung disease pattern into obstructive or restrictive.

quadriplegia: spinal cord damage resulting in loss of sensory or motor function affecting all limbs.

range of motion (ROM):   Movement at a joint.

range-of-motion exercise: Exercise for mobility of a joint. Falls into two categories: active or passive. Active ROM exercise involves voluntary movement of a limb through an arc of movement; passive ROM exercise involves the *therapist's* moving the limb without patient assistance.

receptive aphasia: Diminished ability to receive and interpret verbal or written communication.

reconstruction aide: Aide (exclusively a woman) responsible for providing physical reconstruction to persons injured in war; forerunners of the profession and practice of physical therapy in the United States.

registration: Process by which the state tracks regulated professionals by requiring updated listing of names, addresses, and qualifications. This generally does not involve a review of whether standards of practice are met.

regulation: Administrative or departmental rules issued to carry out the intent of the law.

Representative Body of the National Assembly (RBNA):   Deliberative body for the physical therapist assistant with representatives from each chapter.

resisted exercise: Form of active movement in which some form of resistance is provided to increase muscular strength and endurance.

resisted test: Test that allows the therapist to determine the general strength of a muscle group and assess whether any pain is produced with the muscle contraction.

respiration: Process of exchanging oxygen and carbon dioxide between the air we breathe and the cells of the body.

restrictive lung disease: Pathological reduction of the volume of air in the lungs.

rheumatoid arthritis: Chronic inflammation of the joints, of unknown etiology.

rigidity: Disturbance of muscle tone; manifests as a resistance when the limbs are passively moved.

risk management: Process by which coordinated efforts are made by an organization to identify, assess, and minimize the risk of harm and loss to the organization, employees, and clients.

Rood's approach: Neurological treatment using a variety of sensory stimuli to influence motor behavior.

scar contraction: Dynamic movement of the edges of a scar (wound boundaries) toward each other.

scar contracture: Permanent or relatively permanent lack of mobility of the scar tissue that results in functional and/or cosmetic impairment.

scoliosis: Lateral curvature of the spine; may be idiopathic (of unknown origin), neuromuscular, or congenital (present at birth).

screening: Procedure to determine if there is a need for further services of a physical therapist or other health care professional.

secondary care: Services provided by individuals on a referral basis.

secondary condition: Condition that is potentially preventable and is a direct or indirect consequence of inadequate attention to (or inadequate amelioration of) an impairment or disability.

section: National level of organizational unit of the APTA for members of all classes to promote similar interests. Membership is voluntary.

sensation: Ability to receive sensory input from within and outside the body and transmit it through the peripheral nerves and tracts in the spinal cord to the brain, where it is received and interpreted.

sensory integration (SI): Technique based on the theory that poor integration and use of sensory input (feedback) prevents subsequent motor planning (output). Providing controlled vestibular and somatosensory experiences enables the child to integrate the sensory information to evoke a spontaneous, functional response.

short-wave diathermy: Use of electromagnetic energy to produce deep therapeutic heating effects.

SOAP note: Documentation format taken from the Problem-Oriented Medical Record System; its components are (1) Subjective (what patient/family member describes), (2) Objective (what the PT observes/measures), (3) Assessment (clinical judgment based on evaluation; includes goals), and (4) Plan (of care).

soft tissue mobilization: One of a variety of "hands-on" techniques designed to improve movement and decrease pain.

special interest group (SIG): One of many groups existing at multiple levels of the APTA to enable members at all levels to further organize into smaller specialty areas.

special tests: Tests designed to examine specific joints to indicate the presence or absence of a particular problem.

spina bifida: Congenital incomplete closure of a vertebra.

spina bifida occulta: Congenital incomplete closure of a vertebra (separation of the spinous process) that is not associated with disability.

spinal cord injury (SCI):   Damage to the spinal cord that results in neurological dysfunction.

spinal muscular atrophy (SMA):   Genetic disorder characterized by severe muscle weakness in infancy and progressive respiratory failure.

spirometer: Instrument measuring the various volumes and airflow rates, which are then compared to a normal scale.

sprain: Overstretching of a joint ligament accompanied by a tearing of the fibers, causing pain and instability of the joint.

standardized testing: Type of formal test in which the evaluation procedures remain the same when administered by different therapists and at variable test locations.

Standards of Ethical Conduct for the Physical Therapist Assistant: Principles set forth by the APTA for maintaining and promoting high standards of professional conduct among affiliate member physical therapist assistants.

Standards of Practice for Physical Therapy: Document approved by the House of Delegates of the APTA that identifies conditions and performances that are essential for the provision of high-quality physical therapy.

static balance: Balance maintained while standing still.

statute: Formal written enactment by the legislative department of government.

strain: Tearing of muscle fibers, caused by a sudden contraction of a muscle or excessive stretch to the muscle.

strength: Amount of force produced during a voluntary muscular contraction.

stroke or cerebrovascular accident (CVA):   Neurological problem arising from disruption of blood flow in the brain.

Student Assembly: Component of the APTA whose members are physical therapy and physical therapist assistant students; provides a forum in which PT/PTA students can better understand their roles.

subjective examination: Interviewing the patient about the extent and nature of an injury; a qualitative measurement based on the patient's perception of the problem.

systems review: Brief examination to provide information about the general health of the patient/client, including the physiological, anatomic, and cognitive status.

target heart rate (THR):   Appropriate heart rate to be maintained during the peak period in aerobic training; calculated as a percentage of the individual's maximum heart rate.

tendinitis: Inflammation of a tendon, a structure that is located at the ends of muscles and attaches muscle to bone.

tertiary care: Service provided by specialists who are frequently employed in facilities that focus on particular health conditions.

tests and measures: Specific procedures selected and performed to quantify the physical and functional status of the patient/client.

thermal agent: Agent used to modify the temperature of surrounding tissue, resulting in a change in the amount of blood flow to the injured area.

tone: Tension exerted and/or maintained by muscles at rest and during movement.

total body surface area (TBSA):   Represents the extent of the surface of the body covered by skin. The percent TBSA is used to depict the size of a skin injury (routinely used to estimate the size of a burn injury).

training zone: Individual's ideal range of minimum and maximum heart rates (see **target heart rate**) that must be achieved for that individual to produce an aerobic training effect.

traumatic brain injury (TBI):   Damage to the brain caused by physical means and resulting in neurological dysfunction.

tremor: Alternating contractions of opposing muscle groups.

Trialliance: Organization that consists of the APTA, American Occupational Therapy Association, and the American Speech-Language and Hearing Association that meets to discuss issues of mutual concern.

ultrasound: Therapeutic application of high-frequency sound waves that penetrate through tissue and cause an increase in the tissue temperature to promote healing and reduce pain.

Vancouver Burn Scar Scale: Clinical method for assessing scar tissue. The characteristics of scar that are examined include pigmentation, vascularity, pliability, and height.

venous insufficiency: Deficiency or occlusion of blood flow through a vein.

ventilation: Process of inspiration and expiration; results in an exchange of oxygen and carbon dioxide between the air found in the lungs and the pulmonary circulation.

vicarious liability: The principle by which one individual may be held indirectly liable legally for the acts of another; for example, the liability of an employer for the acts of an employee during the performance of job responsibilities.

well elderly: People 65 years and over who are not experiencing physical limitations or who have age-related changes that are not significant enough to affect function.

whirlpool: Tank of water used in hydrotherapy for immersing a body part or the entire body.

work-conditioning program: Intervention for an individual with a work-related injury, focusing mostly on physical dysfunctions (e.g., strength, range of motion, and cardiovascular endurance).

work-hardening program: Intervention for an individual with a work-related injury, broad in scope to include behavioral and vocational management (e.g., counseling) as well as physical dysfunctions.

World Confederation of Physical Therapy: International organization that represents physical therapy on a global level and consists of physical therapy organizations in member nations.

Index

Note: Page numbers in *italics* refer to illustrations; page numbers followed by the letter b refer to boxed material, and those followed by t refer to tables.